Third l

Health & Fitness in Plain English

How to be Healthy, Happy, and Fit for the Rest of Your Life

NEW Third Edition featuring expanded information, new chapters, and new illustrations

Jolie Bookspan, M.Ed., Ph.D., FAWM

HEALTHY LEARNING™

Including:

- Exercise (what works and doesn't—in and out of the gym)
- Health (heart, bones, cholesterol, body fat, blood sugar, and weight control)
- Vitamins, health foods, nutrition, drugs, supplements, and diets
- Back pain, neck pain, knee pain, rotator cuff, headaches, leg cramps, and ankle sprains
- Fun facts, plus an A-to-Z glossary

ISBN: 978-1-58518-672-3
Library of Congress Control Number: 2008923846

Book layout: Bean Creek Studio
Cover design: Bean Creek Studio
Cover photo: ©2008 Jupiterimages Corporation
Illustrations: Todd Sargood and Jolie Bookspan

Healthy Learning
P.O. Box 1828
Monterey, CA 93942
www.healthylearning.com

Dedication

To my Grandmother, who got her college degree at age 81.

To her, the highest things in life were education and Jack LaLanne.

To my Mother, who kept everyone dancing.

To my wonderful husband and hero, Paul,

who listens to me and tries all my ideas.

The Surgeon General
has determined
that lack of physical activity
is detrimental
to your health.

—Surgeon General's Report on
Physical Activity and Health, July 1996

Contents

Part III—Health

Reviewers

Thank you to the following expert reviewers:

Alan Berg, Ph.D., M.D., House-call Doctor, Philadelphia County Medical Society Practitioner of the Year (2000)

Russ Gazzara, Ph.D., Developmental Neurotoxicologist, National Center for Toxicological Research, FDA

Green Beret Lt. Col. R. Kelly Hill, M.D

David Hsu, Ph.D., M.D., Department of Neurology, Stanford University Hospital

David Josephson, Josephson Engineering

David Koeppel, Writer, Film Editor, Paramount Pictures

Larry "Scoots" Miller, Ph.D., Microbiologist

Alan Moore, M.D., Board Certified, Obstetrics and Family Medicine (osteoporosis chapter)

Rich Ruoti, Ph.D., P.T., P.C., BuxMont Physical Therapy (back pain chapters)

Audrey Tannenbaum, M.Ed., A.T.C., C.S.C.S., Athletic Trainer and Maccabean Games Triathlon Gold Medalist

Marla Tonseth, M.B.A., P.T., Physical Therapist

William B. Young, M.D., Jefferson Headache Center, Thomas Jefferson University Hospital (headache chapter)

Preface

This book explains why health does not mean to stop your life to "do exercises" or to buy special food and supplements, but how to move in real life so that all the ways you walk, bend, sit, work, and play are healthful. Beginners will be able to get started right. Experienced exercisers and trainers will be able to avoid common harmful practices and put better practices to use.

This book gives upbeat ideas for exercise, health, and nutrition; explains the terminology; puts information in the place of myths; gives practical suggestions for healthier weight loss; discusses how to stop back pain, neck pain, knee pain, headaches, osteoporosis, and leg cramps; explains what good and bad cholesterol mean; and shows you how your real life can become your exercise. The book contains answers to fun questions like: Why does your foot fall asleep? Why do your joints pop? Why is your elbow called a funny bone? At the end of the book is a large, annotated glossary. More than handy definitions, it includes word derivations, concepts, and fun stories behind the people and information. Important areas are restated in different chapters for helpful reinforcement and so that chapters can be read alone, or in whatever order suits you.

With the information in this book, you will be better equipped to make sense of the claims and counterclaims in exercise, health, and nutrition. You will be able to fix pain and get stronger and more mobile without having to "do" exercises, or purchase any products. You will see how to be active and healthy for your real life, not just in a gym. You will be able to make informed decisions about your health. You will save money. You will be empowered to get your life back. You'll even have fun.

Happy reading.

Part I

EXERCISE

A vigorous five-mile walk will do more good for an unhappy but otherwise healthy adult than all the medicine and psychology in the world.

—Paul Dudley White

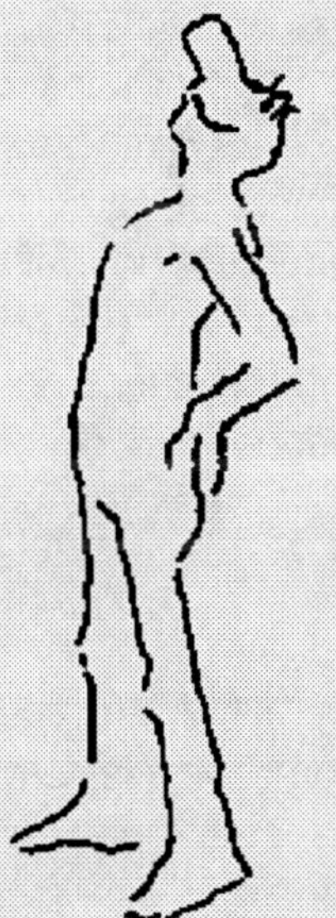

1

Why Should You Be Active?

I don't exercise. What's in it for me? You've got to offer me more than my life to get me on a StairMaster grunting for two hours. I view my body as a way of getting my head from one place to another.

–Dave Thomas, founder of Wendy's

Good physical condition is important for everyone—even if you are not an athlete. Good fitness reduces your risk of many serious diseases, delays several common effects of aging, increases your tolerance to heat and cold, increases muscle, and reduces body fat. Regular exercise, and the wellness it brings, helps you cope with stress and feel better in general. Good physical fitness can improve your safety and comfort during your daily life and recreational activities, and preserve your mobility and independence.

Better Health

An active lifestyle makes major positive changes in your health and well-being. Common Western ills, such as heart and blood-vessel disease, obesity, some types of diabetes, poor balance and repeated falls, and many musculoskeletal problems, are known as *hypokinetic* diseases (*hypo-* means "less than" or "not enough," and *kinetic* means "activity"). Hypokinetic disease is a fancy term for illness related to, or caused by, being sedentary and out of shape.

- Epidemiologic studies show that regular exercise lowers incidence of breast cancer in women, and colon and reproductive tract cancer in both men and women.
- Resistance exercise thickens bones, which is important in osteoporosis prevention (Chapter 22).
- Cardio-respiratory fitness through aerobic exercise reduces your risk of early death from vascular disease, heart disease, and high blood pressure, major killers of both men and women (Chapter 27). Even heavier people who have high aerobic fitness have been found to have lower death rates than lighter out-of-shape people.
- Sudden death from heart attack is more common in an out-of-shape person who exerts past capacity than in those who regularly exercise.

Delayed Aging

Physical deterioration from sedentary lifestyle is frequently mistaken for aging. Getting slower, stiffer, and weaker as years pass is more a result of a lack of regular healthful movement than an inescapable aging process. Although your chronological years increase, you can become functionally younger with exercise.

- Without exercise, muscular strength, speed, and power diminish sharply at any age.
- After about age 30, deterioration would run about 0.75 to 1 percent per year if you didn't exercise regularly. With regular exercise, you can reverse loss and increase capacity.
- Without exercise, the maximum amount of oxygen your body can use to make energy, an important indicator of fitness, would drop about 10 percent each decade from ages 20 to 60. With exercise, the decrease can slow, even stop, up to a point.
- Without regularly moving your body through a range of motion, joints tighten until ordinary reaching and bending can become difficult and uncomfortable.
- Being inactive or injured diminishes your sense of balance. Fear of falling, or the real falls that result, often keep a person from further activity. An unfortunate cycle of inactivity, deconditioning, and further decrease in balance can leave you housebound and weakening.

Regular exercise, stretching, and balance practice slows, even reverses, all this loss, meaning gains equivalent to stopping or reversing years of aging. Older people who exercise, move, balance, and stretch have many of the functional characteristics of a chronologically younger person. They can reach, bend, and move easily. They can walk uneven sidewalks and other terrain. They can carry their own packages, go out, and have fun. The anti-aging effect of exercise to improve strength and mobility is possible for all age groups. Often, physical gains are enough to remove their need for walkers, braces, orthotics, wheelchairs, and canes. They improve self-sufficiency so much that, once again, they can carry out their own activities of daily living—all from regular exercise.

Fewer, Less Serious Injuries

Pushing beyond capacity, which is easy to do when you don't have much capacity, can lead to injury. Lt. Col. Bruce H. Jones, M.D., Chief of the Occupational Medicine Division of the U.S. Army Research Institute of Environmental Medicine, reported on data from army recruits. He found that recruits of lower physical fitness had consistently higher injury rate than recruits of higher fitness.

Good balance skills decrease risk of sprains, falls, and the injuries that come with them. When you are injured or have poor balance, it is crucial to train balance, although it is during those times that people often restrict activity, producing more losses in balance and physical ability. Practicing balance restores independence, improves fitness and mobility, and allows more activity with less chance of injury from falling or dropping things during a slip.

Some studies show no benefit of physical fitness to lower incidence of injury. The reason is that people often exercise and stretch in unhealthful ways, then go back to injurious daily life of bending wrong, sitting badly, and standing and moving in slouched, tight ways. Healthful exercise and stretches needs to be geared to retraining good body mechanics. Rounding your back over your desk is obvious bad posture. It is counterproductive to promote the same rounded and bent-forward postures that create pain syndromes, for example, using the forward-bending motions of abdominal crunches and many Pilates exercises.

Everyone needs physical exercise for general health and injury prevention. Without it, a vicious cycle of inactivity and injury grows. If you are sedentary, begin to become more active, working within your safety and comfort zone to make activity a lifetime habit, rather than a chore to endure and avoid.

Positive Mood

Regular exercise is thought to affect your mood positively in several ways:

- In the short term, vigorous exercise is thought to produce a class of hormones called endorphins. The word endorphin is a contraction of "endogenous (made from within) morphine-like substance." Endorphins improve mood after hard workouts by releasing chemicals that stimulate your brain's pleasure center.

- In the long term, exercise increases many physical abilities so that you can do things you enjoy more often and more comfortably.
- Regular exercise is established to reduce premenstrual symptoms and cramping during menses.
- Regular exercise helps decrease moodiness and sugar cravings by increasing insulin sensitivity. That means less insulin mobilizes to process a given load of carbohydrate and other food. This seems to be the case no matter what time of day you exercise, as long as you exercise regularly. Your blood sugar maintains a steadier level, reducing the swings that produce physical health problems, food cravings, and moodiness.
- Regular exercise is associated with reducing and reversing depression and anxiety. Exercise activates the same growth factor systems in the hippocampus of the brain that anti-depressant drugs activate, far more quickly and without the negative side effects of such drugs.
- Greater physical ability, body awareness, and improved body shape and health with exercise might also make you happy.
- Evidence exists that regular exercise promotes an increased feeling of well-being and ability to face emotional stress.

Better Brain

Regular exercise is documented to improve brain function at all ages.

- Exercise improves brain blood supply and promotes growth hormone and other factors needed for brain cell function.
- Immediate exercise intervention promotes recovery from stroke and traumatic brain injury, and helps prevent disorders like Parkinson's disease, Alzheimer's disease, and depression.
- It used to be thought that new neural connections could not be made after a young age. It is now known that the brain continues development throughout life and needs stimulation of many kinds to do it.

Decreased Incidence of Colds

- Studies report reduced incidence of colds with regular exercise.
- Related work shows that being a regular exerciser is associated with quicker recovery from colds.

- Studies of exercise and immune function show that moderate exercise bouts enhance immune function during the exercise and for a few hours following it.
- Specific research into mechanisms has found that moderate exercise speeds various immune-function cells through the body, and increases levels of leukocytes, a type of white blood cell that fights infection.
- A 2006 randomized clinical trial found that "postmenopausal women who exercised regularly for a year had about half the risk of colds compared to those who did not work out routinely." The women in the exercise group also reduced body weight, body fat, and intra-abdominal fat from increasing their exercise level.

Decrease in immune function is seen with intense exercise coupled with poor nutrition and lack of sleep. Regular brisk exercise with healthy food and sleep improve healthy immune effects.

Enhanced Recovery From Serious Illness

Until recently (sometimes currently), cancer patients, heart patients, and back-pain sufferers were told to rest and stop activity. Inactivity creates new health problems and worsens existing health problems.

- Lack of regular exercise decreases strength, endurance, energy, blood-sugar regulation, and cellular repair and increases fatigue. Cancer treatments of radiation and chemotherapy do the same, and worse. This process is called *iatrogenic* harm, which means injury or illness brought on by medical treatment.
- Medical studies confirm that debilitating tiredness and loss of energy from cancer treatments can be more disruptive to the patient than the original pain of cancer.
- A major cancer report called fatigue "the most important consideration for the patient with cancer." Cancer fatigue can be a problem for months, even years, after treatments end.
- Regular physical exercise is documented to increase survival in those with existing cancer, improving both number of years and quality of life.
- Lack of regular stretching to lengthen muscles tightened in pain and long periods of rest and immobility from any disease can create shortened, tight, resting postures (which create new back pain), shoulder impingement from rounded shoulders, aching pain in the extremities, and other symptoms that can be confused for pain from the cancer. Patients are often then subjected to unnecessary and unhealthful tests and procedures, fear, stress, and more pain.

One of the benefits of exercise is that your body produces more of a compound called heat shock protein. Heat shock proteins (HSP) are families of proteins that do several things, including accompanying and helping other proteins under stress (called chaperoning). Heat shock chaperones keep the other proteins neatly folded when they are being deformed by stress factors such as infection, ultraviolet light, starvation, heat, and other harsh conditions. Heat shock proteins help cell survival and are thought to mobilize immune function against infections and diseases. One of the big areas in heat shock study is cancer. Heat shock proteins have been investigated for their role in activating immune response to cancer, and in cancer vaccine research.

Reduced Fatigue

It may seem backwards that exercising gives energy, while not exercising leaves you tired, but exercise works to reduce fatigue.

- The out-of-shape body doesn't use oxygen efficiently. When your body can't supply the oxygen your muscles demand, you tire easily doing ordinary activities.
- Out-of-shape muscles find simple tasks tiring, while strong muscles can easily accomplish them.
- Weak, out-of-shape muscles can't do the work to hold healthful positioning all day, resulting in slumped, achy, and unhealthful joint angles that rub, strain, or don't work efficiently
- Regular exercise raises your body's level of physical "readiness," making you feel energetic.
- Regular exercise makes many physical changes in your body, including more blood volume and oxygen-carrying blood cells, more blood vessels to carry the blood, blood vessels that are less clogged with fatty deposits, better strength and tone of your various body parts, and other changes that make you feel vital and energetic.

A negative cycle occurs when you are too out of shape to exercise enough to get much exercise benefit. Sedentary behavior leads to feeling tired and weak, which reduces your ability and inclination to exercise. A positive cycle comes when you stick with an exercise program until you become accustomed to regular exercise, and can exercise hard enough to make gains, which, in turn, allows you to do more and feel better and more energetic.

> A brisk walk or other short exercise will make you feel better than a candy bar or stimulant pill, without the unhealthful side effects.

Better Breathing

- It was previously thought that lung function declined steadily with each passing year after age 30. It is now known that lung function can improve at any age.
- Breathing muscles of the chest and abdomen are muscles like any other. You need to exercise them. Regular exercise builds breathing muscles and practices better ventilation.
- Exercising your respiratory system with exercise is important to reduce many respiratory problems, and is part of staying in shape and able to do normal activities without getting out of breath.
- Regular exercise can decrease the "work of breathing," making daily life easier for the general population as well as for those with respiratory conditions, including asthma.
- Exercising the muscles that you use to breathe in (inspiratory muscle training) is known to improve the endurance of the respiratory muscles in people with spinal-cord injury and cystic fibrosis, and is shown to improve exercise capacity in patients with heart failure. It has also been found to help physical training in athletes and combat swimmers.

Better Tolerance to Heat

Exercise in the heat has been described as probably the single greatest stress on the human cardiovascular system. When you improve your physical fitness, your body makes changes that improve your ability to tolerate heat and do activity in the heat.

Blood supply to your heart and limb muscles is crucial for you to move around. You also need to shunt blood to your skin to take heat away from your body to cool you. Because your body has only a finite amount of blood to go around, competition develops.

- A fitter person has more total body fluid volume, greater blood volume, and can pump more blood with each heartbeat.
- The fitter person can supply blood to muscles for movement and skin for cooling, without running short for either one.
- Fitter people increase how much they can sweat for cooling.
- With increased fluids to go around for cooling, body core temperature will not rise as high at the same exercise intensity as in an out-of-shape person.
- The out-of-shape person has less cooling capacity and decreased ability to do activities safely in the heat.

More than any other factor, physical fitness reduces your susceptibility to overheating. If you get out of shape again, you lose your adaptations. Improved fitness, and the improved heat tolerance that comes with it, is not only for athletes who exercise in the heat, but for everyone who wants to be comfortable in the heat.

Better Tolerance to Cold

Physical fitness improves tolerance to exercise in cold environments, although to a lesser extent than in heat. Even so, the structural and metabolic changes that occur with regular exercise appear to keep you warmer in the cold.

- Increased muscle mass, which you get through resistance exercise, increases heat production and storage.
- A fit person can do more exercise to keep warm in the cold.
- A fit person tolerates a lower body temperature than an unfit person before shivering starts.
- Exercise in the cold improves your cold tolerance much more than exercise alone.

Recreational Fun and Safety

A high degree of muscular strength, cardiovascular endurance, and muscular endurance positively affects your capacity for exertion, common to many activities you enjoy for sport and health. You need your exercise reserves for extended efforts like long runs, rollerblading, soccer, biking, swimming, and going dancing all night; and for shorter, more intense efforts, like bowling, rugby, tennis, moving furniture, doing home repair, the changing demands of a weekend hike, carrying groceries and kids, and doing household chores.

- Someone with high cardiovascular capacity can more easily run, hike, bike, skate, dance, or swim a distance that is difficult for someone with less cardiovascular adaptation.
- Better fitness makes daily chores around the house and yard easier.
- Fitter people feel less exertion at the same exercise intensity so they can do more before fatiguing. They carry more, lift more, move more, and have more fun without feeling tired.
- People with higher cardiovascular fitness are less likely to have heart trouble during activities. Programs that say that weightlifting is enough for weight loss programs and cardiovascular activity is not needed is skipping a major health aspect. Fitness is more than weight loss.

- Being in good condition may make the difference between a difficult situation and an easy excursion.

Fat Loss

Exercise burns calories so you can lose weight, or eat more without gaining weight. Regular exercise shifts your body to a mode where it preferentially burns fat. The carbohydrate "sparing" effect extends the supply of the carbohydrates stored in your muscles and liver, thereby extending your exercise capacity.

> The Surgeon General's Report on Physical Activity and Health, released in 1996, defines moderate exercise as using about 150 calories per day, or 1,000 calories a week. This rate translates to about a half hour of medium-intensity exercise per day.

Getting "In Shape" Versus Getting Healthy

Just as not every medicine is healthy, not all exercises and stretches are healthy. Just as smoking "works" for weight loss, but is not a smart or healthy way to do it, many exercises "work" for cosmetic results, but result in long-term injury, and promote bad movement habits. Many common exercises don't move your body the way you need to move in real life, resulting in strains and injuries when going about daily activities.

Some yoga teachers and Pilates teachers have back pain, hip pain, and neck pain from doing common but unhealthful bent-forward exercises. Some personal trainers have herniated discs and body builders with back pain despite all the abdominal exercises they do. Some fitness instructors aren't getting more flexible no matter how much stretching they do, because some the most common stretches are not what your body needs for real-life health, and are not done in a way that is healthful. Many people are stressed, tired, achy, and not in shape, even though they spend hundreds of dollars a month on supplements and pills, gizmos, equipment, trainers, and classes. Many people create much stress over trying to stop their life to make time to go do artificial exercises. Honking the horn and cursing people in your way so you can get to your yoga or "distressing" exercise session on time is missing the point, and not being healthy in real life.

You don't need to go to a gym. Use healthful movement for all the times you bend and reach in daily life, in a variety of ways, and you will get much movement in the way your body needs. This book will show you how to be fit from an active daily "real" life, not just gym exercises. Going to a gym is not fitness as a lifestyle. (Refer to Chapter 8.)

Changing your real life into healthy movement and actions is a big and inspiring area of rethinking and retraining. Instead of sitting slouched then stopping to stretch because your back hurts, sit and stand well so that you do not get stiff and sore in the first place. Instead of lifting packages, babies, groceries, laundry, and everything else incorrectly all day, then stopping to do back exercises because your back hurts, lift properly. You will get built-in exercise, strengthen your legs, and save your back. You don't need to go to a gym; move, balance, and reach in healthy ways in order to do your real life. Instead of thinking you must stop your life to get health and exercise, fill your life with built-in healthy movement. This book will give you hundreds of ways to use your body properly and get fit in your real life, and have true fitness as your real lifestyle.

Fitness is for "real life," not just in a gym. Why do leg exercises in a gym, then bend wrong all day, not using your legs, for all the many dozens, even hundreds of times every day you need to bend to reach and pick things up?

Physical Fitness Is Important to Life

Being in good physical and mental fitness is important to your daily life, comfort, and health, even if you never want to play sports or climb mountains. The many health and well-being effects contribute to safe, healthful, fun, and happy living every day.

2

Different Aspects of Fitness

You've got to be very careful if you don't know where you are going, because you might not get there.

–Yogi Berra

You can be in shape in different ways. You need to know the various aspects of fitness so that you can know where you're going with your health and the results of doing different exercise. Each fitness aspect improves from different types of movement. Without including each, "you might not get there."

Why Different Aspects of Fitness?

Weightlifters may not be lowering their risk of heart trouble if they never exercise their cardiovascular system. Dashing for a bus or doing yoga (or Pilates) doesn't improve ability to go long distances. People who only use an "elliptical" jogging machine may need to add weightlifting for their bones. Taking long daily walks or runs will not build big muscles. Neither will sit-ups take fat off your stomach; for that, you need to burn more calories. Stretching will not strengthen your cardiovascular system. Weightlifting using weight machines can improve muscle and bone strength, but doesn't give you good posture, balance training, or often, the ability to lift real objects in real life. Why?

Different activities make different adaptations in your body, giving you different kinds of fitness. To walk or run long distances, you need to train for distance. To get fast, you need to train fast, not lift weight slowly. Being fit in only one way won't be much help to the other things you need to do. Getting a good run every day conditions your legs and heart in ways that don't transfer to swimming. Good runners may exhaust themselves during long swims, and swimmers during runs, even though both may be aerobically fit. For lifting grocery bags and children, you need a combination of strength, balance, and weight stabilization since no artificial gym-machine framework is doing it for you. You need each aspect for daily life, not just in a gym (Figure 2-1). To improve each element, you need to exercise them. Each factor also needs to work and be exercised together with the others, not as separate systems. This chapter explains each adaptation to different exercise. Chapter 3 gives specifics on how to improve them.

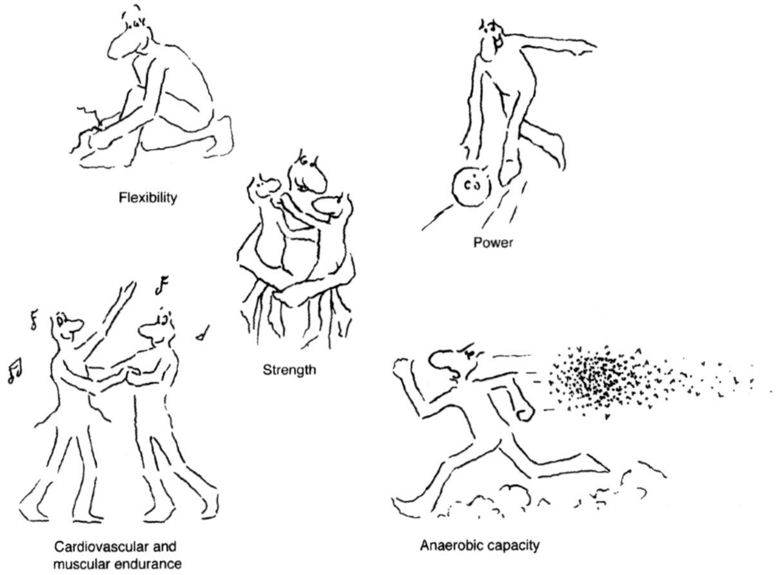

Figure 2-1. You need all of the components to fitness, not just for sports or the gym, but for everyday life and health.

Cardiovascular Endurance (Aerobic Capacity)

Cardiovascular endurance is also called cardio-respiratory endurance or aerobic capacity. It is the ability of your heart and lungs and their interconnected system of blood vessels to supply oxygen and nutrients throughout your body. Your cells burn some of the food you eat to manufacture special fuel compounds in a process that needs oxygen, so the process is called *aerobic*, which means "with oxygen."

Your cardiovascular endurance determines how long you can walk, run, bike, dance, skate, ski, jog, hike, shop, or swim at your chosen pace. It contributes to how tired you will be at the end of doing things you need to do all day. It affects your general health. Improving your aerobic condition makes getting where you want to go easier, and means you can get through your day more easily and with less fatigue. (Refer to Chapter 4.)

Anaerobic Capacity

Not all activities are aerobic. With fast intense activity, your body doesn't have a chance to activate its aerobic system. Your body has to use quick and ready-stored fuel, not oxygen to make some, so it is called *an*aerobic. *Anaerobic* means "without oxygen." You have only enough of this special stored "quick" energy for a few minutes of anaerobic activity. If you continue activity at a pace that is too fast for your aerobic system, your body can't switch over to its oxygen-using aerobic system to any great extent. Your body continues trying to use your stored fuel, but your demand exceeds the supply, and you run out of fuel. Unless you are in good shape, you will have to slow activity.

You use your anaerobic system to run for a bus, get out of your chair, lift packages and children, throw things, hold your breath to swim underwater, go up a flight of stairs, run out of a burning building, and do any short, hard activity. Developing your anaerobic system will make all these activities easier and safer. If your body is not prepared for short, quick activities, you can wind up hurting yourself and missing the bus besides. Your anaerobic system is explained more in Chapter 4.

Strength

Muscular strength is usually measured by the maximum force your muscles can generate in a single or short effort. You need strength to lift and carry weights, packages, children, groceries, and yourself easily, and without struggle. By increasing your strength through lifting weights and yourself, you can move around more easily, and reduce your chance of musculoskeletal injury while doing it.

Elderly and debilitated people who could not previously lift themselves from their chairs become more mobile after strengthening programs, allowing them to walk unaided once again. Many people won't kneel down or sit on the floor because they are too weak to get up. That inability is not a symptom of aging; rather, it is a sign of the need to regain the strength to do it.

Weightlifting is important for health for both men and women at all ages. Even people who don't do activities commonly regarded as strength activities need strength to do daily activities like carrying several 20-pound grocery bags and a 40-pound child. Weightlifting to increase muscular strength also strengthens bones. The pull of muscle against bone thickens the bone. The stronger a muscle, the more it can pull on the bones it attaches to. Weightlifting is a key part of osteoporosis prevention.

> Weight lifting to strengthen muscles also thickens bones, helping prevent osteoporosis.
>
> If you are afraid to sit on the floor because you can't get back up, you may be dangerously weak, and need to regain the strength (and balance skills) to do it.

Extra muscle helps you stay warm in winter and is your chief calorie burner. Building more muscle through strength training means that you burn more calories every day.

Power

In exercise physiology, power is measured by how fast you can be strong. It is a product of speed and strength together. You call on power to lift things, throw things, move things, hit things, dash out of the way of cars, or catch a falling child or package.

Different activities need different amounts of strength compared to speed. To throw the discus and lob a tennis ball, baseball, or football, you take a light weight and hurl it fast and far away. Offensive linemen in American football and forwards in rugby try to do the same to heavy defensive backs and tackles. A higher strength component compared to how fast you move (for example, in bench pressing or lifting any weight) is called strength-dominated power. Swimming, running, jumping, baseball, and tennis use primarily speed-dominated power. You need different amounts of both around the house every day.

Power is not just for athletes. When you increase your power, you can move things and yourself around more quickly and easily, with less chance of injury. It may save your life in an emergency, or help you save someone else's life.

Muscular Endurance

Walking, jogging, biking, skating, swimming, and holding healthful posture when carrying bags, children, groceries, and yourself, involve continuing muscle work against the relatively light resistance of the ground, the bicycle pedal, the water, and the weight of your body and packages. Continuous effort against relatively low resistance calls on muscular endurance.

Muscular endurance is different from cardiovascular endurance. It is the endurance of the specific muscles you are working, not your heart and aerobic system. Untrained muscles do not have muscular endurance. They will get tired before you are out of breath. Trained muscles have specific changes in their cells and how they function that increase endurance capacity. These adaptations don't change muscle size.

Improved muscular endurance makes long walks, runs, rides, and swims easier, and reduces your chance of leg cramps. For carrying things around, and just getting through the day, muscular endurance of your back, hip, and thigh muscles can make the difference between an uneventful day and a tired, achy back or knees that night.

Flexibility

Flexibility is usually thought of as touching toes or doing contortions. In daily life, you need flexibility to reach shelves and cabinets without your shoulder and hip being so tight that reaching up hurts your shoulder, and you lean back to reach up, increasing the inward arch in your lower back. Your hip needs to bend enough to tie your shoes without rounding your back to reach. You need to have enough Achilles-tendon length to keep your heels down when you squat to pick things up. You need functional flexibility to cut your own toenails, scratch your own back, and do all your daily movement activities with healthful joint angles.

Functional flexibility means the ability to stand and move in biomechanically healthful positioning without tightness pulling you into injurious bad body positions. Muscle tightness pulls you into round-shouldered poor posture and makes standing straight and moving in healthful ways feel unnatural. Someone with tight shoulders is more likely to lean back and arch their lower back when reaching upward, which shifts upper-body weight onto their lower spine. Tight anterior (front) hip muscles can create a bent-forward standing position. Often, the lower back will overarch along with it, creating much "mystery" lower back pain. When sitting and bending, tight hips can tip the pelvis backward, rounding the spine. Rounded spine physically pushes lumbar discs to move (slip) outward and puts unequal pressure, increasing disc degeneration. Many conventional stretches increase the problems of poor posture and tight, achy joints, because they reinforce and practice the forward-bent unhealthful posture with which you started. Stretching for health and injury reduction needs reform. (Refer to Chapter 3 for a section on flexibility, and Chapter 6 on stretching.)

Balance

Balance is an often forgotten aspect of fitness. Good balance is essential to preventing falls and the injuries that result from them. A cycle develops when you get out of shape and decrease your balance skills along with all your other "use-it-or-lose-it" abilities. You become more afraid to fall and more afraid to bend or do activities. You do less, lose more balance skills, and so on, losing more and more ability and independence. Many people become housebound or even chair-bound—afraid of falls.

Walking heavily is often a sign of poor balance. Walking heavily is hard on the joints and can contribute to a lot of aches and pains. A slip or misstep while walking with packages, for example, can either be easily rebalanced with good equilibrium skills, or result in a cascade of shoulder, neck, or back strain from sudden repositioning, or a sprained ankle and various impact injuries from the fall. Balance is highly trainable. Ways to improve balance are described in Chapter 9.

Aspects of Fitness

Cardiovascular Endurance. Also called aerobic fitness, it is the ability of your heart and lungs, and their system of blood vessels, to supply oxygen and nutrients to the body. Enables you to run, swim, bike, skate, walk, ski, and dance farther and longer, with less effort. Good condition lowers risk of several diseases.

Anaerobic Capacity. Stored fuel system for short, intense activity. Enables you to run or swim short distances quickly, and exert against resistances from pushing open a stuck door to doing strenuous exercise.

Strength. Ability to move a heavy weight once, or a few times. Increasing your strength makes it easier to lift weights and move yourself around. Strong bones reduce fracture risk.

Power. Ability to move weight quickly. You call on power to push, pull, punch, throw, and lift things and yourself quickly.

Muscular Endurance. Ability to move or support a weight repeatedly or continuously. You need muscular endurance of your legs to walk, jog, and cycle long distances, and go dancing. You use muscular endurance of torso and shoulder muscles to stand and sit in healthful position while reading this book.

Flexibility. Ability to move easily and safely through a range of motion, and to stand, walk, run, and move without hunching or being pulled by tightness into unhealthful posture.

Balance. Ability to keep your body stable and in position without swaying, slipping, or falling. Crucial to preventing falls and near-falls, and the injuries that come with them. Injury and disuse diminish balance.

Mental. Memory, pattern recognition, problem solving, and other thinking functions. It is not true that you must lose mental sharpness with age. With use, you can improve at any age.

Emotional. Several centers in your brain process self-control. They need exercise like anything else and can become strong with regular practice.

Mental Fitness

Decline in mental ability is not aging, but disuse. Memory, problem solving, noticing surroundings, setting goals, organizing, and other thinking functions are all "use-or-lose" skills. They need practice and exercise.

Emotional Fitness

Just as you can't go through red lights every time you just feel like it, or hit someone any time you just feel like it, you don't just eat anything you feel like at any time. It is unhealthy. Some people say any denial is unhealthy. It is like saying you can just wet your pants when you feel like it. Self-control is cleaner in body and spirit. Several centers in your brain process self-control. They need exercise like anything else to become strong enough to do their job.

Our bodies are our gardens, to which our wills are gardeners.

—William Shakespeare

Not Just One

You need all the different aspects of fitness for a healthy, comfortable life. They need to work together, not be exercised separately. Doing "isolation" exercises that develop only one aspect of fitness, or only one at a time, or work "muscle groups" or "body parts" is robbing you of functional movement and setting the stage for health problems. The Chapter 3 explains how to develop and use each different aspect of fitness together.

3

Improving Your Fitness

Speaking generally, all parts of the whole body which have a function, if used in moderation and exercised in labours to which each is accustomed, become thereby healthy and well- developed, and age slowly; but if unused and left idle, they become liable to disease, defective in growth, and age quickly.

—Hippocrates

A little over 2,500 years ago, the Greek athlete Milo realized he could increase strength by using workloads above those normally encountered. He began lifting a young calf every day. The calf's maturing weight provided progressive resistance until, it was said, he carried the grown bull around the Olympic arena. He became a military hero and was undefeated as an Olympic wrestler.

Physical and cerebral ability improves by progressively increasing the effort, a process called overload. Routinely carrying increasingly heavy loads, for example, increases strength. Progressively raising the number of times you lift a weight improves muscular endurance. Progressively swimming, running, or walking farther or dancing longer extends cardiovascular endurance. Increasing your range of motion improves flexibility.

Thin people can be out of shape. Average-weight people can be out of shape. Fat people can be in or out of shape. Even athletic people can be out of shape in activities they don't regularly do. Understanding differences among aspects of fitness was covered in Chapter 2. This chapter covers how to improve different aspects of fitness in ways they need to work together for better health and ability, and to get in the shape you want.

Cardiovascular Endurance

Improve your cardiovascular status through continuous large-muscle activity, like walking, running, skating, dancing, biking, dancing, cross-country skiing, swimming, and active occupations and hobbies. Play active games and sports. If your intensity is low, as in slow walking, exercise class "floor work" of leg lifts and abdominal crunches, or a yoga class, you will not gain aerobic exercise benefit or burn as many calories.

Exercise studies find a close match between how hard your body actually works and how hard you consider the activity. In other words, you can easily monitor your workload. A pace you find to be medium effort usually is a medium load on your system, and is about right for exercising for general cardiovascular fitness. A good rule of thumb is to be able to carry on a conversation. If you are too out of breath to talk, you are working at an intensity that is too high to be mostly aerobic. That is not bad; it means you're working hard. (Refer to Chapter 4.) Keep an easy, moderate pace to make easy, moderate progress.

> Recommendations call for regular moderate exercise to improve your health. What is moderate? Your body is smart. Exercise that feels moderate is moderate. Exercise that feels easy really is too easy.

Anaerobic Capacity

You need good anaerobic capacity or short, intense exertions—dashing to catch a bus, carrying laundry up a flight of stairs, throwing a ball, sliding home in baseball, moving things, or carrying someone to safety. Improve your anaerobic capacity through high-intensity, short-duration activity like sprint runs, rope skipping, swims, and going up stairs.

Work up to being able to do 30 seconds of hard anaerobic work, followed by a short period of aerobic "rest," which is easy, mild activity until your heart rate returns to normal. Then, increase the length and number of times you can work hard. Light to moderate activity aids recovery better than complete rest.

As with aerobic activity, you can tell your intensity by how it feels. You are anaerobic when you are working hard and fast enough to be out of breath, and the workload feels taxing, even uncomfortable. Train for this, and what was previously uncomfortable becomes possible, and eventually easy.

Strength

Strength training is good for you. Done properly, strength activities increase your ability to lift and carry things without fatigue, firm your muscles, increase your ability to do the physical work of your favorite activities, strengthens your joints, and increases your amount of muscle, which burns calories and keeps you warm. Strength activities will "tone," or give firmness to the muscles worked. Strength activities like lifting weights and pulling and pushing your body weight up and down is an important part of osteoporosis prevention. The stress of muscle pulling against bone increases bone density.

Continuously lifting weights, when done at a high enough pace and effort for long enough, can elevate heart rate and respiration enough for cardiovascular gains too. Examples include chopping wood, moving furniture, and other real-life activities involving moving something weighty many times.

How Do You Get Stronger?

Your body makes several adaptations to increase your strength when you start a weight-lifting program. Usually, the first adaptation is a learning effect, which immediately increases the amount you can lift, even before any physical changes occur in your muscles. Then, three physical changes begin. The firing rate of nerves serving your muscles increases; the number of nerve-muscle units, called motor units, that can fire together increases; and you increase the size (cross-sectional area) of your muscle.

For the first three to four weeks, neural factors predominate to increase strength. After that, strength increases in young males primarily by increasing the size of the muscle. Women and older men increase strength more through neural mechanisms than size, even when they make the same strength increases as young men. Obviously, women and older men can increase muscle size through training, but size is not the only predictor of strength. Strong things often come in small packages.

How Do Muscles Get Stronger?

- The firing rate of nerves serving your muscles increases.
- More nerve-muscle units can fire together.
- Your muscle cells get bigger.

To get stronger, you need to contract muscles strongly at close to the maximum they are able to contract. To do so takes fairly heavy weight, which is why most exercise class "floor work" and using light hand weights does not strengthen appreciably. In the same way, light water exercises are not major strength builders, unless you are debilitated from sickness or injury or do large numbers of laps at high speeds, which increases intensity and total work.

Most studies agree the maximum number of times to lift a heavy weight consecutively to maximize strength gain is between 4 and 10. For the recreational lifter, the recommendation is 8 to 12 lifts at a time.

Popular fitness magazines sell protein supplements, stating you need extra protein to build muscle. This claim is rarely true. The Western diet usually provides much more protein than you need, even with heavy activity. You ordinarily do not need to consume additional protein to increase strength or musculature. More on healthy eating is covered in Chapter 18.

More important than doing strength exercises is knowing how to use your muscles to move and position your body for real life. Healthful positioning, also called body mechanics or ergonomics, does not come automatically from stronger muscles. For this reason, many physical-therapy programs that rely on strengthening do not fix major sources of back, neck, and knee pain. For example, strengthening your abdominal muscles does not automatically make them do anything for your back. Many people with strong muscles have unhealthful poor posture and the back pain that frequently results. Chapter 7 details abdominal muscles, and Chapters 20 and 21 cover back pain.

> Strengthening muscles does not make automatic change in their function. Many people exercise their abdominal muscles by rounding their spine forward with abdominal curling exercises called "crunches." They then stand up and don't know how to use their abdominal muscles for their major purpose—to stand in neutral spine instead of swaying in the poor posture of an overly large inward arch. Abdominal muscles do not automatically position or "support" the spine. Neutral spine is a voluntary posture.

Strength building in ways you really move is important to everyone's fitness plan. It is a myth that being strong reduces coordination or flexibility. You can be strong with poor coordination, or strong with no functional application, but not too strong to do the other functions.

> It is not true that if you stop exercising, your muscles will turn to fat. Your muscle cells will shrink, as with any other "use-it-or-lose-it" situation, but they do not transform into different cells.

Muscular Endurance

Muscular endurance is the ability of your muscles to do continuous activity. Examples are pedaling a bicycle, running, swimming, walking, and maintaining healthful body positioning while exercising or sitting, hiking with backpacks, carrying bags or children, or even just while preparing dinner.

Training is simple. Keep going. Hold healthful position even if you are tired. Intersperse easy and hard days, rest adequately, and have fun. The long-duration, low-intensity, large-muscle aspect of training for muscular endurance also increases cardiovascular endurance to varying degrees.

Power

Power is the product of strength and speed. Lifting a weight takes strength. Lifting a weight quickly takes power. You increase muscular power any time you move faster against a given load, get stronger, or both, in varying combinations. To develop power, lift, throw, or move a weight, such an object for throwing, a dumbbell, or yourself, but do it more quickly. Use your brain and good joint positioning to prevent moving in injurious ways. (Refer to Chapter 6 on stretching and Chapters 20 and 21 on back and neck pain.)

To increase throwing power, throw a heavier object than usual toward a specific safe target, faster than usual. Increase swimming or running power by swimming or running hard every few laps. Rest with easy laps. Warm up before beginning power laps. At the pool or waterfront, practice throwing a rescue line or float to increase throwing power. Lift yourself out of the pool without using the ladder. Doing so will increase strength, as well as power when it's done quickly. In addition, it is a functional activity that can potentially increase safety in a boating accident, for example.

Flexibility

If you look at many catalogs for stretching and fitness products, the pages seem to feature mostly people bending forward. If you saw the people walking down the street just as badly bent forward, you might think they needed to purchase some fitness product to fix that problem. Functional stretching is a popular buzz phrase, but it should mean that you are addressing function. That function is the ability to stand up straight and move in healthful positioning.

Stretching has been shown in some studies to prevent injuries or pain, or improve athletic performance. Based on this finding, gyms and fitness events are busy with people stretching—often in tight, unhealthy ways that re-emphasize the rounded-forward postures that caused the tightness, pain, and injuries in the first place. Other studies cast doubt on benefits of stretching for injury reduction, or indicate that stretching reduces muscle tensile contraction. Based on those studies, some athletes say they won't stretch at all. The problem seems to be how people stretch, then how they then go exercise and incur their injuries. Another key issue is how they go about their real life outside of the gym and their stretching routine. How are you sitting right now while reading this book? Is your chin jutting forward or downward? That contributes to upper back and neck pain. Keep chin in instead of overstretching your upper back in unhealthful bad stretches.

Although stretching for flexibility can reduce injuries, many common stretches can produce them. Many people don't have the flexibility they need to stand up straight, but make things worse by forward-stretching their already rounded back and shoulders, making the rounding worse. Stretching joints rather than muscles can destabilize your joints until they don't seat well, increasing wear and tear, and predisposing to injury. Forward-bending stretches, which are the majority of conventional stretches, are among the last things you need after a day bending forward over a desk, steering wheel, household chores, or work area. Good forward and backward ankle flexibility is important for general pain-free walking, and for many sports, particularly swimming, but looseness on the outside of your ankles increases chance of ankle sprains. Chapter 6 covers healthy flexibility and explains counterproductive stretches to avoid and good stretches to do.

> Functional flexibility reduces your chance of muscle and joint injuries and reduces back pain.
>
> Bad stretching from commonly-done stretches can increase your chance of pain and injury by destabilizing joints and reinforcing already poor posture habits.

When stretching, avoid stretches that promote the same bad posture with which you started. A common example is stretching forward through toe touching and abdominal crunches, pulling one arm forward across the body, and all the other forward bending that is counterproductive after a day of sitting and slouching over a desk or steering wheel. During daily life, avoid bending, standing, and sitting with a rounded spine and your chin forward. That stretching is not good stretching. How are you sitting right now to read this?

> Don't stretch hamstrings by bending over to touch your toes from a stand. It mechanically presses discs outward, promoting herniation over time, and promotes poor posture. You already sit hunched over a desk and know that is bad posture. You already know that bending over from a stand to pick up something is a way to injure the back. It doesn't magically become good for you by calling it a stretch.

Size

Lifting weights in healthful ways improves strength, endurance, power, and health. You will firm your muscles. To build large muscles, you need specific and intense work.

Power lifters are strong, yet they look different from bodybuilders. Power lifters train for strength; bodybuilders maximize size and visual effect. Two things bodybuilders do differently when doing honest training without drug use, are to increase volume of work and muscle definition.

> Power lifters and bodybuilders look different even though they both train by lifting heavy weights. They train differently and get different results.

Volume is the product of how much weight you lift and how many times you lift it. To maximize volume, lift more weights more often. You still need heavy weight, but to be able to do more lifts, use less weight than for strength training. Use a weight you can lift 12 or so times before muscle failure stops you. When you can easily do that four times in a row, increase the weight and, later on, try for five times in a row. Definition comes from losing fat under the skin.

> Bigger muscles don't always mean a stronger person.
> Small muscles can be strong too.

Someone with large muscles may not always be able to lift as much weight in a single effort as a smaller person who trained specifically for strength. It is not accurate to make assessments about the strength of women or older men, or anyone, based on muscle circumference.

Balance

Balance is directly and immediately helpful to prevent injury from slips and falls, and to maintain independence and mobility. Do you practice balance? Without practice, balance skills diminish. Balance will also be decreased in an injured limb. A negative cycle develops when people fear moving in fun ways or for independent living because of poor balance, and decrease their activities because of it.

You don't need to go to a gym to practice balance. You don't need fancy rehabilitation equipment. Stand on one foot for increasing lengths of time. Try any time you are standing around—washing dishes, folding laundry, waiting for buses or elevators. Safely try standing on one foot with your eyes closed. Without vision, you have fewer balance cues, providing more of a challenge to the balancing muscles. Throw and catch things standing on one foot. Put on trousers, hosiery, and shoes while standing. Walk on a line, and then walk the line backward. Walk the line sideways. Hop on the line, and then hop the line backward. Hop on one foot for increasing periods of time. Slalom-hop the line, and then slalom-hop the line backward. Stand on one foot, pick up things with the other foot, and pass them up to your hand without holding on.

If you need to begin slowly at the beginning, practice shifting your weight slowly from foot to foot, keeping good leg and back posture. Then try more quickly. Practice in a safe area without risk of falling onto objects, down stairs, or onto hard surfaces. How to improve balance with fun lifestyle instead of specific exercises is covered in Chapter 8.

Mental Fitness

Practice and use your mental abilities and you will keep function at any age—memory of where you left things, names and faces and contact information, draw or paint from memory. Practice and use them and you will keep function. Learn a skill that uses your brain along with your hands. Draw pictures, paint, sculpt in clay, learn a foreign language, learn flower arrangement, origami, practice a musical instrument, learn to build small (or large) projects. Teach your skills to others. Do these activities alone and with family members for healthful, beneficial creative time together.

Emotional Fitness

An important part of emotional fitness is refraining from harmful actions and doing good ones. The emotionally fit activity of self-control was reaffirmed in recent times by the Mahatma Gandhi, and in the West by Martin Luther King, Jr. Emotional fitness is something you incorporate in all your actions. Don't harm yourself by destructive thoughts and actions. Don't harm yourself by sitting in injury-producing bad slouching.

Don't harm yourself with bad exercise. Don't harm yourself with unhealthful food and drink. Don't harm yourself by hunching your shoulders to stress through preparing meals, when you can relax your shoulders, straighten your back, breathe, and use each stoke of washing, cutting, and preparing food as beautiful meditation in the same amount of time. Don't harm others with spiteful words, deeds, and thoughts. Don't cause others fear or pain. Don't cause yourself fear and pain.

Self-discipline is a voluntary exercise. To have inner peace, you just stop tensing your body and saying rude things. To stop slouching, you just use your own muscles to move your spine to healthy position. No special exercise can strengthen you to do it; you use your muscles to sit and stand straight and that gives you the exercise, psychological and physical. To stop overeating, you need to use your brain to recognize that you are doing it and that it is not necessary.

It is not cute or funny or powerful to be spiteful, smug, immoral, or to put others down with words or actions. Banter is not meaningful or enlightened conversation for real daily life. Learn to really speak with, and listen to, the people who matter.

Children, and even adults, need consistent positive examples. It is good and crucial exercise. It is easy to be destructive to yourself and others, while it takes energy (but also gives energy) to be good. Do positive actions. Make your word mean something. Learn gardening. Help the community. Don't litter. Volunteer at a shelter. Exercise your spirit. Increasingly, medical studies show positive medicinal effects of humor and laughter. Exercise your sense of humor. To be happy, you need to practice it. Think a good thought now. If you can't think of one, find one and practice it until it becomes natural to think it when you are stressed, and first thing in the morning when you wake instead of negative thoughts.

How to Improve All Your Aspects of Fitness

Cardiovascular Endurance (aerobic capacity). Long-duration, large-muscle activity like walking, running, skating, dancing, playing soccer, cross-country skiing, swimming. Brisk, fun intensity.

Anaerobic Capacity. Bursts of intense movement activity like sprints, whether on land, in the water swimming or finning, rope skipping, tumbling, martial-arts moves, or on a bicycle. Alternate short, hard exertions with easier ones. Work hard enough to get out of breath, rest briefly, and then sprint again.

Strength. For general strengthening, safely lift the heaviest weight you can lift 8 to 12 times. The weight may be your own body weight for push-ups, pull-ups, getting up and down from the floor, lifting children and furniture, and other fun, functional body exercise. For serious strength building, lift the heaviest that you can for 4 to 8 lifts. Build up how many times you can do this lift.

Muscular Endurance. Do continuous lifts or motions, with relatively lighter weight. Maintain good joint positioning to prevent injury. More on positioning in the two back-pain chapters, Chapters 20 and 21.

Power. Move a heavy or light object (including yourself) quickly. Repeat many times. Use your brain and good joint positioning to avoid injury.

Flexibility. Remember that slouching is a stretch—a bad one. Your back becomes overstretched and rounded. Don't add to that with continued forward stretching. Don't bend over from a stand to stretch your legs. You know that picking things up that way is bad for your back. It doesn't magically become good for you by calling it an exercise. Stretch muscles to restore your ability to stand straight and move in healthful ways. Don't force joints into such looseness that they no longer seat properly. More on flexibility can be found in Chapter 6.

Size. Lift heavy to moderate weight often. Exercise and eat low fat so muscles aren't hidden beneath fat stored under your skin.

Balance. Balance is easily and highly trainable, but often neglected. It is crucial for ease of movement, independence, variety of activity, and preventing sprains and falls. Stand on one foot while on the phone or washing dishes, for example. Increase the challenges with fun and varied balance games. Put on and take off pants, socks, and shoes standing up for combination balance and flexibility. More on balance can be found in Chapters 8 and 9.

Mental Fitness. Practice and use your many various mental abilities and you will keep function at any age.

Emotional Fitness. Negative thoughts and practices can be thought of as junk food for the mind: habit-forming and unhealthy. Brain centers for self-control, positive actions, kindness, discipline, and feeling happy come from practicing those actions.

When you're a child, you're told, "Sit still. Be quiet. Eat everything on your plate."

As an adult, it's suddenly, "Get moving. Don't eat so much. Say something profound."

Now is the time to learn that active and self-disciplined behavior is health, while eating when not hungry and eating junk food is not health. Don't wait to teach good habits to children or to learn them yourself.

Can You Have It All?

To improve a specific sport, you need to develop the systems and movements used in that particular activity. For health, also choose activities that coordinate and mix different aspects of fitness, rather than only isolating one. Real life does not move or work in isolation.

Do weightlifting that uses real life loads to develop strength, endurance, and power. Regularly walk, jog, cycle, swim, row, roller-skate, play, and dance to develop cardiovascular endurance. Do regular stretching, and stand and move with straight positioning to develop healthful, functional range of motion and reduce injury potential. Challenge your balance and your mind to keep you agile, mobile, thinking, and caring.

Check with your health-care providers before starting any program. Use your brain. Then, instead of "doing exercises," enjoy fun movement. It does not have to hurt to be effective. Feeling exertion and tired muscles afterward is satisfying and healthful. If your joints hurt, you are doing it wrong. Stop and change it. You can have gain without injury. You can have it all.

4

What Does Aerobic Mean?

A friend of mine runs marathons. He always talks about this runner's high. But he has to go 26 miles for it. That's why I smoke and drink. I get the same feeling from a flight of stairs.

– Larry Miller

When are you most aerobic?

a. Sitting in a chair
b. Doing 50 sit-ups
c. Swimming 100 yards

The answer is (a). You have more aerobic than non-aerobic processes going on when you are sitting in a chair than when you are either doing 50 sit-ups or swimming 100 yards. To understand why, you need to know what "aerobic" really means and how it relates to aerobic exercise.

Quick Overview

"Aerobic" is not just a type of exercise. It is a way your body makes energy, not only to do exercise, but to be alive at all. *Aero* is a Greek word meaning air, and *bios* is another Greek word meaning life. You need the oxygen in air all the time to manufacture the energy to stay alive, for all your body functions at rest, and for moving around. Using oxygen to burn food to make energy is called aerobic metabolism.

Although not an exact example, aerobic metabolism uses oxygen and the breakdown products of food the way a carburetor or fuel-injection system mixes oxygen with gasoline to combust into energy and combustion by-products. In your body, the combustion is much slower than in automobile engines. Unlike a car with only one energy-manufacturing mode, you have three different energy-generating systems. Only one of these systems is aerobic, the one using oxygen. The other two are *an*aerobic. *An* is a prefix meaning "without." Anaerobic processes make energy without oxygen. They use stored fuels and don't need oxygen.

You use your aerobic system nearly all the time—sleeping, sitting in a chair, or right now while reading. It is why you breathe continuously. When you begin physical activity, you add energy-making ability from your two *an*aerobic systems. All three systems contribute in different proportions during different length and intensity activities. Some activities use more aerobic than anaerobic processes, and so they are called aerobic exercises; other activities use more anaerobic processes, and so they are not aerobic exercises. All three of your systems work to do the same thing—to make an energy-giving molecule called ATP.

Aerobic Metabolism Is Not the Same as Aerobic Exercise

Your body makes energy to stay alive using three systems; one is aerobic, the other two are anaerobic (not aerobic). You use all three systems in different amounts, depending on what you are doing. You need your aerobic system all the time. You are using aerobic processes right now reading this, and when you sleep.

You need a boost from your two non-aerobic systems when you exercise. When an exercise uses the aerobic system the most and gives cardiovascular benefits, the exercise is called aerobic exercise, but the term is often misused.

Your Universal Energy Molecule

A special body molecule called ATP is the universal energy molecule. ATP fuels the activity and life processes of all living things, from bacteria, to plants, to bats, to you.

You can't eat ATP. Your body makes it using the breakdown products of the food you eat. You can make large amounts of ATP using oxygen, and can make a little without oxygen. You don't store much ATP in your body. You mostly make it as you go. It is why you keep breathing—to supply the oxygen to make ATP. The fitter you are, the more you can make, and the more energy you get to do your activities.

You need oxygen to "burn" your food fuel to make ATP. Your body can use only so much oxygen—determined by how fit you are, not by how much you breathe.

If unfit, you can't do as much exercise to use stored carbohydrate and fat fuels. You also can't move as much oxygen to your muscle cells during exercise to burn the food fuel. Getting fit makes you better able to move the oxygen with more blood cells, blood volume, blood vessels, and cellular enzymes.

ATP is short for adenosine triphosphate. ATP is a *tri*phosphate because it has three phosphates. The third phosphate is held on with a lot of energy (a high-energy bond). Breaking off the third phosphate releases the energy. Think of ATP like a toy spring-loaded snake in a can. When you undo the latch, the snake springs out. The latch is the high-energy bond—just a little thing, but holding back much energy. When your body needs energy, it uses a bit of water and an enzyme to undo the latch of ATP, and— zing!—out springs energy (Figure 4-1). You have billions and billions of ATP molecules releasing this energy all the time.

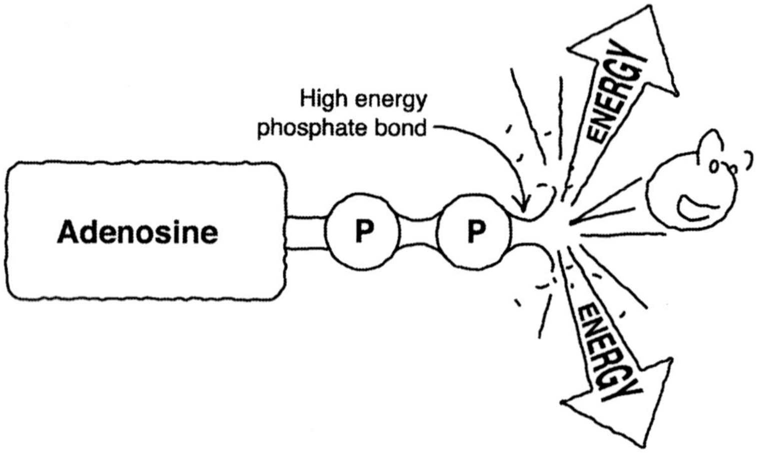

Figure 4-1. You get energy from millions of molecules of ATP by breaking their high-energy bond. You store a little ATP in your body and make the rest all the time using oxygen and the food you eat.

All three of your energy systems (two anaerobic and one aerobic) work toward the same final common event—to make ATP. Your aerobic, oxygen-using system makes large quantities of ATP from fat, carbohydrate, and sometimes protein. It keeps making ATP as long as oxygen is available. That process is a good thing—you need to fuel your body processes even when you are asleep. However, your aerobic system can't make ATP very quickly.

Sometimes, you begin an activity so quickly and intensely that you can't supply your muscles with required oxygen fast enough. The first few seconds are fueled by your first anaerobic system of stored ATP. You don't have much stored ATP, so you run out quickly. If you continue your activity, your muscles have to change over to your second system, also anaerobic, where you make ATP by breaking down glucose and another carbohydrate called glycogen that you store in your muscles and liver. This second system is also limited in how much ATP it can make. After several more minutes of continued activity, your third system, the aerobic energy system, begins to contribute more and more to the energy needs of your cells.

When you exercise above the fitness of your aerobic system, your muscles can't make the switch back to aerobic metabolism to make the energy to do your exercise. Without aerobic metabolism, you have to continue using the quick-and-ready glucose and glycogen. One problem is you can't make much ATP that way, so you get tired. Another problem is that without aerobic metabolism, your body can't remove lactic acid and other products that build up during anaerobic metabolism (more on this aspect later in the chapter). All of these factors force you to slow to a pace that can be supplied with ATP energy aerobically. If you don't slow down, you are soon gasping and burning—anaerobic. In short, the harder and faster you work, the more anaerobic the exercise is. The steadier, or more relatively comfortable, the pace, the more the oxygen supplied, and the more aerobic the exercise is. The more you push your limit, the further you extend the dividing line, and the more you can increase fitness over time, to work hard and remain aerobic.

The more in shape you are, the harder you can work and still be comfortable and aerobic.

	System 1	System 2	System 3
System Name	ATP-CP	Glycolysis	Oxidative
Type	Anaerobic	Anaerobic	Aerobic
Method	Stored ATP	Makes ATP from stored glucose and carbohydrate	Makes ATP from fats, glycogen and sometimes protein
Uses Oxygen?	No	No	Yes
Duration	Very short—seconds	Short to medium minutes	Long—hours
Intensity of Activity	Very high	Very high	Moderate to low

A Closer Look at Your Three Energy Systems

You use your three energy systems for activities of varying intensity and duration, ranging on a continuum from quick power, to speed and strength, to long endurance. Following is a closer, but still simplified, look.

System 1. ATP-CP

The original earth atmosphere was oxygen-free. The first living things made energy using only anaerobic processes. Several kinds of your cells, including muscle fibers, retain that anaerobic ability. Nerve cells can't work anaerobically, so they are sensitive to oxygen shortages. The heart is also completely aerobic. The heart and brain cannot lose or reduce their supply of oxygen and glucose, even for a brief interruption. It is for this reason that your blood must always stay circulating for you to stay alive, and you can only hold your breath for a short period. Muscle cells work both aerobically and anaerobically, so they have a great capacity to vary metabolic rate—more than any other body system.

Extremely brief, high-intensity bursts of activity lasting less than about 10 seconds are anaerobic and use stored ATP in your muscles to give you immediate energy. This type of burst is the realm of power movements, like opening a window, hitting a home run, doing football sprints, lifting a suitcase or grocery bag, putting the shot, leaping for a tennis ball or basketball, or kicking and punching in martial arts.

ATP stores energy until you need it. Biological energy is measured in calories. One mole of ATP can break apart to give you about 7 to 12 calories of energy to spend as you like (a mole is a chemical measurement of an awful lot of molecules—refer to the glossary). ATP gives you energy by breaking off its third phosphate. You still need to make energy, and without the third phosphate, adenosine triphosphate becomes only adenosine diphosphate, ADP, with just two phosphates. The low-energy bond of the second phosphate is of as much use as a nearly run-down battery. You need to recharge it.

As rapidly as you break up ATP for energy using this system, another stored molecule called creatinine phosphate (CP) puts it back together. CP sits in your muscles until you need it to give up one of its phosphates. CP sticks one of its phosphates onto ADP to make ATP again. Because ATP and CP work together, the ATP system is also called the ATP-CP system, or phosphagen system. You now need to make more creatinine phosphate (CP).

Your supply of CP is limited. When you are doing intense exercise and run low on CP, you must slow down enough to be aerobic again, using oxygen. Oxygen then helps make and replenish your ATP and CP stores, a process taking only a few minutes. The energy repayment comes mostly from the calories in your next meal. Being in shape with good aerobic ability increases the rebuilding of anaerobic energy stores, aiding the anaerobic recovery process. Someone seriously ill, for example in heart failure, builds ADP because they cannot get enough oxygen to restore it to ATP. That situation is bad.

How to Improve Your Anaerobic Capacity. Anaerobic training, like sprint running, swimming, and jumping, increases the levels of enzymes that are part of the ATP-CP cycle. Short intense lifting (for example, bringing heavy boxes of laundry up from the basement, or moving furniture up and down flights of stairs) can contribute toward this system. Your body makes these enzymes. Eating these enzymes directly in a supplement won't work to increase performance, no matter what the advertising for the products claims. All enzymes are proteins and are mostly destroyed by digestion if eaten. That is the job of digestion. They won't automatically reassemble back into enzymes on the other side of the intestinal wall. (Refer to Chapter 14, "Nutrition Myths.") Power and speed-specific exercise builds this system.

System 2. Anaerobic Glycolysis

When you continue activity past the point where your CP stores run low, your muscle cells switch to energy system 2. This system breaks down glucose to make ATP. Breaking down glucose is called glycolysis (lysis means "breaking down"), pronounced gly-COL'-ih-sis. This system needs no oxygen, so this process is alternately called anaerobic glycolysis.

Anaerobic glycolysis can make ATP quickly, just not very much of it. For comparison, glycolysis can make about two molecules of ATP for each molecule of glucose, while your aerobic system can make 36 ATPs. (Actually, glycolysis makes four molecules of ATP, but uses two ATPs to do it. Everything takes energy.)

When Do You Use Glycolysis? Glycolysis lets you do longer activities than those using your ATP-CP system, but not as long as you can with aerobic energy-making processes. Since glycolysis can make ATP quickly, it allows more intense activity than aerobic processes. This process is the strength and speed domain. Efforts of one to three minutes, like a 400-meter run, a 100-meter swim, climbing a hill carrying a load, or carrying someone out of a burning building rely on anaerobic glycolysis. Since this system is anaerobic, you can do some of these activities holding your breath, like swimming underwater. The extent of glucose and glycogen use by your muscles depends on whether your exercise is continuous and long, or intermittent and exhaustive, and varies greatly with intensity.

Glycolysis and the Food You Eat. Carbohydrate can be turned into energy without oxygen. Your body can store a fair amount of glucose by chaining glucose molecules together into molecules called glycogen, which you store mainly in your muscles and liver. When you need more glucose for glycolysis, your body breaks apart the glycogen. Glycogen is broken down to glucose in all cells, but this process is most active in muscle and red blood cells. Your red blood cells have no oxygen-processing ability (no mitochondria) and only use anaerobic glycolysis for their energy all the time. Muscle cells use glycolysis when you exert yourself.

Restoring your muscle and liver glycogen stores after hard exercise depends on how much carbohydrate you eat and how soon after activity you start eating. The optimum time for restocking is in the first 30 minutes after exercise. The second restocking "window" is in the next two hours or so. If you don't eat much carbohydrate in this time period, you won't have as much glycogen, even as long as five days later, than you would have if you ate right away (Figure 4-2). You want this muscle restocking so that you will have quick and ready energy for daily life and the next exercise you do. The small amount of stored carbohydrate holds water in your muscles, making the muscles firmer and more shapely. Low-carbohydrate diets deplete your muscle carbohydrate. Your muscles lose their water, and you seem quickly smaller and lighter, but it came from your muscles, not fat.

Increase your muscle glycogen stores by eating healthful amounts of complex carbohydrate right after exercising. Don't overdo or the extra will have to store as extra fat that you may not need. You also need to exercise regularly enough to convince your muscles they have a reason to store more carbohydrate. Exercise, not food, principally trains this system.

You might see claims that to burn fat you must not eat carbohydrate after exercise. If you don't restock your carbohydrate stores, you will not be able to exercise as hard. Losing weight and what is healthy are often separate things. Also, claims about burning fat can be misleading because the substance that is "burned" during exercise is not spare body fat, but dietary fat that forms in the bloodstream from meals of all kinds. Don't be misled by diet claims of restricting healthful food. Don't eat junk sugar either because advertising says that you need it right after exercise. Just eat small simple meals getting carbohydrate from fruit and vegetables, and do good honest exercise for health and weight control.

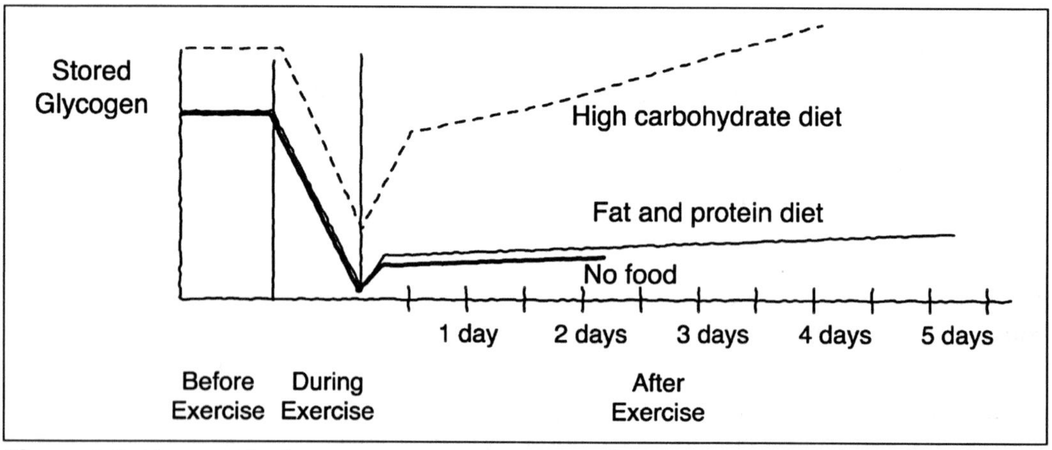

Figure 4-2. How much glycogen energy you can store for your next activity depends on how fit you are, how hard you work, how soon after exercising you eat, and how much carbohydrate you eat.

Lactic Acid. Breaking down glucose to make ATP for the fuel to be alive and to move takes 12 chemical reactions. The end-product of glycolysis is pyruvate (or pyruvic acid). After pyruvate forms, it can go two ways. Without enough oxygen to carry off the hydrogen ions that form when you are working anaerobically, they stick onto the pyruvate, making it into lactate, or lactic acid (Figure 4-3).

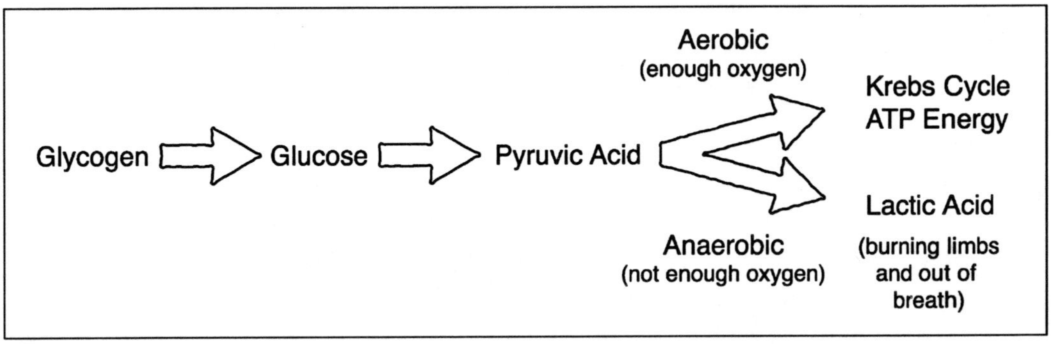

Figure 4-3. When you break down stored sugar to make energy while working hard (anaerobically), the process stops with lactic acid because t enough oxygen is not present for how hard you are working. When you work aerobically, the lactic acid doesn't build because it turns into pyruvate, which you use for more energy.

Your body produces lactic acid all the time. That process isn't bad, and you don't feel it below certain levels. Lactic acid has important functions to increase exercise capacity and serves as a fuel for your heart. Lactic acid is also made into glucose in the liver through another cycle called the Cori cycle. Your body then processes it, using oxygen, so that it doesn't build up more than you need. When you work above your aerobic capacity, more lactic acid is produced than you can process, so levels build. The extra acid products stimulate receptors to cause a burning feeling, which indicates those muscles are working anaerobically. You can open and close your hand widely 10 times as fast as you can to feel this effect.

The better shape you are in, the more lactic acid you can process and use. Improving physical condition makes a number of body changes that supply more oxygen to your cells to remove it. Breathing in more oxygen (on a tank, for example) won't work. Your body can't use it, unless you are at a high altitude or sick. Exercise lets you use more oxygen. With exercise, you grow more lung capillaries to take up oxygen, more red blood cells to carry the oxygen, more and bigger blood vessels to convey it, and more enzymes in the cells to uptake and change oxygen into energy. Feeling a burn with intense activity doesn't necessarily mean you are out of shape. Olympic athletes gasp and pant after their events, too. It means they are giving their top effort.

Various remedies are sold to reduce lactic acid on the premise that you can work harder without the pain stopping you. Most involve stopping to take the pill or potion. The pain diminishes, not from the potion, but because you stopped working. Some experiments have been tried with making the blood more alkaline to offset the acid produced. Results are marginal to nil for most exercisers. Nothing works better than just getting in better shape.

You can reduce lactic acid in two ways. You can lower your intensity to where available oxygen can supply your needs, so oxygen can turn the lactic acid back to pyruvate by carrying off the hydrogen ions and combining with them to form water. You can also get into better shape and be able to work at a higher level and still process the lactic acid into pyruvate. In both cases, the pyruvate becomes available for your third, and last, system—your aerobic system.

> A burning feeling in working muscles is lactic acid building and stimulating your pain receptors—a signal that you are working above your aerobic capacity. Working at a lower level reduces lactic acid to a level where you can process it. Getting into better shape lets you work at a higher level and still process it.

System 3. Aerobic (Oxidative) Metabolism

When your activity continues for long durations, and intensity is low enough to be met without your anaerobic systems, your body signals your cells to begin the gradual change back to your aerobic system. Endurance events are primarily aerobic and use oxygen (oxidative metabolism) to produce energy. Aerobic metabolism can make a great deal of ATP to carry through long events. Reptile and amphibian hearts and lungs are not developed enough to use aerobic (oxidative) metabolism. They rely on glycolysis. Lizards, for example, can't go long distances.

Aerobic metabolism uses stored carbohydrate, fat, and protein (if necessary) in two interesting pathways to make ATP. The first pathway is the Krebs cycle, and the second is the electron transport chain. For more detail on these pathways, refer to the glossary. You make most of your ATP in the electron transport chain. The electron transport chain takes the hydrogen ions formed in the energy-making process and, by combining them with oxygen, makes lots of ATP instead of allowing the ions to stick onto pyruvate. The extra ions turn pyruvate into the burning lactate. With lactate, you can't get into the Krebs cycle, so you lose a large portion of your ATP production opportunities. Having oxygen makes the difference between stopping your energy-making processes with lactate (while you gasp and rub burning limbs) or restoring lactate to pyruvate, so the pyruvate can enter into aerobic energy-making processes.

The Difference Between Aerobic Metabolism and Aerobic Exercise

Your aerobic metabolism goes on all day and night, even when you are sitting or sleeping, making a distinction between aerobic metabolism and aerobic exercise. Not everything that predominantly uses your aerobic system is aerobic exercise. What does aerobic exercise mean in light of the fact that you are aerobic even when you are sleeping?

The word "aerobic" describing a type of exercise was coined by Dr. Kenneth Cooper, the "Father of Aerobics." The intensity must be high enough to give a cardiovascular training effect, or it is not aerobic exercise. Often, the intensity will be high enough for you to be breathing hard, making you use the anaerobic systems as part of your exercise.

If you are out of breath and your heart is beating faster, you are more anaerobic than aerobic. Although you are breathing in plenty of oxygen, your body can't deliver and process it fast enough. Lactic acid builds. That process is not bad, and it does not mean that you are not exercising or benefiting; it just means you are not processing energy in your muscles using only aerobic metabolism. Your brain and nervous system are still using aerobic metabolism, but your muscles are not, so it is considered anaerobic exercise. When you exercise aerobically, oxygen changes lactic acid back to pyruvate, which can be used to make ATP. With low fitness levels, you have to stay at a low level to stay only aerobic. Staying at that low level doesn't make the exercise better because it is all aerobic. If you pushed a little harder, you could raise the level to where you can gain more exercise.

What About Walking? Slow walking mostly uses your aerobic system. It does not invoke much of your anaerobic systems because it is such low intensity. In this case, energy is supplied aerobically, but it is not much aerobic exercise. Faster walking may qualify as aerobic exercise depending on how high you raise your heart rate and how long you walk. Walk so that you feel you are moderately exerting yourself for at least 10 to 20 minutes a few times each week to start gaining health benefits. Walk longer and more briskly, and add other forms of exercise for fitness benefits.

What About Running, Swimming, and Biking? If you go very slowly, you may have aerobic metabolism but not much aerobic exercise. It also won't be very aerobic if you do it so fast that you are out of breath and have to stop. Then you are exercising primarily *an*aerobically. It does not mean that you are not getting good exercise, just make sure that you can last long enough to give you cardiovascular (aerobic) and other exercise-training effects. One way to achieve these effects is to move in intervals. Go hard and fast, rest a short bit, then go again before your heart and breathing slow to below your training level. Working in intervals is a nice way to train both systems, and get more aerobic benefit. Both systems need the other to help recovery. To swim, bike, run, or jog aerobically without intervals, try a pace that you can maintain for at least 10 to 20 minutes, and that feels comfortably hard.

What About American Football? Football games may be long, but the actual exercise is short—a few tens of yards and tackles for most players. It does not mean that football is not a hard sport, just that it is not an aerobic one.

What About Sit-Ups? During short, anaerobic exercises, you use stored ATP, CP, and glycogen. Swimming 100 yards is not long enough to switch back to primarily aerobic exercise, and is why doing the 50 sit-ups mentioned at the beginning of this chapter is not aerobic, and is metabolically less aerobic than sitting in a chair, where all your processes are just about 100 percent aerobic. Sit-ups also practice the same bent-forward posture that causes so many problems, and loads the discs of your spine in unhealthful ways. Sit-ups and crunches are unhealthful, counter-productive exercises that do not work your core muscles they way they need to function in daily life. Chapter 7 shows functional, effective, and healthful abdominal and core exercise.

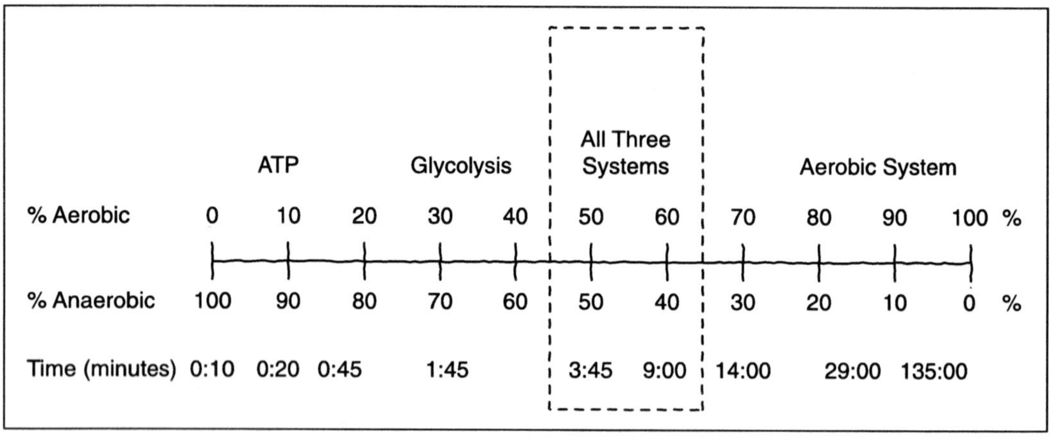

Figure 4-4. You have three energy systems—ATP-CP, glycolysis, and aerobic. Each system contributes in different amounts during different intensities and durations of exercise.

What About "Fat-Burner" Classes? A fad exercise class is the "fat-burner." Fat-burner classes are lower intensity than regular exercise classes, yet advertising for these classes states that participants burn more fat. The reasoning given is that during high-intensity exercise, glycogen is the primary fuel, but with lower-intensity activity, more fat is used as a primary fuel. A half-knowledge of "aerobic metabolism" yields a wrong final result.

Fewer total calories are burned in these classes than in more vigorous classes because the intensity is lower. Fat would supply a greater percentage of the energy in a low-intensity class, but not as much in total would be mobilized over the same period of time. High-intensity activities, done for the same time, burn more total fat and calories.

That does not mean that overweight, beginning exercisers must start with high-intensity exercises. Prolonged low-intensity exercise is a way to get started getting used to exercising. Even regular exercise at only 50 percent of your maximum ability helps reduce risk of high blood pressure, diabetes, and cardiovascular disease.

Eating for Aerobic Exercise

The in-shape body wants to preserve muscle carbohydrate stores as long as possible, because more carbohydrate allows exercise to continue longer. Preferentially using fat instead of glycogen is called glycogen sparing, and is a training adaptation that delays fatigue. That does not mean that eating fat will make you exercise better, but that your body uses it. A trained endurance athlete's body will begin the change to fat-burning from glycolysis, sooner than an out-of-shape body.

Since the main energy fuel your body draws on for aerobic exercise is fat, it is popular to market foods that are high fat and call them foods that "give you energy." Eating fatty food is not the way to get energy. Healthy food with a good portion of carbohydrate is the dietary fuel that supports exercise so you can draw from your fat stores. Regularly exercising aerobically, like swimming, biking, and skating, gets you in better shape so you can better use your fat stores. (Refer to Chapter 3, "Improving Your Fitness," for more on how to get in shape, and to Chapter 14, "Nutrition Myths," and Chapter 17, "Ergogenic Aids" for more on foods that do and don't help physical ability.)

An Aerobic and Anaerobic Bike Ride

You now know enough to follow the three simplified metabolic pathways through a sample physical activity—a bike ride. You're sitting quietly, oxidatively aerobic. You decide to go for a bike ride. You stand and walk to get your bike, with the help of some ATP-CP stored in your legs. You lift your bike in another short use of ATP-CP, and carry the bike out the door and down the steps, rapidly shifting to anaerobic glycolysis.

You begin your ride, first an easy warm-up, and then up a nearby hill. As you increase the pace, your bodily processes increase speed to manufacture more ATP for energy. You breathe faster to take in more oxygen to help make ATP. Your body has a limit as to how fast it can deliver oxygen to your cells and how fast your cells can process oxygen in oxidative energy production. In your uphill ride, your energy demand exceeds the oxidative supply. Your cells rapidly switch to a mostly anaerobic glycolytic system. You begin to breathe heavily. Had you regularly worked out more, and gotten in better shape, the energy demand would be within range of your aerobic system. You would now be comfortably supplying your leg muscles with oxidatively stoked energy, not likely to run low soon.

Your cells are switching to your energy-production processes that don't need oxygen. These processes can make energy for only short periods of time. Without enough oxygen to carry off extra hydrogen ions that attach to the pyruvate that forms from anaerobic metabolism, the pyruvate becomes lactic acid. Hydrogen ions accumulate, dropping your pH to the acid. Your legs burn.

The terrain changes and the hill levels off. You drop intensity and slow your pedaling. After several more deep breaths, you "pay back" what is called the oxygen debt to your anaerobic system and allow oxygen to turn lactic acid back into pyruvate. You settle into a comfortable aerobic pace. After 10 or so minutes of continuous pedaling, you are about half aerobic and half glycolytic anaerobic. After another 10 to 20 minutes of exploring, the aerobic percentage might have risen to about 60 to 70 percent or so. If your fitness level is high, it can climb higher, a response of a well-trained body to help spare muscle glycogen and delay fatigue.

At the halfway point, you turn and pedal back, now mostly aerobic. At the hill, you enjoy the coast downhill. Your energy needs are still supplied aerobically, even more than during your uphill and level-terrain ride, although you are now doing almost no exercise. During the aerobic portion of your ride, your body has been busy replenishing much of your stored muscle CP for your ATP-CP system, but not glycogen. For restocking glycogen, you need to eat and drink.

You went too far downhill and missed the turnoff. You turn around and pedal back uphill with a rush of ATP-CP. Seconds later, your body shifts to primarily anaerobic glycolysis, but not as much glycogen is stored as before. These few minutes seem harder than the first strong pedals at the start of your ride. You turn off at your street, and lift your bike up the steps in another ATP-intensive effort.

You put your bike down and take off your jacket, using all three systems. Sitting quietly after your ride, you are primarily in aerobic metabolism. You get a snack of raw walnuts and fruit to begin restocking muscle and liver glycogen.

If you had decided to go grocery shopping by bicycle, you would have included a stop halfway. Your system would have remained at a higher calorie-burning rate while you shopped, since it takes time for heart rate and other functions raised in exercise to return to regular levels. You would have added more anaerobic moments of lifting grocery bags into your knapsack or bike baskets, and then increased efforts of all three of your systems to carry the extra weight while bicycling back. Grocery shopping by bicycle can be functional, practical interval training.

5

What Does Warm-Up Mean?

If you spend too much time warming up, you'll miss the race.

—Grand Heidrich

Getting warmed up for exercise doesn't mean stretching or deep breathing. Some common activities done for warm-ups in exercise classes are not warm-ups.

What Is a Warm-Up?

"Warm-up" means doing enough muscular work to raise your body temperature. Just about any preparatory activity is often called a warm-up, but the term literally means to raise body temperature—to get warmer.

You are like an automobile engine that heats with use. Not all the fuel you put into your car goes to move the car. Much of the fuel energy used to move the engine and connected parts is lost as heat. In you, about 75 percent of all the energy you use to make your heart beat, for digestion, and for every other body process, turns to heat. Human energy inefficiency works in your favor to heat you to about 98.6 degrees F (37 degrees C) at rest. That "inefficiency" is good. If your body didn't work that way, your chemical processes wouldn't go as quickly, and you wouldn't be able to move around as easily. Muscular work using large muscles converts more mechanical energy into heat, further raising your temperature.

"Warm-up" is not synonymous with any preparation for exercise. It specifically means to raise your body temperature, up to a point, making exercise safer.

What Is Not a Warm-Up?

You won't raise body temperature with deep breathing, arm-waving, or small muscle activity. Rising up and down on your toes, or alternately bending and straightening your elbows, or stretching, does not contribute enough heat energy to warm your body. It does not mean that these actions do nothing to start you moving those areas, just that they are not an entire warm-up.

Stretching is not a warm-up. Warm up first using large muscle exercises before major stretching.

Why Warm Up?

Warming up changes your body in several ways that make exercise healthier. By raising resting body temperature, your muscles become more pliable and can work faster. Warmed-up muscles can stretch more and endure more force without tearing. Increased body temperature improves diffusion of oxygen, carbon dioxide, and metabolites to and from tissues. Blood viscosity lessens, and blood vessels widen, slightly reducing resistance to blood flow in muscles, including the heart. Abruptly beginning intense activity without adequate warm-up can leave you without enough blood and oxygen to your heart. In a study of men with chest pain accompanying exercise because of narrowed heart blood vessels, warming up increased the length of time they could walk before onset of chest pain.

Benefits of Warm-Up

- Muscles can work faster.
- Blood viscosity lessens.
- Muscles become more injury-resistant.
- Muscles can stretch farther without tearing.
- Necessary chemical reactions in your body speed up.
- Blood vessels widen, reducing resistance to blood flow.

- Blood and oxygen can get into your heart and muscles more easily.
- Carbon dioxide and waste products can get out of your tissues more easily.

How Does a Warm-Up Work?

Your body's chemical processes are sensitive to small temperature increases. The enzyme reactions in your cells that produce energy and control body functions speed up proportionally as your body temperature rises. A 10-degree C rise would double the rate of enzyme reactions. This doubling is called the Q10 effect. Your internal temperature could never change 10 degrees without severe health consequences. The idea is that the few degrees that a warm-up raises your temperature uses the Q10 effect to boost athletic ability.

Who Doesn't Need a Warm-Up?

You won't benefit by warm-up exercises if you are a lizard. Lizards are cold-blooded, meaning they can't change body temperature on their own. They have to lie in the sun to warm up. Their internal temperature changes as their environment changes, so they are called poikilotherms (POY'-kill-oh-thurms), which means "variable temperature."

Warm-blooded animals, including humans, maintain a remarkably constant internal temperature at rest, so we are called homeotherms (HOME'-ee-oh-thurms), a word meaning "same temperature." Even though we are warm-blooded, scuba divers are a group that may not benefit by warm-up activities, but for different reasons. Warmer body temperature allows more nitrogen to get in and out of you. Lower temperature inhibits nitrogen uptake and elimination. Studies found that divers who spent their entire dives cold were less likely to get decompression sickness. A diver starting a dive warm would absorb more nitrogen. If that diver then chilled, which is common during a dive, eliminating that additional nitrogen slows, increasing decompression sickness risk.

Other activities benefit from warm-up. The more strenuous the activity, or the more range of motion you need, the more likely that warm-up may help.

How Do You Know When You're Warmed Up?

You're warm when you break a sweat. A common recommendation is that is takes 5 to 10 minutes of exercise to warm-up, and needs to include light jogging or cycling. However, a dozen push-ups and lunges, properly done, will quickly increase whole body-muscle temperature and put joints through a range of motion.

What to Do

You can warm up for activity in three ways:

- Active direct warm-up
- Active indirect warm-up
- Passive warm-up

An active direct warm-up is the same activity as the intended exercise, but at lower intensity. For example, fast walking warms you for jogging. Slow jogging warms you for running. Slow cycling warms you for faster cycling. Slower swimming (not just sloshing) is a good warm-up for pool training. An active indirect warm-up uses any large muscle activity, such as push-ups and lunges.

A passive warm-up uses a sauna, steam, or conventional hot bath. Your body temperature rises with passive warm-up, although passive warm-up does not give all the circulatory benefits of active exercise. Hot, steamy showers give people with arthritis or other injuries a head start on muscle heat helpful to reduce pain and increase range of movement enough to start exercising actively. Drink a little extra water to avoid dehydration.

After raising body temperature, review the motions you use for your activity. Go through the range of motion slowly. Then repeat each successive motion faster and fuller in range until reaching the full activity, for example, kicks for martial arts, tennis serve, bowling approach, swing and release, dance moves, golf swing, and so forth.

Points for Warm-Ups

- Start with large muscle movement.
- If anything hurts or doesn't want to move where you're moving, check why and change it.
- Break a light sweat.
- Review the movement for which you are warming up.
- Have fun so that you'll look forward to the next time.

6

Innovations in Stretching

One learns to itch where one can scratch.

—Ernest Bramah

For many people, stretching means bending forward to touch the toes, or something to do before or after exercise. Many of these same people don't have the flexibility to comfortably lie flat without a pillow under their head or knees, or to stand straight, with their back and heels against a wall and the back of their head comfortably touching the wall without craning their neck or lower back. Their back and shoulders are too rounded. Their chest and hip are too tight. The average person is often too tight to just stand up straight (Figure 6-1). Consequently, they stand, walk, and do all activities at joint angles that impinge, grind, rub, and stress, using muscles that strain at painful points. This condition is called functional tightness.

It is not a mystery when you don't become more flexible or prevent pain syndromes, and injuries through conventional stretching routines. The idea of stretching needs to be reframed as restoring healthy length to your muscles, so that you no longer stand, sit, bend, and move all day with strained, tight, unhealthful positioning.

Unhealthful stretching is ingrained in popular fitness. Start with the ideas in this chapter to retrain your muscles and brain to stretch in ways that restores and retrains healthy positioning, rather than distort it, during all you do.

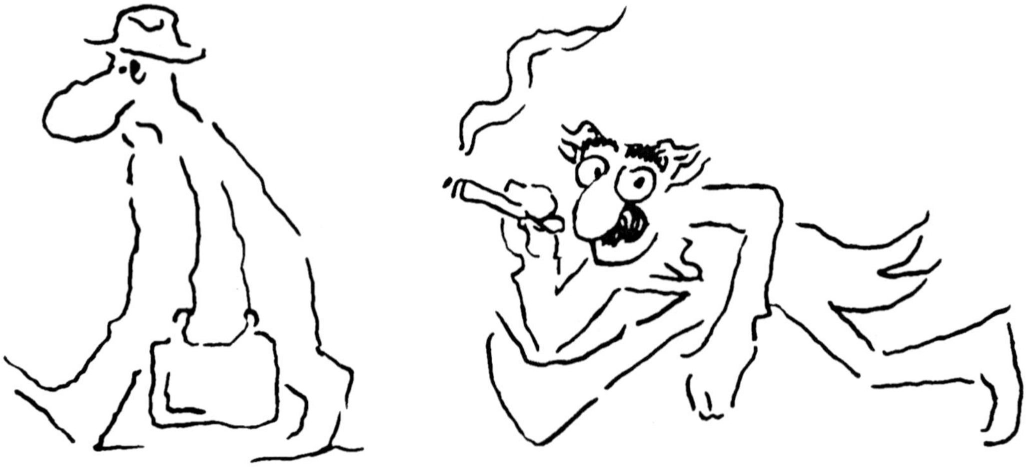

Figure 6-1. An overstretched back and tight chest are so common they look normal. The bent forward postures that result can lead to several pain and injury syndromes.

Three Top Stretches to Change

HIP

The front of your hip at the crease where the leg meets the body should be able to straighten completely to let you stand upright. If your anterior hip is tight, you may feel natural to stand bent forward. With the hip tilted forward, it is common to increase the inward curve of the lower back attempting to stand straight. The resulting overarching, called hyperlordosis is a major cause of mystery lower-back pain. (Refer to Chapters 20 and 21.)

Tight front hip muscles are sometimes a hidden source of shoulder pain. During overhead activities, if the hip is tilted forward, the shoulder has to overrotate to reach (Figure 6-2 left). The repetitive strain on the shoulder during weightlifting, tennis, football, and overhead activities, like combing and washing hair and reaching shelves, can produce shoulder pain that is hard to rehab if you do not also stretch the tight front hip muscles and retrain neutral spine positioning (Figure 6-2 right). See Chapter 7 and 21 to learn neutral spine.

Good Hip Stretches

Most conventional stretches of the lower body involve bending the leg forward at the hip, which contributes to the problem. Instead, you need to extend the leg and hip the other way so that the front hip stretches enough to allow you to keep neutral spine when standing and walking.

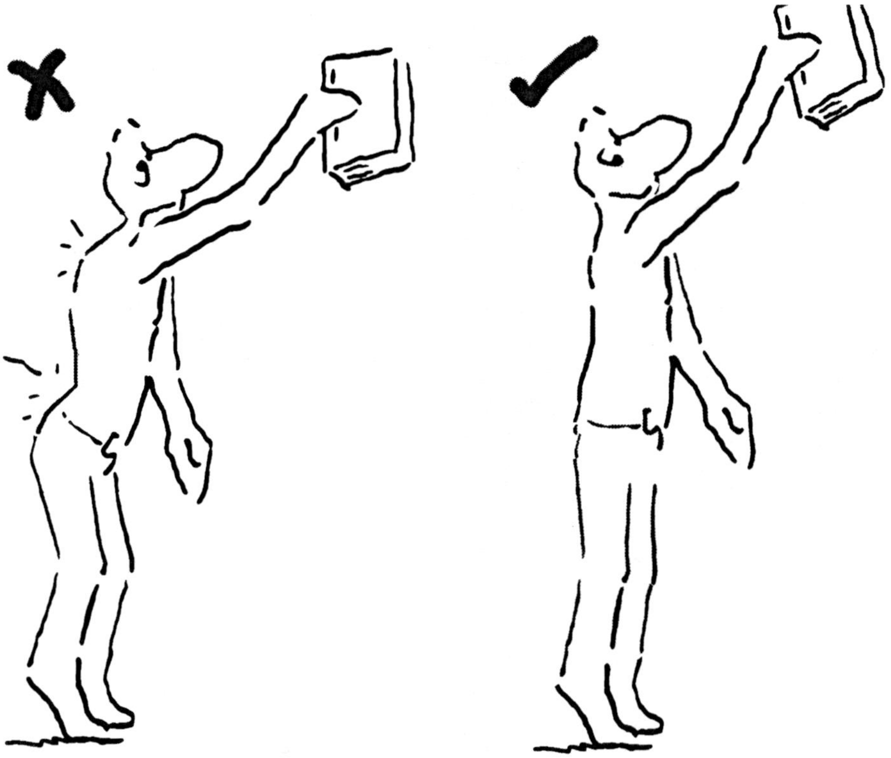

Figure 6-2. Tight front hip muscles can tip your hip forward when standing, making feel normal to overarch the lower back (left). Tight shoulder muscles promote more overarching in your lower back and are hard on the neck when reaching overhead. Note the level belt reflecting neutral spine at right.

Lie Over a Bed. A quick way to stretch the front of the hip is to lie over a bed or bench.

- Sit at the edge of a bed.
- Lie back with your upper body and hips on the bed and legs dangling to the floor.
- Make sure the edge of the bed is right under your hips, not lower (at the thigh) or higher (at the lower back).
- If your lower back hurts, you are arching. Press your lower back against the bed and if you regain neutral spine, the compressive pain should stop right away. If not, stop and check what you are doing.
- Feel the stretch at the front of the hip where the leg meets the body and through the thigh.

Lie Face Up Over a Pillow. A similar, but smaller, stretch as Lie Over a Bed can be done by lying flat on your back, with your hip on a pillow. The pillow raises only the hip to stretch the front muscles.

Lie Face Up Over an Exercise Ball. When stretching face up over an exercise ball, don't put the ball under the lower back. Roll the ball (safely) under the hip to stretch it. Before rolling the ball down to the hip, position your arms ready to place on the floor overhead. Raise both arms to your ears as you lean back over the ball. Point fingers back toward the ball as you place them on the floor, and roll the ball downward past your lower back all the way under your hip.

Quadriceps Stretch. A common stretch for the thigh and front hip is to stand and hold one foot behind you. It is often done in a way that gives little stretch to the front hip. Tuck the bottom of your hip under (Chapter 7) instead of letting the bottom of the hip tilt backward and the lower back arch. As soon as you return to neutral spine, the stretch will increase and be felt in the front thigh and hip.

Lie Face Down Stretch. This move is a big, good-feeling stretch for the hip and thigh.

- Lie flat face down on any comfortable surface. Feel both front hipbones touch the surface.
- Extend one leg out to the side to any comfortable distance. Keep the knee and toes facing front. Don't roll to any side. Feel both front hipbones touch the surface.
- To get more stretch, prop gently on elbows.
- To increase the stretch further, bend the back knee to lift the foot.
- If your lower back hurts, you are arching. Tuck the bottom of your hip under until you are in neutral spine (Chapter 7).

Active Front Hip Stretch—The Lunge. Refer to Chapter 21 on fixing back pain for more on the lunge for active hip stretch and strength.

- Stand with one foot in front and one in back.
- Point the back foot straight and forward, not turned out. Lift that heel.
- Bend both knees and lower straight down. Make sure to tilt the hip under, not push it forward. When you do, you will feel the stretch move to the front of the leg.

SHOULDER

Tight front chest muscles pull the shoulder where the upper arm attaches, making round-shouldered posture feel natural. The upper arm rotates so that the thumbs face inward (toward each other) rather than forward (Figure 6-3). Check for thumbs facing each other on people you see. Check yourself.

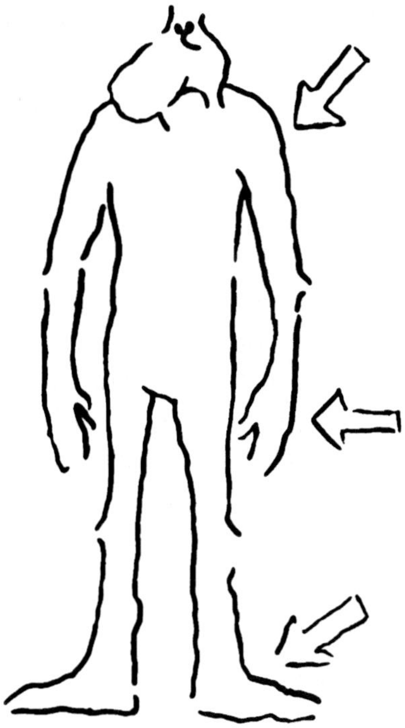

Figure 6-3. Tight chest muscles promote round-shouldered posture and arms that rotate inward. Tight hip and calf muscles and Achilles tendons contribute to walking "duck-footed" or toe-out. This habit can wear on your ankles, knees, hips, and big toe.

Bad Shoulder Stretches

People chronically overstretch their upper back and posterior shoulder all day by sitting, standing, and walking with rounded forward posture. Then the only "fitness" stretching they do is more forward motion during toe touches, sit-ups, leg lifts, and chest exercises. Damage builds as the overstretched posterior shoulder and tight anterior (front) muscles cause poor bent-forward posture, shallow breathing, upper-back pain, and shoulder injury. Two common shoulder stretches you don't need are pulling your arm across the front of your body, and pulling both arms up behind you.

Posterior Shoulder Stretch Over Your Body. Bringing one arm across your body in front is one of the most common stretches—and one of the least necessary. You probably already have overstretched the back of your shoulders by slouching all day over your desk, steering wheel, and other work. Sitting and standing with rounded shoulders wears on the neck and shoulder joints and is a common source of upper-back and neck pain. One of the most unnecessary things you can do is to further stretch the back of your already overstretched shoulder. Going to a gym to do it does not magically make it healthy.

Pulling Arms Up Behind You. Clasping your hands behind you and pulling your arms upward is not a useful stretch. It does not stretch the front chest muscles in the way needed for healthful joint positioning and making straight posture natural; however, it does press forward with high force on the front of the shoulder joint.

Not Overuse, but Misuse. Swimmers, pitchers, and other "overhead" athletes routinely practice these two counterproductive shoulder stretches for a greater range of motion, which can improve swimming speed. The price can be shoulder instability and susceptibility to long-term injury. When pain develops, they are often told it must be the repetitive strain of the swimming or pitching, or their sport, and they must stop the sport. Meanwhile, it was not necessarily the sport, but the bad stretching. They stop the muscle-building activity of swimming, but continue the injury process. Much of the problem is unhealthful stretches, not the range achieved. You can have a mobile strong shoulder without developing instability or injuring the shoulder joints and surrounding cartilage and soft tissue with good stretches.

Good Shoulder Stretches

The best way to stretch your shoulders for health and to restore ability to stand and move in straight position is to stretch the front chest (pectoral) muscles (Figure 21-4). It helps straighten and "unround" your shoulders and upper back. The following is a check for how well you can straighten your shoulder positioning for healthy standing and sitting:

- Can you put your hands on your hips and bring your shoulders back?
- You should be able to pull your shoulders back without tilting your shoulders forward, or arching your lower back, or jutting your head or chin forward.
- When you can pull your shoulders back easily with your hands on your hips, try pulling your shoulders back with your hands clasped together behind your back. Keep chin in and shoulders back.

HAMSTRING

Bad Hamstring Stretches

Stretching hamstrings by sitting and leaning forward to touch toes, or standing and bending over to toward the floor is an unhealthy stretch. Even with your back straight, forward bending stretches are a large contributor to lower back pain. It may stretch your back and legs, but sitting and standing bent forward and bending over forward puts high forces on the discs of your lower back, pressing them outward in a process that leads to herniation.

You already know that sitting bent over your desk, steering wheel, and computer is unhealthy for your back. If you go to the gym and sit bent over to touch your toes to stretch, it is the same bad bending. It is not magically different or healthy because it is called a stretch, a yoga pose, or a Pilates exercise. Modern lifestyle predominantly favors being bent forward, overstretching your back and tightening the front of your body until it becomes natural to slouch forward and uncomfortable to stand straight. Lower-back discs become pressed outward from all the forward bending. It starts feeling "normal" to stand and move with your back rounded in unhealthy position.

Stretching bent forward, sitting or standing, is also not the most effective way to stretch your hamstrings, even though it is a common stretch, and has been done for many years. Many things that are common and traditional are also not healthy, like smoking and hostility. A common alternative is to lie on the floor and lift one leg. It can be a good stretch when done functionally. Use it to learn healthier positioning. Don't bend the other leg and round the back. It is a more functional stretch to lie flat (Figure 6-4).

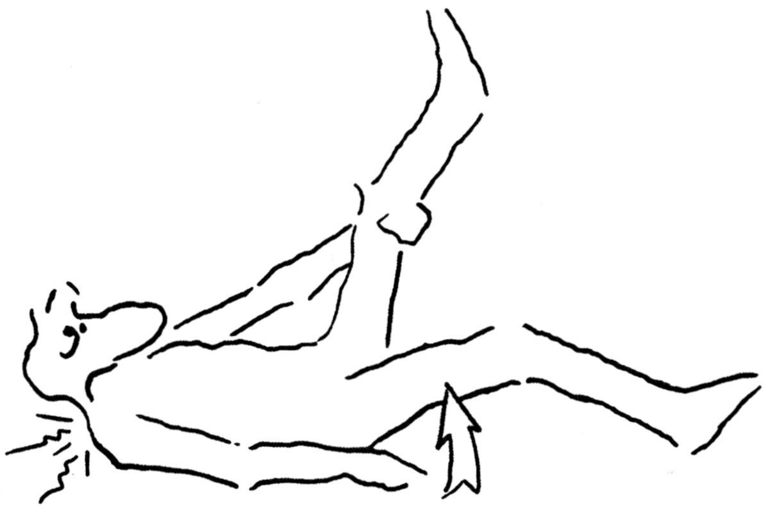

Figure 6-4. When the muscles in front of your hip are tight, the tight leg will come up when you raise the other instead of lying flat. Don't deliberately bend the knee since it keeps the hip tight. Instead, rest your leg, head, and shoulders straight and comfortably flat on the floor.

Good Hamstring Stretches

Figure 6-5 shows two good hamstring stretches. Learn the standing hamstring stretch for better functional stretch (Figure 6-5, left).

Standing Hamstring Stretch

- Instead of propping one heel on a low support, stand about arm's length from a wall. It will feel too close, but it is this distance that will focus stretch to the hamstring.
- Keep your standing foot facing straight forward, or the stretch will be greatly reduced.

- Press the raised heel against the wall.
- Keep the raised leg straight in front of you, not out to the side.
- Keep your hips straight across the front, not tilted toward one side.
- Stand straighter to lengthen the hamstring.
- Keep your body upright and chin in.

Lying-Down Hamstring Stretch

- Lie on your back and raise one leg up without lifting your head or shoulders from the floor.
- This stretch keeps your back straight and the pressure off your discs.
- Experiment with arching your back.
- Don't let your behind lift from the floor.
- To stretch the hip of the other leg, keep the other leg flat on the floor.

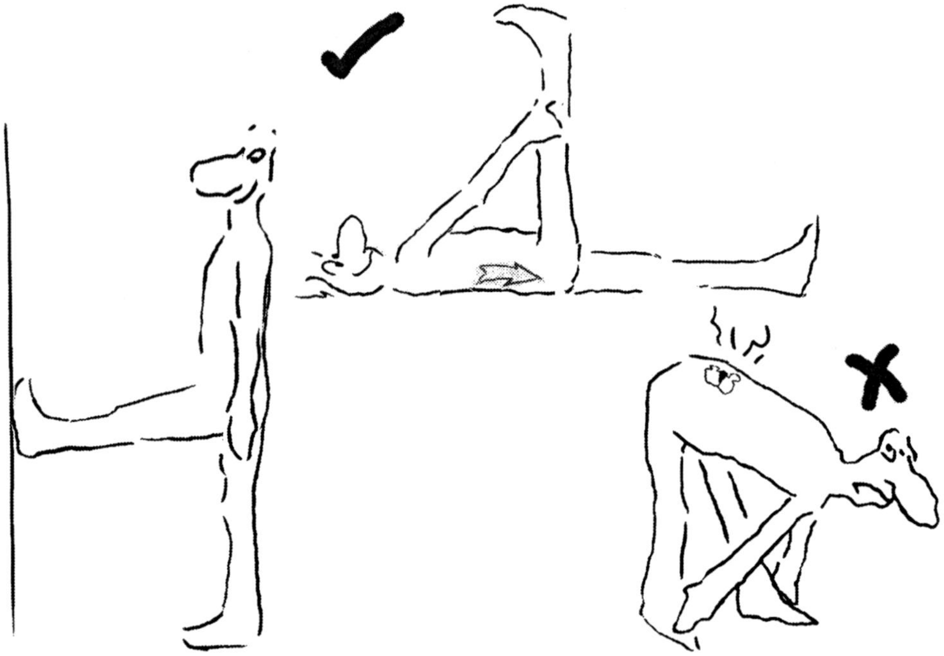

Figure 6-5. *Left:* Press the lifted heel against a wall. Keep your standing foot facing directly straight, not turned outward even a small amount. Stand straighter to get more stretch. *Top:* Lie flat without rounding the back or lifting the hip. *Right*: Avoid bent-forward hamstring stretches sitting or standing.

Stretches That Promote the Original Problem

People hunch forward all day, then do more forward bending for exercise. Their weakened, overstretched back and neck ache. They call that "tension" and do more forward bending to "fix it."

You wake up and sit hunched at the edge of the bed, bend over the sink to wash, sit round-shouldered at breakfast, while commuting to work, and at a desk. You lean and bend wrong all day by bending at the waist. At the gym, you do crunches and toe-touching. You bend over the dishes, the lawn mower, and the vacuum cleaner, and slump to watch television. You go to sleep for the night with your head pushed forward by pillows. You are mystified when your back, neck, and shoulders ache. You call it stress. You go to someone and say, "My back hurts. Can you give me a stretch to fix it?" They suggest bending over to touch your toes, or bringing your chin to your chest, your knee to your chest, sitting on the floor and leaning over to touch your toes, sitting in a chair and leaning forward with your chest on your thighs, touching your elbows in front by rounding your back, curling up in a ball, or other stretches that promote more rounding and more pressure on your back and discs. What you need is to stretch the other way, and stop stretching forward.

> When your muscles are so weak and tight that good posture feels unnatural, that means you need to strengthen and stretch to be comfortable, not slouch to be comfortable.

Doing more of what caused the original problem is not what you need. Just doing a stretch doesn't fix a problem. You need five things:

- Know what healthful posture feels like (refer to Figure 21-9).
- Have the body awareness to know to move out of bad position to straight healthful position.
- Have the flexibility to be able to move the part to the proper position.
- Have the muscular strength and endurance to hold the body part in the proper position all the time, even when you are doing other things.
- Consciously hold the right posture. Like manners, it doesn't automatically happen by itself.

> As a child you were told, "If you make a funny face, it will stick like that." If you spend your daily activities with your head and shoulders hunched forward, your body will eventually tighten up and stick like that. "As bent the twig, so grows the tree."

Are You Stretching What You Think You're Stretching?

Many common stretches are ineffective, such as overhead stretches that don't stretch the shoulder, quadriceps stretches that don't stretch your quads, back extension that doesn't extend the back, and toe touches that don't stretch the hamstrings. This section outlines alternative stretches that are much more effective.

Shoulder

Check to see if you stretch your arm overhead by arching your lower back and leaning back. Many "shoulder stretches" in this way add to mysterious lower-back aches and never fully stretch the shoulder.

Try the following:

- Stand up and reach your arm overhead, noticing if you let your lower back increase in arch and lean the upper body backward.
- With your arm in the same overhead position, flex your trunk, as if to start doing a "crunch" to straighten your torso and return to neutral spine (Figure 7-1, right). Don't round the upper body; just pull to straight position.
- Check if your arm is now lower. Before restoring neutral spine, it was likely that you were not reaching overhead from the shoulder fully, but by leaning backwards.
- Raise your arm completely, elbow to ear, without arching the lower back. Feel the stretch in your shoulder, not lower back.

Quadriceps (Front Thigh) and Hip

The same mistake is common as with the shoulder stretch. Check to see if you increase the inward curve in your lower back.

Try the following:

- Stand on one leg. Hold your other foot behind you. Allow your lower back to arch and the front of your hip to tip forward. You won't feel much stretch in your thigh.
- Still holding your foot, tuck the bottom of your hip under to neutral spine (Figure 7-1, right) as if you started doing an abdominal crunch to reduce the lower back inward curve to a straighter position.
- Don't let the knee pull in front of you. Feel the stretch move to your thigh.

Refer to Chapter 7 on abdominal muscles to learn more on how to restore neutral spine while reaching overhead or moving your legs.

Spine

Lying face down to do extension stretches for the spine will unload the discs and help "unround" rounded posture. Often, this stretch is done so that only one easily movable vertebra in the lower back moves during a backward extension stretch, with the rest of the back getting little stretch.

Try the following:

- Lie face down, and prop your upper body gently on your elbows. Notice where your back is bending. Is it mostly from one "crease" in your lower back?
- Press your forearms down and toward you against the floor. Distribute the stretch evenly up your back, making a graceful C-shape curve throughout.
- Don't crane your neck back from one hinge point. Keep chin in gently, lifting up from your chest.

Hamstrings

The sitting hamstring stretch is often done with little, sometimes no stretch on the hamstrings. Many people can touch their toes and still not put much, or any, stretch on their hamstrings because they bend from the hip and back, rather than their hamstrings. Others have tight hamstrings and don't understand why, since they stretch all the time. For flexibility, use the two stretches in Figure 6-5. To learn how to sit in healthier functional way when you sit on the floor, this section tells how to change a sitting hamstring stretch.

Your hamstrings are three muscles in back of your thigh. Hamstrings attach to your sit bones—the bumps you can feel when you sit. Most people sit with their back rounded and hip tilted under, so that their sit bones tilt to the front, shortening their hamstrings.

Try the following:

- Sit on the floor, knees bent out to the side cross-legged, and let your hip tilt back with your back rounded. Straighten your torso by holding your shins with your hands or putting your hands on the floor behind you and pushing yourself up straight. Does your hip move to allow you to straighten? Many people are too tight in the hips to get the necessary movement. When your hip can move, even a little, let it rock back and forth until it moves easily.
- Straighten your legs in front of you. If your hamstrings are tight, your hip will tilt under too much and your back will round again. Put your hands right behind

you and press them against the floor. Lift your ribs and straighten your back to lengthen your hamstrings. This exercise alone should give you more stretch on the hamstring than you get by leaning forward, which puts unhealthful pressure on the discs.

- Let your hip rock under again, and feel the stretch on your hamstrings immediately decrease. Make sure not to stretch this way. (Refer to Chapter 20 on back pain for why hamstrings stretches contribute to mystery back pain.)

> Most people don't have the hamstring flexibility to sit properly without their hip tucked under and back rounded.
>
> Instead of stretching their hamstrings to sit properly, they sit rounded because tightness makes it more comfortable that way.

Stretch Your Muscles, Not Your Joints

Ligaments are fibrous bands that hold your bones together, like the latch on a briefcase. Typically, ligaments are not supposed to stretch much. They retain their length, within a range, to hold your bones in position, so the bones glide past each other along anatomically healthy paths.

Ligament damage from improper stretching instruction is common. When injury or chronic improper stretching forces ligaments to lengthen, they do not readily go back to their former length. Technically speaking, they are *plastic*, but not *elastic*. Stretched ligaments hang shapelessly loose like worn-out underwear. What is so bad about that?

Stretched ligaments don't hold your bones in line, allowing them to rub and grind at unhealthy angles. The friction contributes to degenerative changes over time and all the pain and disability that accompany those changes. Ligament instability predisposes a person to sprains and dislocations. For example, too much looseness on the sides of your ankle increases your chance of ankle sprains. Laxity and instability are not the same thing. Damaged shoulder capsules may slip out of place from forces that healthier joint capsules tolerate. People with unstable joints need strengthening for the supporting musculature, but more importantly, they need retraining exercises involving knowledge of joint positioning to control their own joint position to offset the potential for injury.

Several well-known stretches hold the joint at an angle that puts too much weight and pressure on ligaments. The hurdler's stretch is an example. When sitting on the floor with one knee bent and the lower leg turned outward, if you don't rotate inward from the hip, you need to get the sideways twist from the knee. Similarly, pulling your arms high up behind you to stretch the chest and shoulders loads the front–and weakest—part of your shoulder capsule. Don't stretch the joint like that; it is the muscles you want to stretch. Use the stretches shown in Figures 21-4 and 21-5 instead.

Avoid constant pressure on joints over extended periods of time. An example is continuously sitting with a rounded back. Slouching overstretches the long ligament running up and down the back of your spine called the posterior longitudinal ligament. A chronically overstretched posterior longitudinal ligament weakens your back, and can lead to disc trouble. (Refer to Chapters 20 and 21 on back and neck pain.) Habitually standing with your head forward stretches the back of your neck, with similar results. Full squatting on your toes with heels up can pry knee ligaments apart, particularly if you have heavy legs. Continuous, long-term heel-up squatting can damage the small discs of cartilaginous cushion in your knees, called meniscus. The bad knees of professional baseball catchers come from chronic squatting up on the toes, rather than keeping the heels down.

- Ligaments normally are not supposed to stretch much.
- Stretched ligaments don't hold your bones in line, allowing them to rub and grind at unhealthy angles.
- Avoid putting weight and pressure on ligaments, such as in the "hurdler's stretch" and pulling your arms high up behind you.
- Avoid positions that place constant pressure on joints over extended periods of time, such as slouching and standing and sitting toe-touching for hamstring stretches.

Don't Damage Joints

Your joints are places where your body crams many structures into little space. For this reason, it is easy to do things that squash, tear, and abrade your joints. Joint cartilage and ligaments have a poorer blood supply than other body parts. Low blood supply means slow repair that may not keep up with each small, destructive incident. Damage usually occurs slowly without your knowing it is happening and can, over time, injure your joint to the same degree as a single accident. Chronic mistreatment slowly thickens a joint with fibrous scar tissue. Scarring makes the capsule less mobile and more uncomfortable as small abuses gradually accelerate the normal wear and tear of aging.

An example of a common stretch that can damage your joints is the "plow" and shoulder stand—lying on your back and shoulders with your legs in the air, weighting your neck (Figure 9-1, middle and right) which can not only damage the joints of the spine, but the discs between the vertebrae, and promote bone spurs. Another example is standing and sitting toe-touching, which weakens back muscles and joints and pressures the discs.

- You can squash, tear, abrade, and scar your joints when you stretch badly.
- Examples of stretches that overweight your joints are the "plow," duck walk, standing toe touch, sit-and-reach toe touch, and straight-legged dead lift.
- Damage can occur slowly without your knowing it and can injure your joints over time as much as a single accident.

Stretching Without Strengthening

Being highly flexible, by itself, does not make you a better person, or more fit. It can create problems. A joint must be able to move, but not so much that it moves out of place, rubs adjacent structures, or jangles loosely during daily movement. Joints that are too loose and not strong can become unstable and not seat well. Like any two surfaces in your car or other machinery that don't seat well, your joints will suffer early wear and tear. Flexibility and instability are not the same thing.

- By itself, being flexible is not synonymous with an unstable joint.
- Stretching a joint's attachments so that the joint itself rubs and doesn't seat well, without training the musculature how to hold it in position, can result in chronic pain.

Stretching and Warm-Up

Much is made of warming up first. You should not be so tight that moving through the normal range needed for daily life strains or tears things—for example, reaching overhead, bending correctly to retrieve things from the floor, and stretching the chest muscles to restore resting length to the upper body (Figures 21-4 and 21-5). Use the stretches in this chapter and in Chapter 21 to restore needed resting length for daily life and for exercise. For more vigorous movement, warm up. (Refer to Chapter 5.)

What about yoga and stretch classes that begin right away by bending right over to touch the floor? In most classes, it is stretching without a warm-up. It does not magically become all right because it has a mystical name.

Increasing Range With Neuromuscular Facilitation

To make your stretch receptors work for you to increase flexibility, try this easy technique. Lie on your back, one leg up in the air and the other flat on the floor, not bent. Hold the back of the lifted leg with your hands and press your leg against your hands firmly, counting to three or four slowly. When you relax the press, you may find you can pull your leg into a further stretch. This technique usually works with all stretches. First, push away from the stretch to fatigue the muscle, and then relax and pull the stretch in a bit further.

Another way to do this stretch is to lie on your back, put your hands on the front of your thigh, and try to push your leg down with your hands. Resist with your leg. When you relax, you may find you can pull the hamstring into more of a stretch. This stretch can be done on all muscles. First, push the opposite muscle while resisting, then relax and pull the muscle you want to stretch without resisting.

What to Avoid

- Conventional forward-bending stretching is the last thing you need after a day of sitting.
- Stretching shouldn't mean doing strange contortions; it should address the posture you need for daily life so you can stand up straight and bend properly.
- A common belief is that tight hamstrings cause back pain. Based on this idea, many pain sufferers are told to stretch back their hamstrings. They do it by bending over forward and sitting bent forward. With the back straight or rounded, both ways are a major cause of back pain. (Refer to Chapters 20 and 21.) If you feel you must lean over forward to stretch out tightness and pain in your back, it is likely that you stand with too much inward curve (hyperlordosis), which compresses the lower spine. (Refer to Chapters 7, 20, and 21.)
- Avoid the "plow," and other shoulder-stand positions where you put your weight on a bent-forward neck and back.
- Avoid sitting with a rounded back and a forward head.
- Don't push or force back stretches, and don't let anyone help you stretch by pushing or forcing.
- Don't tighten, strain, grunt, force, and contract an area by pulling the area taught, then call it a stretch. "Stretch" means to lengthen and relax the area.

What to Do

Stretch the Way You Need to Move. More forward stretching when you are already round-shouldered adds to the problem. Make your stretches functional, so you can stand and move comfortably straight.

Do The Purpose of the Stretch; Don't "Do" a Stretch. Don't follow a rigid list of rules, then stretch in a tight, strained manner. Know the result you are trying to achieve, and move in that way. You will then accomplish the purpose or desired result instead of spending time "doing a stretch" that misses the point.

Stretch What You Think You're Stretching. When stretching one part, don't crane other parts so that you lose the stretch. When stretching your shoulder or hamstring, for example, don't let the stretch come from your lower back. For back-extension stretching, make an even arc backwards with your entire spine, rather than just "folding" at one easily moved joint.

Functional Stretching for Daily Life

Many of the declines in mobility that come with doing less are often confused with aging. A stiff and rounded upper back, for example, is not necessarily aging, but practice. Are you sitting rounded forward reading this right now? Do you spend your day rounding over your desk and steering wheel, then go to the gym and bend forward for crunches, leg lifts, Pilates, and toe touches? Do you bend your neck down to do biceps curls? No wonder it is hard for you to straighten out. How long will you practice unhealthy bent-forward position before you get stuck that way? You don't need to stretch in the same way that is not healthy when sitting at your desk. Instead, practice functional healthy stretching during daily life.

Resources for More Information

Stretching Smarter Stretching Healthier
Dr. Jolie Bookspan
ISBN 0-9721214-6-3
www.DrBookspan.com/books
Almost 200 humorous drawings guide you step by step.

7

Abdominal Muscles—What They Really Do May Surprise You

Thought depends absolutely on the stomach, but in spite of that, those who have the best stomachs are not the best thinkers.

—Voltaire

Your abdominal muscles have something to do with posture, but exactly what? Most people want "ab" exercises but have no idea what the exercises really do or how they translate to real life. The most popular conventional abdominal exercises of abdominal crunches (flexes, half-sit-ups) and Pilates don't work your abs the way they function in real life, are tough on your discs, and promote the same bent-forward posture that causes pain syndromes. Using abs doesn't mean sucking them in or making them tight. Then, how do you use them? Did you know that your abs need to do the most for you while you are standing? How can you do that?

What Do Muscles Do?

Muscles pull bones closer together to bend the joint between the bones. All muscles originate on a bone, cross a joint, then attach to another bone on the other side of the joint. Like a marionette—when you pull the string, the attached part moves closer. In your body, the string is the tendon that attaches muscle to bone. To move your arm, for example, your biceps muscle in front of your upper arm contracts to pull your lower arm bone closer, bending your elbow.

What Do Abdominal Muscles Do?

Abdominal muscles connect from hip bones to the rib bones. The joints they cross are your lower spine. When you use your abdominal muscles, they pull your ribs closer to your hips, bending your spine forward and pulling the lower front of your pelvis upward. The amount of inward curve in the lower spine becomes smaller (Figure 7-1, right). The way abdominal muscles need to work in life is to prevent an overly large inward curve, sometimes called a swayback. When you are standing, if you don't use abdominal muscles to pull forward enough, you may increase the curve by slouching the upper body backward, or letting your hip tip forward in front and out in back (Figure 7-1, left). That posture is not normal. It is a painful bad posture called hyperlordosis (swayback), and a major overlooked cause of chronic lower-back pain during standing, walking, running, and reaching overhead. It is easily preventable, not by strengthening the abs, but rather by using them, the same as moving any other muscle to move a body part.

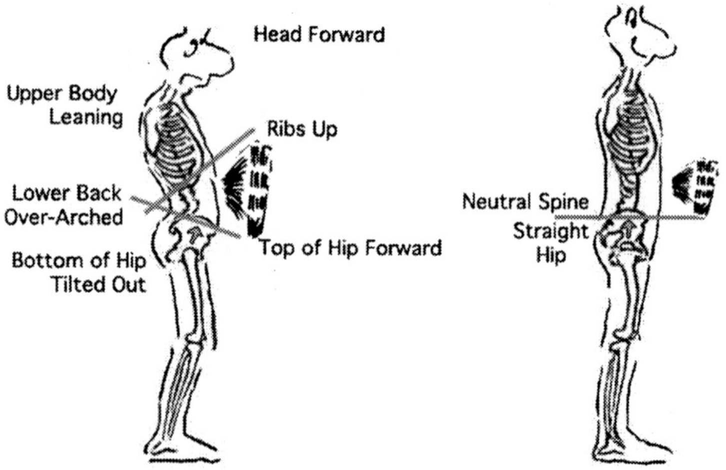

Figure 7-1. The job of abdominal muscles is to pull your ribs and front pelvic bones toward each other. When you don't use them, your torso sways backward and/or your hip will tilt forward. The increased lower spine curve is called hyperlordosis (left). When you use abdominal muscles to pull to neutral spine, the lower spine curve becomes small, and the hip is level from front to back.

How Do Abs Prevent Lower Back Pain?

Abdominal muscles do not prevent back pain just by being strong. They have to actively do something. For example, you may have a strong arm, but that does not make you hold it up in the air. Your arm moves when you make it move. Your abdominal muscles work like a guy-wire, which holds a tree from tipping backward. Your abdominal muscle guy-wires hold the right distance between your ribs and hipbones in front. When they are too long, they let your rib cage tip upward and backward, and your hip tilt downward (Figure 7-2). Both actions increase the small, normal inward curve to the lower spine. A small curve belongs there. A large curve painfully pinches and pressures the lower spine. Abdominal muscles do not prevent the large curve automatically. They only pull forward when you know to use them.

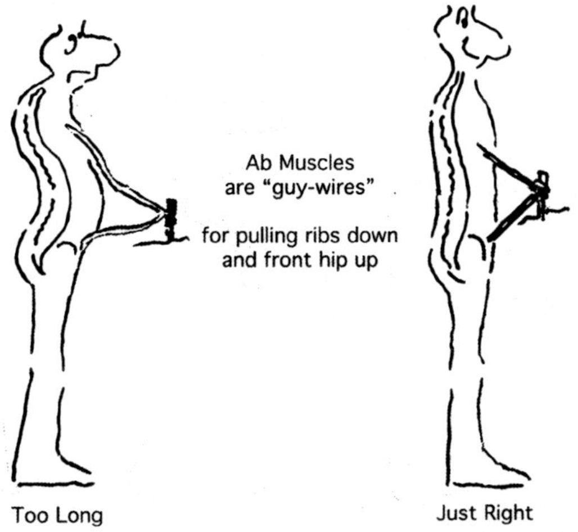

Figure 7-2. *Left:* Your several abdominal muscles function like a guy-wire between your ribs and hips. When the wire is too long, it allows the ribs and front of the hip to be too far apart. *Right:* When you use your abs, you pull just enough to comfortably hold neutral spine.

Using your abdominal muscles doesn't mean sucking them in or making them "tight." It is not a case of: "Press your navel to your spine and contract your gluteal muscles." You couldn't move normally that way, and couldn't breathe in fully or normally. Dr. Stuart McGill, a major figure in spine research, published in the January 2007 issue of *Archives of Physical Medicine and Rehabilitation* that "drawing in" the abdominal muscles, also described as "press the navel to spine," is detrimental to health of the lower back, and that tightening the abs impedes normal movement. McGill concluded, "There seems to be no mechanical rationale for using an abdominal hollow, or the transversus abdominis, to enhance stability." Tightening or clenching the muscles also doesn't change your posture. The main function of using all your several abdominal muscles means holding neutral spine, not overarched lower spine. In that way, your upper body weight doesn't press downward onto your lower back.

Using abs does not mean sucking them in, or tightening them, or "pressing to your spine." It means moving your torso into neutral spine and away from an overly arched lower spine (called swayback and hyperlordosis). Overarching shifts upper body weight onto your lower back.

In life, your abs need to work isometrically—at one length—to hold your torso upright, instead of leaning your body weight backward onto your low back. Yet people do crunches, which are not functional for daily life , and also promotes a rounded forward posture in someone who likely spends much of their day already hunched over a work area. They may be mechanically promoting the back and neck pain they think they are working their abs to prevent.

What Is Neutral Spine? What Do Abs Have to Do With Neutral Spine?

Exercise programs and trainers frequently talk about neutral spine, but what is it? In general, the line from the bump at the top of your hipbone in back (medical abbreviation is PSIS) to the bump at the front of your hipbone (ASIS) will be approximately horizontal when you are holding neutral spine (Figure 7-1, right). (Refer to Chapter 21 for more information about neutral spine.)

If you tip your hip forward (slouch) so that the front of the hip (ASIS) tilts downward, and the back of your hip sticks outward in back, the small normal inward curve of the lower back increases (Figure 7-1, left). It is overarched, (hyperlordotic). It is not neutral spine. Another way to see the anterior hip tilt when the spine is overarched is to check the line from the ASIS to where the pelvic bones meet in front, called the symphysis pubis (PS). When you hold your spine in neutral, the line from ASIS to PS will be vertical (Figure 7-1 right and Figure 21-6). The same vertical line can be drawn from the top of the leg bone to the center of the crest of the hipbone. Someone standing in anterior tilt will have the center of the hip crest forward of the top of the leg bone.

Another way to increase hyperlordosis is to lean the upper body backward. The hip may be fine and level, but if you slouch and lean your upper body backward, you overarch the lower spine and pinch it under your upper body weight. Watch for this kind of overarching when standing, lifting arms overhead, and carrying loads in front.

> Most people hunch forward for a few "ab exercises," then stand and move in overly arched lower-spine posture without using their abs. Their ribs lift up, hips drop down, and their lower back overarches, pinching the joints called facets, and painfully pressing upper-body weight downward onto the lower back.

The muscles that hold your torso and hip straight in neutral spine are your abdominal muscles. You have to voluntarily, consciously use them, the same as moving your arm or leg. If you don't deliberately use abs to position your spine, you may fall into whatever bad positioning habit you are used to—sticking out in back, or leaning the upper body back, or both at once. Using neutral spine is an all-day, built-in, abdominal-muscle exercise. It includes no tightening and no forward bending that promotes other pain and problems.

Strengthening Does Not Change Hyperlordosis to Neutral Spine

Doing strengthening exercise has no effect on an overly large lower-spine arch if you don't apply the strength the rest of the day to stand and move in neutral spine during all your activities.

You can have very strong abs and never use them to do anything for your back. Doing crunches will not heal your back. You must learn how to use the strong abs to hold your weight up with neutral spine and good body mechanics.

Using abs during a specific exercise doesn't automatically make you know to use them during life. You need to consciously use your abs to control your torso posture during all your activities. Stand and sit well all the time, and you'll exercise your abs without working out. (Refer to Chapters 20 and 21 on back pain and prevention.)

> Strengthening the abdominal muscles will not fix painful hyperlordotic posture. Plenty of people with strong muscles stand terribly. It is like having brains and not using them.

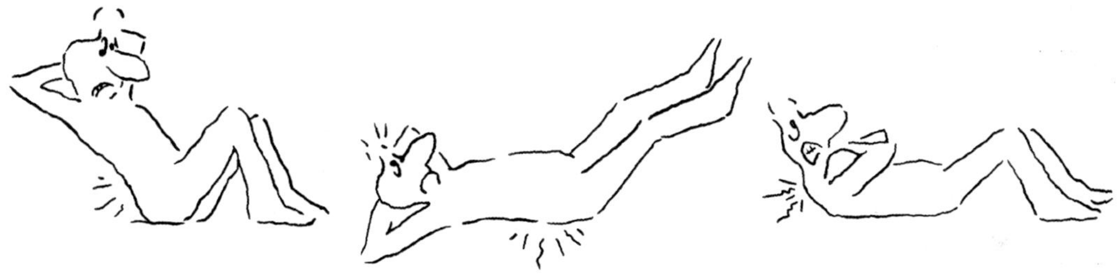

Figure 7-3. "Crunches" and other forward-bending exercise in ab and Pilates classes are common but do not work your abs the way you need them for real life. Do you do anything in life that looks this way? Do you want a forward bent position to become natural when standing?

What's Wrong With Crunches and Pilates?

- Crunches and other forward-bending exercise do not work your abs the way you need for real life.
- They promote poor bent-forward posture, even when done properly.

The most common abdominal-muscle exercise involves trunk flexion, also called trunk curls, or crunches, and hip flexion pictured in Figure 7-3. These exercises are not functional. They don't use your body the way you need for real life. Doing crunches and other forward-bending exercises does not automatically make your back held in neutral spine for the rest of the day. Unless you consciously control your torso angles, nothing to support your back happens, no matter how many crunches you have done.

How to Feel How to Use Abs Functionally

To understand how your abdominal muscles move you to neutral spine and how to use the abs during exercise and daily life, try the following:

- Stand with your back against a wall
- Keep heels, hips, shoulders, and the back of your head against the wall
- Put one hand at the bottom of your ribs. Put your other hand on the center-front of your hip. (Refer to Figure 7-1 for placement.) Hold these two points with your fingers.
- Draw your two hands toward each other, still holding on to where the abs attach at the top and bottom. Your torso should curl forward. Your lower back should press toward the wall. Don't flatten your lower back; just feel how to reduce the arch.
- Step away from the wall. Hold your ribs and hip bone, and let the distance between your two hands increase, showing the slackening abs. Lean back and let your ribs pull up and your abdomen curve outward. You may feel your body weight fall onto your lower back. This position demonstrates what not using your abs allows—an arched back and your weight pressing your lower back.
- Pull your two hands toward each other, and your torso upright to a straight position, showing use of your abs to reduce an overly arched lower spine. Don't curl forward. Only flex enough to stand straight. Check yourself against the wall. This position is the way you need your abs to stand properly. Use it when reaching overhead and carrying loads. Do not let the hip tilt or the upper body lean back. You will keep the load on the abdominal muscles instead of the lower spine. The results will be no more lower-back pain with standing, and better posture.

What Exercises Work Abs the Way You Need Them for Real Life?

Other than standing, carrying, and reaching properly all day every day, what can you do to train good abdominal muscles for posture, activities, and good looks? The ab exercises commonly seen in gyms make you good at bending forward. However, your abs need to work isometrically in real life, not by bowing you forward. Exercise your abs to challenge them to hold neutral spine that you can transfer to postural control when you sit, stand, walk, run, and carry packages, so you don't arch backwards. You can benefit by exercising your abs in the manner in which they normally should work. That approach means radically different exercises than you commonly see in gyms and on exercise videos.

- Hold the push-up position (called the plank) without sagging and arching in the middle or hiking up your bottom. Tuck your buttocks under and straighten your spine. As soon as you tuck the hip as if doing a crunch, you will feel the effort shift to your abdominal muscles. If you do not reduce the lower-back arch, this exercise loses effectiveness and does not transfer any skill to real life. It is pointless to "do exercises," then return to bad habits, and to do exercises that do not retrain your daily actions. Instead of "doing" a push-up or plank, use them to retrain your abdominal muscles for real life.
- Hold the same tucked-hip plank, but in the low push-up position. Hold as long as you can. Work to increase the time.
- While holding a plank position, turn to one side, lifting one arm to the sky so that you balance on one arm and still hold your body straight without drooping in the middle. That position uses your oblique abs the way you need them for posture—to hold your posture without sagging under packages, shoulder bags, and children carried on one hip. Do this retraining exercise on both sides.

Most people can't hold a plank with neutral spine and tucked hip for more than a few seconds. No wonder their posture sags badly during the day. They don't have the strength and functional use of their abdominal muscles to stand in healthful position.

> Having stronger abs, by itself, doesn't do anything. You can have a "six-pack" and still stand and exercise with a large, unhealthful arch in your lower back, which slowly injures the area and causes much lower-back pain.

Holding Neutral Spine When Using Weights

To get started:

- Lie on your back with your knees bent and feet on the floor. Arch your lower back up, lifting your ribs high so you know what it feels like. Put your hand on the floor under the arch of your back. Press your back against your hand so that you feel how to use your abs to control your torso and reduce the arch. Don't lift your hips, just use your abs. You'll feel your abs working right under your skin, since ab muscles are shallow.
- Put both arms by your ears, with hands on the floor overhead. Did your back arch again? Press it back down. Feel your abs contract to hold your torso straight without allowing your back to arch.

- When you can comfortably do this exercise, hold hand weights, making sure your lower back does not arch from the floor. Your abdominal muscles work hard on this exercise to control your posture against challenge. Holding the hand weight also works your arms and latissimus dorsi muscles along the side of your back. You get several exercises for the price of one. Remember that your life is multi-segment, not isolated movements, so it is helpful to exercise as you need for real life. Your shoulder should not hurt. Make sure the pivot point is your ab muscles, not your lower back or shoulder joints.

To Learn Neutral Spine for Real Movement

- To make this exercise functional, extend your legs so that your knees straight, as if you were standing up. Keep your abs working so that your back does not pull into an arch.
- You may need to stretch your hip-flexor muscles so that you can straighten your legs without your lower back being pulled into an arch.
- Think of all the exercises involving lifting weights overhead, where people should stand straight, as you have practiced, but don't, and pump the weight up and down with the force crashing down on their lower back. When you do standing weight lifting, control your posture with what you learned with this lying-down training exercise.
- Try pulsing the weight fairly quickly—an inch higher and lower up and down without touching the floor. Each time the weight lowers, your back will want to arch. Don't let it. This exercise simulates all the daily life activities where you need to keep healthful position as you carry or lift things.
- Increase the weight slowly and safely as you improve your abs so that they can maintain your low back in good neutral posture.

It is not true that you must bend your legs to protect your back. If it were true, how are you supposed to stand and walk around in real life? Your abdominal muscles hold neutral spine, not your knees.

Don't hold your breath, tighten your muscles, or do other things that unsafely raise blood pressure. Just learn healthful muscle movement in the ways that you need to move in life.

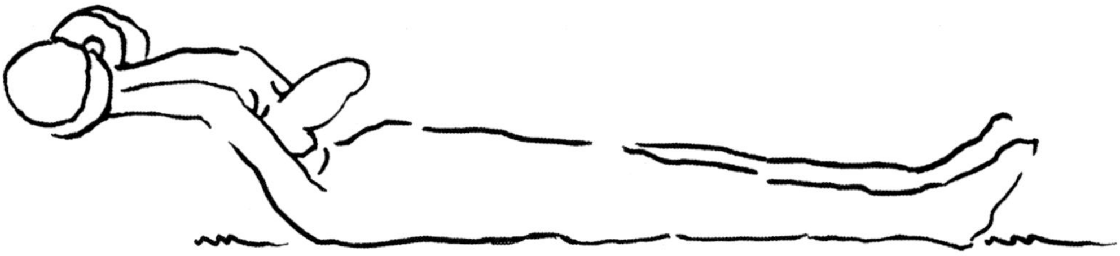

Figure 7-4. Your abs normally work isometrically—at one length—so you can stand, sit, walk, and exercise without overarching (hyperlordosis). In this isometric ab exercise, you don't allow your back to arch, which contracts your abs the way needed in life to hold neutral spine when standing for posture control and normal function.

Controlling Torso Posture When Standing and Using Resistance

- Stand up and reach overhead. Did your ribs come up and your back arch? First, learn to stop doing that with the isometric abs exercise shown in Figure 7-4. Keep your hip tucked under you to neutral spine. Reach overhead again. Wave your arms around. Keep your torso from increasing the arch in all you do.
- Tie the middle of a commercial stretchy band, surgical tubing, or stretchy clothing securely to a doorknob, pole, or pipe at about waist height. Leave both ends free. Turn around with your back to the tie. Pick up one end in each hand. Lift both arms overhead, holding neural spine, not allowing your lower spine to increase in arch. Step away until you feel tension on the band. Don't let your arms become pulled behind you. Try various arm exercises, throwing, punching, paddling, and realistic motions while controlling your torso position with your ab muscles. This approach simulates the loads you carry in daily life. Keep your lower back from overarching.

Using Abdominal Muscles for Throwing, Punching, and Other Arm Activities

When throwing and punching properly, you use your arm for only a small part of the power. Your torso and legs should power most of it. If you just fling your arm. shoulder and back pain can eventually develop. When swinging a tennis racquet, for example, by not using your abs to pivot, you may shift more pivot angle and load to the shoulder.

- Using the stretchy cord tied as described in the previous section, turn your back to the wall, still holding both ends of the stretchy cord. Keep your arms in front of you and overhead. Don't let the cord pull you into an arch or pull your arms behind you. Feel how to stabilize your body, using your abs.
- Simulate throwing a ball or a punch by first contracting your abs.

- Turn sideways, and hold your torso stable against the sideways pull of the stretchy cord. Do side curls or walk around and keep your torso stable against the changing pull of the band.
- Have a friend hold the other end of the band and pull you in odd directions while you practice torso stabilization. This approach simulates walking a dog, and carrying a squirming baby and packages while trying to get in the door.

> Backpacks and heavy shoulder bags don't make you arch your back. Not using your torso muscles to counter the pull so that you stand with good posture is the problem.
>
> Carrying your bags could be a built-in ab exercise.

Abs for "Lat Pull-Downs"

- Leaning back while pulling down decreases work of the "lats," the large latissimus dorsi muscles of your back and sides, in the line of the muscle fibers.
- When pulling down, do not lean back or increase the lower-back arch.
- Instead, flex the torso to neutral spine, and you will immediately feel the effort of the pull shift off the lower back and onto the abdominal muscles.

Should You Work Your Abs Every Day or Every Other Day?

It is common for people to debate fiber type and fatigue, and conclude whether to exercise abs daily or intermittently. Flurries of articles are written on this topic. What is missed is that you need your abs working all day every day. Doing specific moves for an hour and not using your abs for daily life is like couples being nice in a counselor's office for an hour and then screaming at each other the rest of the day, justifying that behavior by saying harmony was already done for a time each day (or alternate days) and it is too tiring to do it all the time. Plenty of guys have six-pack abs and don't use them for daily life the way they need for posture and back-pain control. Like your heart beating, you need your abs working all the time. If you worked your abs all day all the time to control your posture, you wouldn't need to go to a gym to do funny little crunches, either every day or every few days.

How Do You Flatten Your Abdomen?

No exercise selectively removes fat from any target body part. That myth is called "spot reducing." If spot reducing worked, people would have thin mouths from talking, speed skaters would have little legs, and the repetitive act of chewing and swallowing lots of food would make your face thin.

> Stand, sit, and reach using neutral spine all the time, and you'll get free, built-in abdominal exercise without working out.

Resources for More Information

The Ab Revolution™: No More Crunches, No More Back Pain (Third Edition, expanded)
Dr. Jolie Bookspan
ISBN 0-9721214-2-0
www.DrBookspan.com/books

8

You Don't Need a Gym for Real Fitness—Fitness as a Lifestyle

Men have become the tools of their tools.

—Henry David Thoreau

What Is "Fitness as a Lifestyle"?

To many people, fitness means stopping their real life, changing clothes, driving to a gym, and doing arbitrary and often uncomfortable motions that have no similarity to real-life movement. They then stop and go back to their real life—slouching, bending incorrectly, using poor posture, walking heavily, sitting round-shouldered, taking elevators, driving everywhere while sitting slouched, and avoiding movement.

Going to a gym a few times a week is not fitness as a lifestyle. How you live your life outside the gym is lifestyle. Many people who exercise in a climate-controlled gym become unable to heat-regulate when exercising outdoors. They work on a treadmill or elliptical trainer but sprain their when ankle out walking because they haven't trained balance and stabilization. They work with weights to isolate arms but never learn how their entire body stabilizes a weight, then hurt their back opening a window at home. They sit hunched in bad posture while waiting for exercise class to start. They lift weights using machines, and do not train how to stabilize real loads. They may be in good shape, yet at risk of falls from poor stability and balance. They get back strain carrying their groceries, children, and exercise equipment. At the gym, people do squats with a trainer, paying to learn proper form and upright back, then bend over incorrectly to put the weight down when they're finished, pick up their gym bag with bad bending, and sit slouched on the way home where they don't apply their squat training for good bending around the house (Figure 8-1). They have no idea why their back hurts.

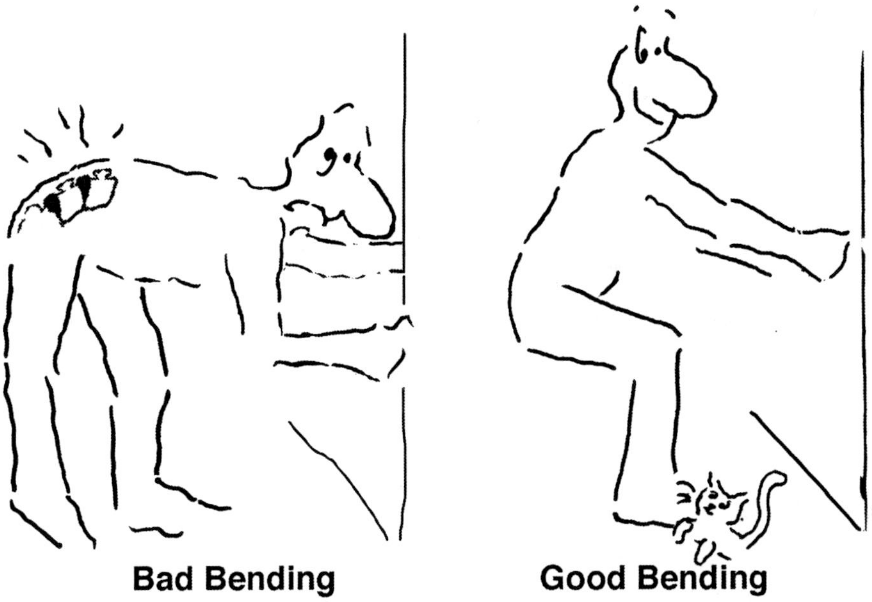

Figure 8-1. *Left:* Bad bending pressures discs outward and hurts back muscles. *Right:* Good bending strengthens legs, and stretches your hip and Achilles tendons. Keep both heels down. Don't overarch the lower back.

In modern life, exercise is something you go and specially "do," then damage and ignore your health the other 23 hours a day. Fitness has become "fast food"—stripped of value, sweetened, mass produced, and unhealthy.

Exercise should not be something you change clothes and go "do" (if you can make time), but all the ways you sit, bend, reach, lift, and move all day in real life, using muscles to hold the positioning that prevents body aches and joint wear and tear, and comfortable easy movement. Fitness should relate to how you sit at the desk, walk, do chores, and how you move all day every day. It doesn't mean stopping and "doing" exercises. Are you using your upper-back muscles right now to not round forward or jut your chin forward reaching this?

Fitness as a lifestyle is how you live, standing in healthful position to cook healthful food, carrying groceries and children without rounding your back forward or increasing the lower-back inward arch, breathing and smiling when people get in your way, going outside in the sunshine, and vacuuming for an ailing neighbor.

Exercise Without Going to the Gym—Fitness as a Lifestyle

- Make daily chores your exercise. Get fresh air, sunshine, balance, and real exercise by going to work or grocery shopping and carrying packages on a real bike or walking on real ground, instead of driving, then rushing home or to the gym to "do" exercise, illogically spending money on an artificial machine, exercise cycle, or treadmill.
- Make adventure your exercise. Take reconnaissance or architecture-observation walks around your neighborhood. Carry packages for people. Help your local club lug things around. You might learn things, meet people, and work out all at once.
- Make romance your exercise. You can walk in the park to feed geese as easily as going out to eat a fat dinner. Carry each other piggy-back (observing good body mechanics). Walk all over town to find just the right flowers for a surprise. Walk to the post office often to mail frequent, friendly notes. Volunteer to help the community together. Dates are more memorable when you do fun things, not just sit and eat.
- Bend properly. You know you shouldn't pick things up by bending over at the waist; you already know you should bend knees and keep your torso upright. Done properly, it is important exercise for your legs, burns calories, and prevents back and knee pain (Figure 8-1, right). You probably do several hundreds of bends a day just doing housework, picking things up, tying shoes, arranging papers, and getting things off shelves. Those motions could easily be equivalent to going to a gym and doing squats and lunges for an hour. You already may have done that during a normal day.
- Start a garden of any size. Getting outside to dig, bend, stretch, think, and create in the fresh air is health as a lifestyle. Learn to grow fresh vegetables without chemicals. Use healthy bending with one foot in front of the other and feet side by side. (Refer to Chapter 21.) Breathe. Smile.
- Pick up litter for discipline, exercise, and dignity through keeping your neighborhood areas clean.
- Try a parcours, or make your own. Parcours (pronounced: par-core) is a French word meaning "course" or trail. A parcours is a path with obstacles at varied intervals. You navigate using your body and brain, similar to steeplechase. Some parcours are formally designed municipal parks. Some are impromptu collections of trees, walls, buildings, windows, and rocks. On a rainy day, you can make your own parcours in your house. In ancient times, a course might involve days of travel. Today, several cities around the world have public courses used by people of all

abilities and ages. Modern fitness programs use it, with names like free running and various brand names like Parkour™, but the idea is not new. Stations may be a log to walk across, rings to swing on, various height and shape objects to stretch on and around, a place to see how far or high you can jump, something to balance on, a ladder or wall to climb over or under. To get to the next station, you can walk, run, bike, skate, or whatever you can do. Parcours length varies from a block to miles. Some people make a day of it with picnics and rests between stations. Others make a quick lunch run over part or all of the course. Parcours uses the body in natural ways to build strength, spirit, and balance. It can be healthier, better training, and more fun than doing artificial repetitions of an isolated exercise.

Bending Properly Is Major Fitness as a Lifestyle

Bending correctly in daily life is the way to physical ability and health, instead of stopping life to do a bunch of exercises. Much time and money is spent for treatments and gadgets for back and knee pain and tight Achilles tendon. Healthy bending prevents the commonest sources of all of these ailments.

- A major predisposing factor of knee and hip arthritis is weak thighs.
- A major risk factor of hip osteoporosis is lack of weight-bearing exercise.
- A major risk factor of falls is weak legs and poor balance.
- The Achilles tendon gets a natural stretch with each time you bend correctly with heels down, and loses this constant normal source of stretch without good bending.
- The most important contributor to making a lumbar disc degenerate, or slip out of place (herniate), and press on nerves causing sciatica, is bad bending forward.
- The biggest contributor to upper-back and neck pain is keeping the upper body rounded and bent over forward.

If you would like to reduce risk of falls, osteoporosis, bad discs, sciatica, achy upper back, and arthritis, get a built-in Achilles tendon stretch, and get strong shapely legs all at the same time, just use your legs with good body position for daily healthy bending. Why go to the gym or to physical therapy to do knee bends to strengthen your legs, then spend your "real life" weakening your legs and degenerating your lower-back discs with bad bending, and say, "I don't have time to exercise."

Imagine how good your legs would look if you did 400 squats and lunges a day, and how many calories you would burn. Using your legs would strengthen them and reduce risk of both osteoporosis and arthritis. It has been found that a major predisposing factor of knee arthritis is weak thighs. If you want to use fitness as a lifestyle to make a quick big improvement to your fitness and health, bend right.

How many times a day do you bend for ordinary household and work activities? It is more than you think. The average sedentary person bends an average of 100 to 200 times a day just getting things out of the refrigerator, dishwasher, closets, washing, and doing other little things around the house or workplace. The average, non-sedentary (but still not-active) person bends 200 to 400 times a day. The average fidgety and active person bends over 500 times a day.

You can now realize how many times a day you are hurting your back and missing free exercise by bending over in unhealthy ways (as in Figure 8-1, left). Leaning over all day is also a factor in neck pain. If you only burned half a calorie each time you bent properly, keeping your body upright, and bending knees, you would get a lot of exercise. You would not have to change clothes or go to a gym or pay a trainer. You would not have to take pills because you make your back ache. You would not have to do anything except live your life. You life is supposed to be healthy. You are not supposed to stop your life to go "do exercise." It is a sad thing to see people do squats and lunges in a gym, then bend over incorrectly to put their weights down, and bend incorrectly again to pick up their things to leave. One way to bend correctly whenever you bend is to use the half-squat (Figure 8-1, right):

- Stand comfortably with feet apart and side-by-side.
- Bend both knees.
- Keep both heels down touching the ground.
- Keep your upper body upright.
- Keep and your weight back over your heels to keep your weight on your leg muscles and off your knee joints (Figure 8-1, right).
- Don't stick your behind far out in back (Figure 8-1, left).

Healthy bending saves your back and gives much exercise without going to a gym, and helps, rather than hurts, your knees. You will get free, built-in exercise just bending right in life instead of spending money to go to a gym or buy equipment to exercise your legs. More on the half-squat and the lunge for good bending can be found in Chapter 21 on fixing back pain.

The following is a fun way to change mindset to exercise as a lifestyle. Count how many times a day you bend and how many times you can choose to harm yourself or help yourself. If you would like to try "fitness as a lifestyle," think of it in the following instances:

- Bending to make the bed
- Picking up laundry
- Looking in the refrigerator,
- Loading and unloading the dishwasher
- Picking up your shoes
- Opening a lower cabinet
- Lifting a child or pet
- Feeding a child or a pet
- Picking up things from the floor
- Picking up hand weights to do exercise
- Putting down weights after exercising
- All daily activities

Upper-Back Strengthening Through Fitness as a Lifestyle

Notice all the times you round and hang forward over tables and work areas that you can easily reach by standing upright. Check your upper-back positioning when standing over counters, sinks, grocery bins, vacuum cleaners, cribs and baby-changing tables, and when setting food tables. Don't let your body weight hang over and forward. Stand upright, chin in, and just tilt your head downward in relaxed manner to see what you are doing. Relax shoulders downward. Smile. Breathe.

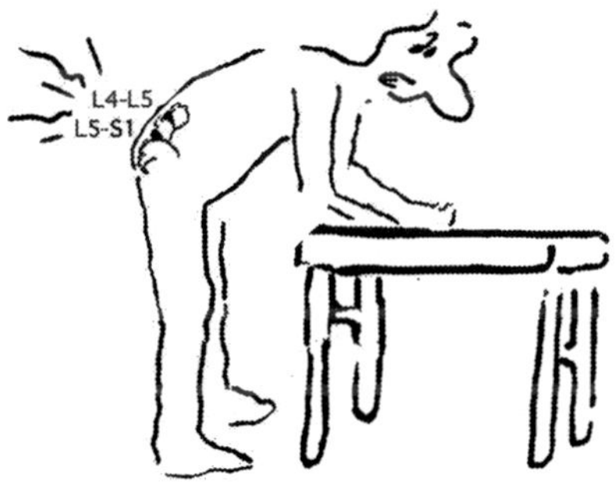

Figure 8-2. Chronic forward bending (flexion) is a main factor in herniating discs.

Abdominal Muscle Use as a Lifestyle

Lifestyle use of abdominal muscles does not mean doing crunches during commercials, or holding abs tightly so that normal breathing is limited. Abdominal muscles hold your lower spine in neutral position when you use them for that purpose. Neutral spine is not an automatic position for many people. When you don't train your spine position, the lower back can increase in inward arch. The phrase "neutral spine" is often used. What it means is not to let the pelvis tip, or the upper back lean backward. Consciously preventing the increase in arch and holding neutral spine uses the abdominal muscles as explained in Chapter 7.

To carry chairs, babies, grocery bags, furniture, and any loads in front of you, don't lean back. Leaning backward shifts the weight of the load off your core muscles and onto your lower spine. When reaching upward, and lifting overhead, don't lean backward or let the front of your hip tilt forward (Figure 8-3). Get free, built-in exercise for your abs and save your back by standing straight with neutral spine during daily activities.

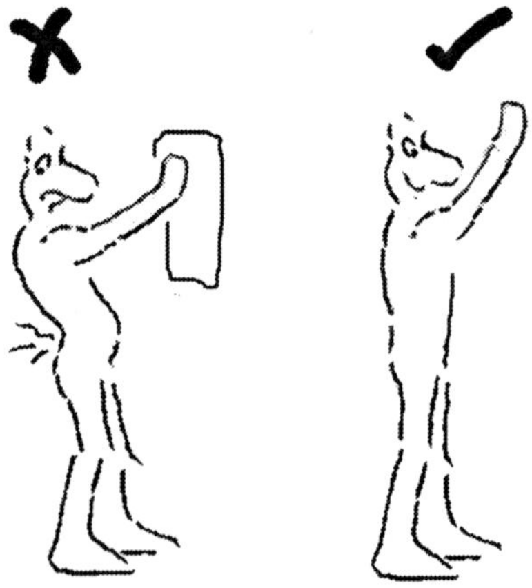

Figure 8-3. Don't lean backward to carry, reach, or lift things, which increases the inward arch of the lower back (left). Using neutral spine (right) gives lifestyle abdominal exercise.

Your Chair

If you need to use your arms to get out of your chair, your legs are probably too weak. This condition is not the result of aging as much as deconditioning. A good starting exercise is to just get up from a chair without arms, and without leaning far forward:

- Stand from a sitting position by pushing off your full foot, including heels. Don't slide forward onto your toes.
- Don't use your arms to push out of the chair.
- Keep your knees parallel over your heels. Don't let your knees sway inward.
- Lift straight up without leaning far forward, and without jutting your neck and chin forward

- Notice how you have to use far more leg and hip muscle, and the pressure of holding your body weight comes off the lower back and knee joints.
- Sit down lightly, using leg muscles to decelerate. Don't lean forward; just lower yourself, using leg muscles. Don't flop down. Notice if you reach for the arm rests, or other support, out of habit. Use your leg muscles instead. Work up to 20 or more times.

This set of tips is not a bunch of strange rules for sitting, or a weird, contrived exercise. It is just basic concepts for normal healthful positioning. It is missing the idea to do 10 squats in a gym, or 10 good chair-sits, then go back to unhealthful movement each time you sit in real life. Have comfortable healthful movement all day. Sit and rise easily. Doing so is fitness as a lifestyle.

Developing Sense of Balance With Lifestyle Exercise

Your ability to stabilize your ankles and balance while walking anywhere, particularly over uneven ground or ice, can make a large difference to your health, your joints, and your ability to live an active, independent life.

After a three-year study of more than 300 senior citizens, researchers at the University of New Mexico concluded that people were at twice the risk of suffering an injurious fall if they could not balance on one leg for at least five seconds. If you do your own check of people at any age, you may find the same problem.

Inactivity decreases your balance skills. Balance is "use-it-or-lose-it." Leg and foot injury also decreases your balance skills. In both cases, balance retraining is crucial to recovery. Poor balance after injury creates a vicious cycle of "wobbling," poor positioning, weakness, poor ability to stabilize the limb, and disuse. Poor balance from inactivity creates a vicious cycle of reducing activities that require balance, which are most activities of independent living, and losing more balance skill.

You can easily improve balance with normal lifestyle movement. Get started carefully, in a safe manner, away from nearby objects, with supervision, if needed.

- Stand to put on your pants, shoes, and socks. Take them off standing too. Get a free hip stretch and balance workout.
- Stand on your toes. Keep weight on your big toe and second toe, rather than teetering on the outside of your foot. Then try standing on the toes of only one foot. When you get good, try balancing with eyes closed.
- Stand on one foot then the other for increasing periods of time. Try it when you are on the phone and washing dishes.
- Walk on uneven ground.

- Practice getting up from the floor and back down in a smooth manner. Then repeat without hands. Then repeat holding a package, then with a friend pulling on the stretchy band, as described previously.
- Go ice skating, roller-skating, and dancing.
- Try Tai Chi. In Tai Chi, you practice shifting weight slowly and standing on one foot.
- Do some regular home or work activity while balancing on one leg—filing, cleaning, picking things up, reading, opening mail, or juggling.
- Get out of chairs without using your hands. Get up and down from the floor without using your hands. Use good leg and back posture. Breathe.

Body Weight in Lifestyle Exercise

It is not the case that you cannot get stronger without lifting external weights, and that body weight is not enough for strengthening. Often, the weights used in exercise classes and physical therapy are lighter than the resistance your muscles get from moving your own body during a real-life activity.

Think of people in exercise classes who lift small hand weights, then bend over incorrectly to put the weights down and bend over incorrectly again to hoist up a 20-pound handbag. Knee-pain patients in rehab centers may lift two- and three-pound weights strapped on their ankle while sitting, or they pull stretchy bands with their leg. They then get up and walk away with injurious body mechanics, letting their knees and ankles sag inward because they are not using their leg muscles to stop it. The unhealthy sagging grinds away joint cartilage and prevents full use of the leg muscles. They don't understand why their knees, ankles, and feet still hurt even when they "do their exercises."

It is crucial to health and independence to be able to lift and move your own body weight. Following are things to start with, to strengthen without a gym or equipment. The main purpose of these activities is not to "do" them as an exercise 10 times, but to use them to retrain your muscles how to hold your body in healthy position, then use that healthy positioning for all daily life. The following body-weight exercises do not require a gym or changing clothes. When they become too easy, do them carrying functional weight, such as packages, children, books, and other common things.

- Hold a push-up position, called the plank, without arching your lower spine (as described in Chapter 7). The point of the plank is to learn to hold your spine straight without sagging under your body weight. Holding a plank with the hip lifted up in the air, or the lower back sinking under body weight like a hammock, shifts body weight to the spine. That position is not the normal lower-back curve. It is injurious overarching. Done poorly this way, the plank does little to strengthen.

Done well, the plank is excellent to strengthen your abdominal muscles, back, hip, and also the wrist. The wrist is neglected in fitness, and the resulting weakness is a common source of injury. Try the plank (safely) every day. If you can't hold up your own body weight, you may have serious weakness.

- Use the half-squat for daily bending (Figure 8-1). The point is to use this healthy bending all the time instead of bending incorrectly.
- If you can't sit and rise from the floor without your hands, you are too weak and tight for ordinary daily life.
- Practice getting up from your chair (safely) without using your hands or leaning forward.
- Stand to put on your hosiery, pants, and shoes.
- Hang from a chinning bar, a branch, a pipe, a doorjamb, or any secure overhead. Don't worry if you cannot do full pull-ups, just hold on and hang. When you can do that, hang for as long as you can from a bent-arm position, and begin trying to raise yourself (do a pull-up). Maybe you will need to start by stepping up on a box to help raise yourself, and letting yourself slowly lower without using the box. Work up to full pull-ups. If that exercise is easy, use fewer fingers to hold on.
- Try the quick handstand (Figure 8-4). Crouch down, facing away a wall. Lift one foot high up against the wall. With that foot pressed securely, raise the other foot to the wall for a quick and easy handstand. Step back down easily when you want to go down. Build up the amount of time you can stand. Try small dips until you can do full upside-down push-ups. Practice shifting weight from hand to hand. If things fall from your pockets, you will be able to retrieve and repocket them, still upside down with one hand.

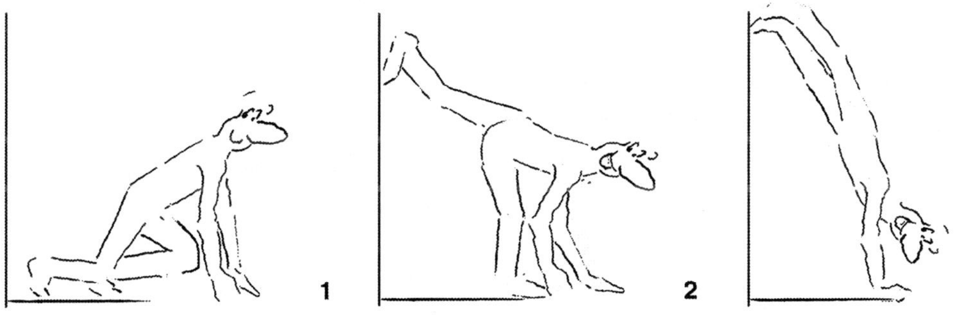

Figure 8-4. Quick and easy handstand to improve strength, wrist and upper-body bone density, balance, agility, circulation, and more.

Exercise With Babies and Young Children

Do you have no time to exercise because of the kids? This section shows ways to have fun, healthful exercise together.

Parent-child classes that strap children in a stroller, restricting their movement, while you do counterproductive forward-bending exercises like crunches and leg lifts (Chapters 7 and 9) go against the goals of fitness. Don't deprive children of the movement they need for health. Hold and lift the kids as the weights, instead of doing unhealthful exercises or using artificial store-bought weights and resistance bands.

A common incorrect notion is that lifting babies and children causes back pain. Based on this belief, some parent-child exercise programs leave the babies strapped in strollers while the parents lift small hand weights. It is not lack of strength that causes the pain, but incorrect lifting by bending over forward (Figure 20-2, left) and leaning backward to carry and lift children overhead (Figure 20-5, left). Lift children properly around the house all the time for pain prevention and built-in weightlifting that provides strengthening, friendly bonding, and exercise.

Parents and children both need movement, interaction, and contact with each other. Babies without continuous human touch cannot develop normally, physically, or socially. Hold them. Touch their skin and make sure they can feel yours in healthy ways. Face them. Hold their gaze. Talk to them as you lift them up and down. It is contrary to health, and it is not fitness, to strap them in the equivalent of a wheelchair facing away from you without two-way human communications.

- Lift babies overhead up and down, three sets of 10. They love that. Don't lean your upper body backward to lift them upward since it increases the inward curve of the lower back creating too much arch, called hyperlordosis. Hyperlordosis (too much lordosis) is a major cause of mystery lower-back pain. (Refer to Chapter 7 on abs and Chapters 20 and 21 on back pain.)

- When you lift children from the floor, crib, or table, don't bend over forward, with a straight or round back. Bend your knees, keeping your torso upright, as taught in Chapter 7 on abs and Chapters 20 and 21 on back pain.

- Is the baby getting bigger and heavier? Good. The increasing weight will increase your strength.

- Do squats and lunges holding your baby. Up and down and up and down. They love the ride.

- Babies have a natural grasping reflex, similar to the grip of world-class climbers. Don't squander that gift. Plop them on your leg and do leg lifts front, back, and side. Do push-ups with them on your back. Let them grasp your hands as you lift them up and down.

- Do "monster" push-ups—put the baby on the floor, face up, and straddle him with your arms. Each time your face lowers to the baby's face, blow raspberries, say hello, or do a peek-a-boo.
- Do "peek-a-boo" back extensions—lie facedown, face-to-face. Lift your upper body from the floor using back muscles, not hands. Hold your arms far out to the side. When you lower to the floor, cover your eyes with your hands. Lift back up and open your hands wide to reveal who it is.
- Bend properly for the hundreds of times a day you need to bend with young children around the house. Teach them to be active as they grow.
- Take kids of all ages skating, biking (use whatever helmets and sensible safety is needed), and to various fun activities. Interact with them.
- As much as possible, carry babies in your arms or in a simple sash or carrier with good body mechanics, rather than using a push-carriage. Children old enough to walk should walk more often, not ride in a "wheelchair" all the time. Let them move, skip, hop, or jump alongside you. Race them. Tire them out so that they go to sleep easily at night.
- Children love to move. Don't set them up for a sedentary lifestyle by only telling them to stand still, then pay for exercise classes.

Exercise With Older Children

- Do sports with older children. You may find you like their karate or swimming or trapeze lessons, and they may like your activities, too.
- Involve children in gardening at any level to teach them lifetime physical skills, knowledge, confidence, cooperation, discipline, caretaking, and purposeful activity. Babies can sit with you and play in the earth. On a small level, children can start with sprouting beans and seeds on a plate (Chapter 19) and can plant a windowsill of seasoning herbs for healthier cooking. Older children can grow healthful chemical-free food and flowers for the table and as an option instead of unhealthy offerings at bake sales. They can learn that good body positioning during movement is healthy, natural, and good exercise.
- Bicycle to the store to grocery shop with them. Older children can ride their own bike, learn to choose healthful food, and help carry packages home.

- Build constructive family time that is active. No-cost games of tag and tumbling can be done indoors and outside. Make fun active games. For example, tear a sheet of paper to different size pieces and throw them in the air for children to catch as many pieces as they can as they flutter downward. They can try catching only with one hand or just one color of mixed papers to increase eye-hand skills. They can then try while standing on one foot. Have them pick up all of the pieces when finished for good bending practice.

- Have them help you notice and evaluate your own posture and positioning when you exercise. Put them in charge of knowing and fixing positioning. Teach each other how to remind each other in helpful and pleasant ways.

- Have kids help with cooking and cleaning, rather than overloading yourself to do everything alone while they miss the discipline, good habits, and exercise of helping you. Make it fun to be together. Start them young so that they have always known how.

- Enjoy time with your kids of any age outside every day. Developing children need sunlight on their skin and eyes to develop immune function, bones, and other health aspects.

- It is common in many countries to have positive sayings and helpful ideas posted in public areas, workplaces, and schools, and even printed on product and food packages. The sayings urge ways to keep thought and actions happy. Teach positive "mental tools" that you believe in, not just clichéd mottos, that children can call upon in moments of stress in school and life to do good instead of destructive actions. It is important mental exercise.

Lifestyle Exercise Reduces Effects of Aging

Much of the loss of strength and balance over the years is from disuse not aging. Many people do not use their legs for the hundreds of times each day they need to bend. They bend incorrectly, throwing their weight on their spine. Their back hurts and their legs and hips tighten and weaken. Eventually, they find they are unable to sit comfortably on the floor, and more worryingly, cannot rise from the floor, or even from their chair without using their hands. This condition is debilitating weakness, and a dangerously unhealthy cycle of use or lose. It is not aging. In cultures where sitting and rising from the floor is a daily activity, people of 90 have the strength and balance to do it. They do not suffer the rates of falls, osteoporosis, arthritis, and cardiovascular disease of less-active populations.

Go Outdoors for Fitness as a Lifestyle

A sharply rising number of asthma cases in Western society has been linked to inactive lifestyles spent indoors. These findings were released in 1996 at the annual meeting of the American College of Allergy, Asthma, and Immunology in Boston. Many factors contribute, including long sitting indoors, which decreases breathing function (refer to Chapter 1), household chemicals, which concentrate indoors, indoor allergens, lack of activity, and lack of sunshine. Get at least a little movement every day outdoors in the sunlight.

Meditation and Relaxation as a Lifestyle

People often meditate by staring at a candle but tense their shoulders preparing dinner and driving, hold their breath to lift things, and are easily distressed when someone cuts in front of them. They may stress to make time to take expensive meditation or yoga classes, and sit in bad posture while there, then return to stress and bad posture on the way home. People use the catch phrase "mind-body," and then sit in poor posture not using their body, and losing their mind.

Sitting quietly, starting at something (or nothing), or counting is the first five minutes of the first lesson. After this simple start, you are supposed to use the concentration and focus to do everything else. The fact that some people take years to master the first five minutes, or spend their life doing only this minor introductory part is another story.

All exercise is supposed to train focus and concentration, as are all household chores and work. Lifestyle meditation is done raking leaves, preparing dinner, chopping wood, during personal interaction, and during all exercise training.

Use meditative action for all you do. Can you stay healthy and keep your blood pressure from rising in real life when the phone is ringing and the babies (of all kinds) are screaming, or when nothing is happening externally to make you focus and get things done? Instead of only practicing meditation sitting, get up and get healthy by turning away negative thoughts, staying on track, standing up straight, and breathing easily when doing housework, during interactions with others, and all exercise you do.

Social/Emotional Fitness as a Physical Lifestyle

- Get exercise by cleaning the house of junk and clutter. Bend correctly to clean the closets. Take the extra clothing, toys, and household items to a shelter. Carry the bags with healthy positioning to the people who need it.
- Make a healthy meal with family or alone, without television or phone. Carry the meals to shut-ins and isolated elderly in your neighborhood, and the homeless on the street.
- Volunteer at a soup kitchen. Do grocery shopping, cooking, and vacuuming for those who are too sick or disabled or alone to do it for themselves. If you think you

don't have time because you have young children, take them with you to help carry things and to teach them healthy ideals, and how thankful they can be for the home you provide.

Interacting with family, co-workers, and the world at large should not be an excuse to do unhealthy behaviors out of habit (like smoking, overeating, drinking too much, and arguing) and then blame it on stress. The bad habits are even more stress on your body and mind. If something is wrong, see about fixing it in a good way. Make your home healthy for yourself. In the world, if someone cuts in front of you, smile, breathe, and wave them through. They may have a dying child at home. Be good to such a person even if he is a lump with no manners. It is not between you and them.

Health for All of You as a Lifestyle

Your physical body is not the only part of you that needs exercise. Exercise your sensibilities. Exercise your smile muscles. Exercise your imagination. Exercise your mental abilities. Exercise your funny bone. Exercise your love of life. Many things improve with exercise as a lifestyle.

Make Lifestyle Fitness Natural and Healthful

Look through this book for something that will make your life happier. Lie face down on a comfortable surface, propped slightly on elbows to read it. If you can't lie comfortably that way, that usually signals tightness that makes daily movement unhealthy and uncomfortable.

Conventional fitness has become unhealthy. Healthful natural, comfortable body movement has become foreign as more people think that exercise means artificial sets of repetitions on a machine or using equipment. How are you sitting as you are reading this? Pull your chin comfortably in, instead of jutting forward, or downward. Stand up, breathe a grateful breath, and walk away from the chair for a few minutes, contemplating a new, healthy, fun life of natural movement.

9

Making Bad Exercises Into Good Movement

Always do right—this will gratify some and astonish the rest.

—Mark Twain

At a 2005 military medical conference, it was reported that the source of as much as 62 percent of casualties to our troops is not the battlefield, but the gym. Part of the problem is good exercises done in injurious ways, and part is the exercises themselves. Some of the most commonly done and accepted exercises are injurious or ineffective. They may give cosmetic results, but injure joints and soft tissue, and reinforce bad positioning and posture. They may work the muscles they claim to work, but not in the manner you need in daily life. Many exercises done to rehabilitate the injuries don't retrain how to move in real life, and have a higher-than-expected failure rate. Exercises that "work" are not always good for you.

Neck Exercises

Neck Exercises That Hurt and Damage

Common exercises put the neck into a position that creates pain and damage. Poor neck posture of holding the neck tilted forward often brings on "hanger-shaped" pain across the top of the shoulders, between the shoulders, and under the shoulder blades, It can press the nerve that runs down the arm, making pain and numbness in the arms and hand. Over years, a forward-head posture and slouching the upper body and neck can herniate the neck discs. Tight front muscles, overstretched upper-back muscles, and continually allowing the forward-head posture will make a forward position feel normal. Common exercises reinforce this posture.

- Classic exercises that press your neck into weighted, forward positions are the overhead bicycle, where you churn your legs in the air with your weight on your shoulders and neck, and the shoulder stand and plow (Figure 9-1), where you lie with your legs over your head and your weight on your shoulders and neck. These exercises force the neck forward, pressing discs rearward and outward, and overstretching the long ligament that runs down the back of your spine.

- The vertebrae of your neck are not shaped for rolling in circular motion (circumduction). They tend to grind. Neck rolls (head rolls) are tough on your neck over time, and better avoided. By contrast, your shoulder, hip, and knuckle joints of hands and feet are shaped for circular motion.

- Don't let anyone roll, push, manipulate, or pull your neck. If you have a disc that is ready to bulge or herniate from years of forward-head positioning, it may be pushed the last amount needed to start pain and serious injury. Cases of paralysis from "assisted stretch" pushing the neck and lower back, and death from stroke from manipulative massage to the neck from neck artery tearing have been recorded.

- Other exercises that reinforce forward-head posture include pulling your neck forward for conventional abdominal exercises, craning and tensing your neck while lifting weights, and tilting your neck forward while lifting or pulling a weight behind your neck. Lift in front instead. Stand, don't sit, for healthier and more functional exercise.

- Jutting the chin forward is common when looking upward, and in some yoga and exercise moves. It adds sizeable compressive loading on the back of neck vertebrae plus shearing force on the discs. In some yoga styles, jutting the chin forward is taught as proper form. However, shearing force on the discs is severe when you jut the chin forward then raise it. Shear is a structural strain when one layer shifts sideways (or front to back) in relation to the other. Damage may take years to accrue until visible on X-ray. Don't jut your chin forward, especially not when looking upward. Keep chin in, and get the upward gaze by straightening your upper body and chest.

> You are better off without the shoulder stand and "plow" stretch. They reinforce forward head posture, overstretch the posterior spinal ligament, promote bone spurs, and put herniating forces on the discs of the neck.

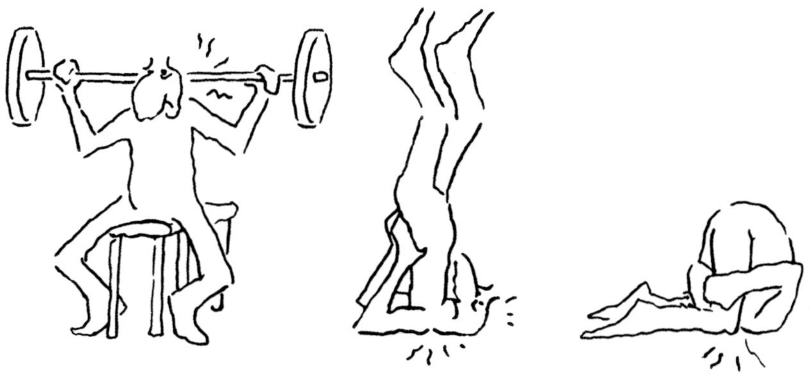

Figure 9-1. Common exercises promote forward-head posture. A forward head can create several upper-body pain syndromes. Why practice it in a gym?

Good Neck Exercises

- To strengthen the upper-back muscles that hold neck and head posture, lie facedown, arms out at your sides. Gently lift your upper body from the floor without using your arms to push off. Hold, lower, and repeat. Don't tilt your chin forward. Chin in. Get the lift from your upper back, not solely one joint in your neck. Work up to 10 lifts. Don't do anything that hurts.
- For a healthy neck range of motion, don't roll your head in circular motion. Use the trapezius stretch shown in Figure 21-5. Keep your shoulders down and back. Don't add stretching the neck forward. You do that all day. No need to add it as a stretch.
- To correct poor head posture during sitting and standing, comfortably pull your chin in until your ears and the corner of your jaw center over your shoulders. Look forward, not up or down. Don't think of it as something to do for 10 counts. Do it once–all the time. Learn to hold the good posture all day. Test yourself by standing with your back and heels against a wall to see if you are straight with the back of your head comfortably touching.
- When looking upward during stretching, yoga, and activities, keep your chin in not forward, and get some of the range from your upper back. Don't just pinch back at one neck joint.
- For more good neck strengtheners, stretches, and posture exercises, see Chapter 21.

Military Press, Shoulder Press, Overhead Lifting

In the military press or shoulder press, you lift a weight overhead. It is functional exercise for people who lift daily objects overhead, play volleyball, lift babies and children, shoot hoops, open windows, and do other overhead activities.

The military press is often cited in orthopedic literature as causing frequent, serious shoulder and neck injuries. It is also frequently a source of mystery lower-back pain. However, most people need to lift things overhead as part of daily life, and often use the overhead press during recreation. It is good to learn how to keep the movement healthy, and how to transfer that healthy positioning to lifting laundry, groceries, babies, and other daily weights. Lifting things overhead is a practical daily life activity. With good positioning, you can avoid hurting your shoulder and lower back when putting things up on shelves or opening windows.

If you hold your head and neck tilted forward when you lift your arm for weight lifting or overhead reaching, it can impinge the four muscles and tendons that make up the rotator cuff. The "forward head" posture rotates the acromion over the humeral tubercle (shifts the shoulder bone over the knob at the top of the arm bone). When you raise your arm, the soft tissue of the rotator cuff is squeezed between. Over years of lifting weights and gear overhead with slouching shoulders and forward head, you can abrade your rotator cuff until it tears.

- Before lifting, do the pectoral stretch (Figure 21-4) and the trapezius stretch (Figure 21-5) to restore muscle length for comfortable healthy positioning.
- Keep your chin in, not jutting forward or upward. Pull the chin inward with neck muscles, not by leaning backward and tilting the entire upper body backward
- Keep the corner of your jaw in line over your shoulder. Holding your head forward of the centerline of your body can interfere with normal shoulder motion when lifting overhead. With each overhead lift, you can be impinging your shoulder. Learn to feel straight position by standing with your back against a wall. The back of your head should be able to touch the wall comfortably. (Refer to Chapters 20 and 21.)
- Don't round or bend your spine forward when lifting.
- Don't overarch your lower spine (increase the inward lower back curve) when lifting upward. Keep the small inward curve of the lower back without exaggerating it. Don't let your hip tip forward, or your upper body lean backward. Both increase the arch (Figure 9-2, left). Increasing the arch, called hyperlordosis, pinches the facet joints and surrounding soft tissue. Tuck the bottom of the hip under and pull the upper body straight to neutral spine (Figure 9-2, right). Maintain neutral spine, not by tightening or "sucking in" your abs, but by preventing the lower back from increasing in inward arch past neutral spine (Chapter 7).
- Sitting while lifting a weight is tough on your back. You sit all day already. It is better for the back and more exercise to lift while standing.
- Use dumbbells instead of a barbell for varied hand placement and arm rotation, and more individual arm stabilization.

- Avoid bending forward at the crease of the leg when standing upright. Stand in neutral spine without sticking your hip out in back. (Refer to Figure 21-9 for the wall stand test to tell how you stand.)

Transfer knowledge of healthful positioning to use in every overhead lift, from pulling off a shirt, to putting away groceries, to lifting children, putting things on shelves or overhead racks, to lifting weights. You will get better exercise and prevent injury.

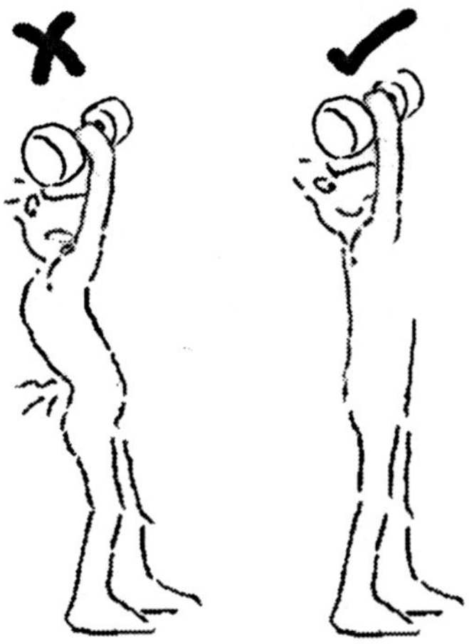

Figure 9-2. *Left:* When lifting overhead, don't lean back or tilt the hip out in back and forwarding front. *Right:* Hold neutral spine.

Overhead Arm Exercise

Overhead arm position is needed for many stretches, exercises, and movement in the home and at work. You may exercise with your arms overhead to stretch, dance, pitch and throw, paddle, do yoga, and other activities. Overhead weight-lifting exercises include the military press, overhead squats, dumbbell press, and others. Check to see if you lean your upper body backward to raise your arms (Figure 9-2, left). Arching your lower back while leaning back pinches and loads the lower back, and reduces the stretch on the shoulder.

Do you arch your lower back to raise your arms? Stand sideways and look in a mirror while raising your arms. See if you lean your upper body backward, and/or tip your hip forward. Another way to tell:

- Stand with your heel, hips, upper back, and the back of your head against a wall.
- Raise your arm to touch your fingers to the wall behind you.
- Notice if you have a large space between your lower back and the wall, or if your ribs are lifted upward. (Refer to Figure 21-9, drawing #4.)

- Notice if you stick your hips out in back, or do the opposite and push your hips forward. Both increase the lower-back arch, which increases load on the joints and soft tissue.

Increasing lower-back arching may occur automatically, and may seem "natural," but it is not healthy. To reduce the overarching:

- Press your lower back toward the wall to decrease the space. Don't flatten your back. Decrease enough to bring the spine to neutral position. You may feel a stretch in your lower spine and front hip.
- Bring ribs back down to level, and tuck your "tailbone" under you to straighten your hip. (Refer to Figure 21-9 to change from arched (drawing # 4) to neutral (# 5).)
- The motion is like doing an abdominal crunch while standing up. This motion is also called a "pelvic tilt." Don't bend your upper body forward; just flex the lower spine enough to reduce the overarching and return to neutral spine.

Try reaching again:

- Reach as high as you can overhead.
- Notice if you lift your ribs upward and lean your upper body backward.
- Hold neutral spine, using Drill #2. Feel the straighter position and how the reach needs to come from your shoulder instead of your lower back (Figure 9-2, right).
- Keep your shoulders relaxed downward. Don't crane or tense your neck

Watch other people when they reach overhead for exercise and daily life, and notice fitness magazines picturing overhead moves. See how often they arch their lower back to lift and reach. It is important to be able to tell when positioning is unhealthy, not just follow a bunch of strange rules about how to stand and exercise.

The next time you are in the shower washing your head, notice if you lean backward. Restore straight positioning. Feel how the pressure is reduced in your lower back. The muscles that work to flex your lower spine to reduce overarching are your abdominal muscles. By preventing unhealthy arching each time you reach up, you will get built-in abdominal exercise and better shoulder stretch, and stop the source of much mystery lower-back pain.

Squats

The squat can be done by standing and bending both knees to a half-squat position that looks like sitting in a chair (Figure 9-3), or sitting fully with hips close to your heels (various names, including full-squat). It can be done with body weight alone, or holding a weight at the chest, overhead, or at the sides in each hand.

Safety of the squat stirs debate. Some people insist it is good for your body and knees. Others insist the squat damages the lower back and knees. It depends how it is done. You can achieve the advantages without harming yourself.

Benefits

- The squat is a multi-segment, full-body, functional activity, meaning it works many body parts simultaneously, in the way you need them in life. It is better than isolating "muscle groups." From standing, to lifting bags, to getting out of bed, to climbing stairs, to most everything you do, your daily activities are multi-segment.
- Rising from low positions is needed daily by heavy and pregnant people. Rescuers, builders, military, farmers, and others squat heavy loads for daily work.
- Use your squat training to remind you to move in healthful way in daily life. You know you shouldn't bend over at the waist to pick things up; you should bend your knees properly, keeping your back upright, as in the squat.

Use the half-squat for daily bending: to do squats for exercise, to pick up clothes from the floor, to retrieve pet dishes from the floor, to look in the refrigerator, to get the laundry, to lift children, to sit and rise from a chair, and so on. You will get a far better workout for your legs and prevent injurious forces on your discs if you use a half squat instead of bending over forward.

You need strong legs for your daily life activities. Doing regular leg exercise dramatically reduces the effects of aging. You may have seen aged people too weak to rise from a chair unaided. This result is not as much from aging as avoidable deconditioning. These people benefit greatly from weight training, and are able to dramatically improve their mobility and independent living.

> If your leg muscles are so weak that you can't bend right for all the times around the house where you need to bend, strengthen them. Don't use weak legs as an excuse to bend incorrectly, hurting your back and knees.

Keeping Half-Squatting Healthy for Your Knees

Practice with a mirror if you can, standing sideways to see yourself fully. You should have no knee pain with good bending. If it hurts, check what you are doing:

- Stand with feet side-by-side, comfortably apart.
- Point both feet in the same direction as your knees.

- As you bend your knees, keep both heels down touching on the floor.
- Watch your knees. They should not move forward (Figure 9-3, left). Keep your knees over your feet (Figure 9-3, right).
- Use your leg muscles to deliberately pull your knees back so that your weight shifts back over your heels. Shifting your weight back keeps your weight on your leg muscles and off your knee joints.
- Look down and see if your knees cover the sight of your toes. If you can't see your toes because your knees are forward, blocking the view, pull your knees back (keeping them bent) until you are still squatting but can see your toes.
- If you let your weight flop as you bend your knees, the knees will come forward. Don't allow your knees to shift forward. Pull your weight back toward your heels. You will feel your thigh and hip muscles working.
- Keep your knees from drooping inward. Use the muscles on the outside of your thigh to keep your knees over the line of your feet.
- Keep your upper body as upright as you can.
- When returning to the upright position, don't "lock" your knees straight, which means straightening them hard and fully against the end range, then resting your weight on the straightened joint. Keep your knees (very) slightly bent. You don't need to stand in a pronounced bent-kneed stance. It is not true that you must bend your knees to protect your back. If that were true, how can you stand straight to walk away?
- Each time you use good half-squat bending with heels down, you will get a built-in Achilles-tendon stretch. If you have trouble learning to maintain knees over feet, practice this habit by putting the front of your knees against something like a doorway, to prevent them from moving forward while you practice bending.

Use the same good positioning for going up stairs. Keep your heel down and your knee back over your foot, not leaning forward. Press off your heel. If you have knee pain on the stairs, and begin using your leg muscles in this way, you should feel the pain reduce or stop.

Keeping Full Squatting Healthy for Your Knees

When full squatting, keep both heels down touching the ground. Keeping the heels down gives a built-in Achilles-tendon stretch and shifts weight off the knee joint and more to the leg muscles. If you are too tight to sit in full squat, which is a typical way to sit in many parts of the world, you are probably too tight for normal function and are missing a routine daily stretch that keeps legs and feet healthy.

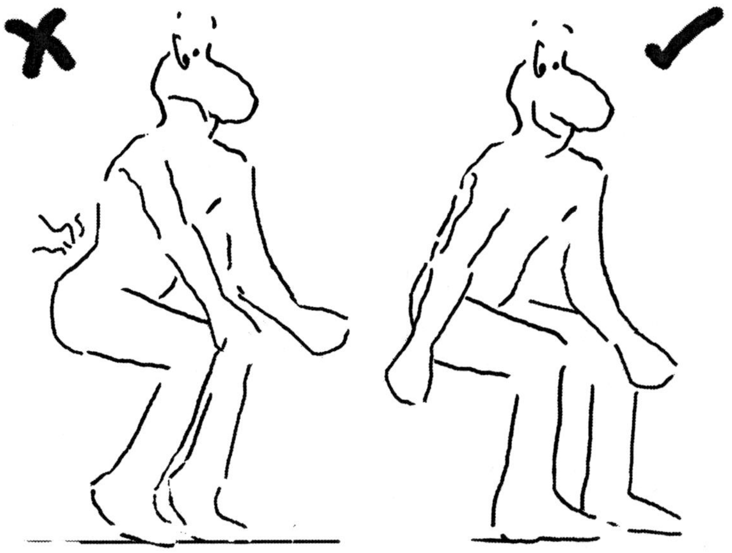

Figure 9-3. Left: Don't overarch the lower back or raise your heels. Right: Good half squat keeps neutral spine and heels down.

Full squats put higher pressure on your knee cartilage. Rising from a full squat twists the leg bones against the cartilage while exerting pressure. To help protect the knee, keep your heels down touching the ground. Don't lift the heels. Keeping weight on the whole foot, not just the front of the foot, shifts weight onto the leg and hip muscles and off the knee joint.

Knee problems are occupational injuries of baseball catchers who squat with heels up. Once injured, the nonvascular cartilage is difficult to heal. The inflammation may subside, but other times the tear acts as chronic irritant, inflaming the area until you have surgery. This problem can be avoided with proper knee posture during squats.

Keeping Squatting Healthy for Your Lower Back

Notice if you stick your hips far out in back by overarching (Figure 9-3, left). Overarching the lower back is not neutral spine. Overly arching the lower back shifts weight onto the spine joints and compresses them in a bent-backward position, eventually increasing incidence of back pain and joint damage.

If you cannot squat without sticking out in back or leaning your upper body far forward, it is a sign that your thighs are weak, your Achilles tendons are tight, you are not using your abdominal muscles, your balance is poor, or all four.

Preventing overarching does not mean you should round your back, which is accepted as damaging when lifting. It means to keep neutral spine. Why do many fitness and lifting programs teach to overarch and tilt the hip out in back? It is well known that the opposite problem of tucking under too much rounds the back and increases pressure. It is sometimes assumed that doing the opposite, increasing the inward lower-back curve too much, will counteract that. Exaggerating the arch initially seems to "work," since by over-arching when lifting, you can lift more because you shift some of the work off your muscles and onto your lower spine. The muscles do less, so it seems easier. Competition lifters use overarching to lift more, regardless of the injuries it can cause later on. People don't power-lift for their health. They do it to lift more than the next guy.

- If you overarch, tuck the bottom of your hip under, curling just enough to bring the spine to "neutral." A small, inward curve remains when you have neutral spine, but not a large one (Figure 9-3, right).
- With neutral rather than overarched spine, you will feel far more leg- and hip-muscle use. The pressure of holding your body weight comes off the lower back and knee joints.
- Raise your upper body to be less bent forward, while staying in the squat.
- When you use neutral spine instead of overarching, you should notice the difference right then how it uses your leg, hip, and abdominal muscles more, and your lower spine less.

It is not news to say to keep neutral spine. Tilting the hip so that the spine has a large arch and the bottom of the hip sticks out is not neutral spine. Neutral spine still has a slight inward curve to the lower back, but not the large one of sticking far out, that lets you do more at the price of slowly, eventually injuring the spine.

Leg Machines

Leg Press and Sled Machines

One way to get some of the benefits of the squat is to use a "leg sled." The leg sled is like a leg-press machine while lying down. In one kind of sled, you lie on your back and push the weight directly upward with the bottom of your feet. In another, you sit or semi-recline, pushing the weight away and/or upwards.

- Both kinds of leg sleds use mostly the same lower-body musculature as the squat, but lack the upper-body stabilization and balance practice of the squat. With machines, you usually can lift more weight, since you do not have to stabilize the weight with body muscles. The machine does the stabilization, and you only need muscle use to lift the weight. Using machines is not as functional as squatting.

- In the squat and some sleds, your feet are fixed (unmoving) on the floor or footplate. You push the legs to move your body and the weight away. In other leg sleds and presses, your body is fixed or still. You press the weight and your feet move away. The joint actions and the forces on your joints are different.
- Keep knees slightly bent at the end of the press, rather than "locking" your knees straight.
- Press with your heels and full foot, not just toes. Keep heels down against the place where you put your feet.
- When sitting or lying in a press or sled, do not let your back round as the weight comes back toward you, or as you push your legs away. Resisting weight with your back rounded is a common factor in herniated and degenerated disc.
- When sitting, lying down, or standing to resist weight, don't let your back overarch (increase in inward arch, increasing normal lordosis to hyperlordosis). Keep neutral spine.

Leg-Extension Machines

In the leg press, previously described, you push the weight with the bottom of your feet. In another machine, usually called leg extension, you sit with the weight at your ankle, moving your lower leg up and down in an arc. Both machines work the thigh by straightening and bending the knee against resistance. The two leg machines seem similar; yet they are different on your knees. It is debated how much difference these two different leg exercises make to the health of your knees.

- Pressing the weight away with the bottom of the feet (leg press) is generally thought to be better for your legs without as much burden to your knees.
- The leg press is also more similar to the motions your legs need to do in sports, except for kicking things, and is used in all daily-life movements like walking, running, climbing up and down steps, and getting up out of a chair or bed.
- Lifting a weight up against the ankles by sitting and straightening the legs (leg extension) is thought to be tougher on the knees upon full straightening.

Lunge

The lunge is a functional exercise. Bending the knees with one foot in front of the other is one of two healthy ways to bend for all daily bending around the house and workplace. The half-squat with feet side-by-side is another. The lunge can be done with body weight, or holding barbells, dumbbells, packages, and children.

- Stand with one foot far in front of the other.
- To get a better hip stretch and stop pressure on the medial knee (the side facing the other leg), don't turn your back leg and foot outward. Keep your back foot facing directly forward. Lift the back heel.
- Keep upper body upright and straight. Keep hands off your front knee.
- Bend both knees and lower straight downward. Don't touch your knees to the floor.
- Lower and rise several times, and then switch legs. Keep feet still, not stepping forward and back.
- Use stationary lunges to teach good knee position, rather than stepping forward into lunges. When lunging by stepping forward, check to make sure you do not slide the front knee forward when lowering, but keep it over the ankle.

Keep the Lunge Healthful for Lower Back and Knees

- Don't allow a large inward curve in your lower back. Don't tilt your hip so that it tilts out in back. Tilt the bottom of your hip under to neutral spine. One way to feel and do the hip tuck is to put your hands on each hip, thumbs in back, fingers in front, then roll your hip down in back so that your thumbs roll down in back. Don't push the hip forward, or lean your upper body backward. The moment you tuck the bottom of the hip under to straighten the hip, you will feel the stretch move to the front of the hip.
- Look in a mirror (standing sideways) when you lunge to see if you keep your body straight and upright.
- Peek downward to see your front knee and foot. You should be able to see your front toes all the way through the bend. If your knee slides forward covering your toes, you are shifting weight to your knee and off your leg muscles. This approach is one of two common ways to increase knee pain while bending. Letting the front knee sway inward is another.
- Keep the front knee steady over your front ankle, not sliding forward or inward. You will strengthen and stabilize your knees and legs instead of hurt them. You will feel more muscle use when you keep healthful positioning.
- Don't lean or slide forward. Lower straight down.

You don't need to go to a gym to do lunges. Use the lunge and half-squat for daily bending to reach and do things around the house and workplace—vacuuming, picking things up, getting things into and out of cupboards, and so on. It will add up to many lunges every day, as built-in as fitness as a lifestyle. Good bending gives free exercise and stops a major cause of several chronic-pain syndromes (muscle strain, disc degeneration, disc herniation, and sciatica) at the same time. If you use the lunge and squat around the house and workplace for all the bending you do, instead of bad bending, you will stop a major source of back pain, and get hundreds of free leg exercises a day. (Refer to Chapter 20.)

Getting Started Strengthening the Legs—Ski-Sit

An introductory exercise for your legs that uses body weight for resistance is called the "ski-sit" (Figure 9-4).

- Stand with your back against a wall.
- Lean against the wall, and "walk" your feet away from the wall.
- Slide down until you are in a position as if you were sitting in a chair, suspended in space.
- Make sure your knees are directly over your ankles, not past them.
- Hold as long as you can.
- Note that your back is upright and you are using your legs.
- Train your brain to remember this upright posture for your bending, then go on to use good bending for lifestyle exercise all the times that you bend.

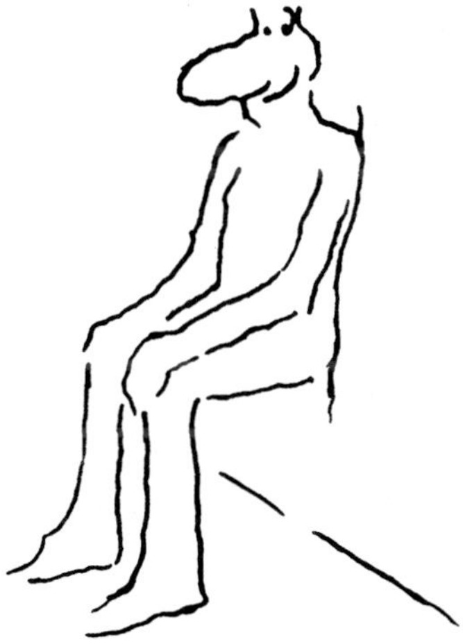

Figure 9-4. The ski-sit can get you started doing something for your legs. Use it to get the idea that good squatting posture keeps back upright and knees in line with your feet. Then use good squats for daily-life activity.

> Do you think you can't exercise your legs without equipment? You have body weight. Practice sitting down and rising from the floor using proper mechanics. Vary how you do it for more exercise. This regimen can become a life-saving exercise in later years.

Getting Started Strengthening the Back and Arms

An introductory exercise to get started strengthening your upper body is dumbbell rows.

- Figure 9-5 shows an easy way to start strengthening your back and arms.
- To progress, hold a push-up position on your hands and toes, instead of using a bench. Hold the push-up position, and lift a hand weight with one arm while standing on the other arm. Don't let your lower back "hammock" into an arch. Use a pelvic tilt (Chapter 7) to restore neutral spine.

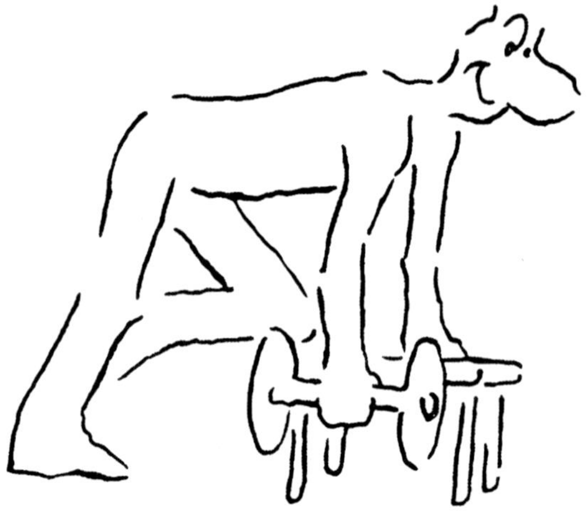

Figure 9-5. Introductory upper-body strengthening.

Step Aerobics

Knee injury is common in bench stepping. How can that be, when benches are used for knee rehabilitation? Specific kinds of stepping were originally thought to help rehabilitate injury involving the meniscus (the shock-absorbing cartilage "washers" between your upper and lower leg bones). With bad mechanics, stepping is injurious to the meniscus, and to another knee problem—a poorly tracking kneecap that grinds with each step.

Normally, your four quadriceps muscles pull equally on your kneecap when you use them to straighten your knee, making your kneecap slide up and down in a narrow track in the front of your knee. Stepping can develop the outer quadriceps muscles more than those muscles on the inside. When the stronger muscles on the outside pull more than the weaker muscles on the inside, it may make the kneecap track poorly, and rub and grind in its groove, causing pain.

When using a step that is high, the high degree of knee bending brings the kneecap in contact with your upper leg bone (femur), even in knees without tracking problems. Some rehabilitation exercises use a lateral step up, so you step to the side rather than the front, avoiding the compression on the kneecap. Stepping to the side, but letting the leg wobble without stabilization, can also increase forces that bring on pain.

A common guideline in step aerobics is to only allow stepping up in a forward or sideways direction. Stepping down is limited to backwards or sideways, never allowing the exerciser to step down forward. Guidelines state it is too hard on the knee and too prone to injury, both to the knee and from ankle sprains. However, in actual daily life, stepping down forward is done on stairs, steps, curbs, hills, and other terrain all day. It would make sense to train good leg placement for these activities in a class calling itself "fitness."

Healthier Stepping

- Sliding your knee forward past your toe, and pushing off on the ball of the foot when stepping up transfers body weight more to your knee joint, and away from the leg muscles. Keep your knee over your foot when stepping up.
- Step up onto your whole foot, pushing through your heel, not just the ball of the foot. Leaning forward on the toe makes the exercise seem easier, but the point of stepping is to use your muscles.
- Check to see if you step up or down, allowing your knee to sway inward. Inward sway twists the knee joint and presses unequally from side to side. Keep your knee over your foot. Use thigh muscles to position your knee without wobbling. When you do so, you'll often find that it keeps the arches in your feet from rolling inward and downward, flattening them.
- Don't step down and land with a straight knee. Bend your knee for shock absorption. It is easier to throw the jolt onto the joint than to use the thigh muscles, but it is bad for the joint and you get less exercise. Bend your knees and use thigh muscles with any step down, not just in an exercise class.
- Check to see if you step down heavily. Shock transmits to the joints of your ankle, knee, hip, back, and neck, and can strain your calf muscle and Achilles tendon. Step down lightly for better shock absorption. Slow your descent using the muscles in

the leg still on the bench or upper stair. You will exercise your muscles more and burn more calories.

- Standing and moving with feet facing toe-out (duck-foot) or turned inward (pigeon-toe) is a common bad habit that is often ignored as normal or not changeable. Stand and step up and down with your feet parallel, not turning toe-in (pigeon-toe) or toe-out (duck-foot).
- Use the same good foot, knee, and posture mechanics going down all stairs and steps, not just in exercise class or on stair machines.

For healthier stepping, train and apply good knee and leg movement for real stairs and hills, not just step class. Also avoid bad forward-bending stretches, crunches, and other counterproductive movement as part of step class or other exercise class.

Foot and Ankle Exercises

You need strong, flexible musculature of your feet and ankles, then you need to use the strength for healthy movement to prevent injury. Strengthening alone, and doing repetitions of an exercise, will not change many of the causes of injury.

- Your feet have posture. Many cases of "flat feet" and "pigeon toes" are not unchangeable hereditary conditions, but allowing poor foot and ankle posture.
- Standing, walking, and exercising with poor foot and ankle posture changes how you distribute your weight across your ankles, knees, and hips. Those habits create extra pressures, shock, and wear.
- Allowing your arches to roll in and flatten can contribute to foot, knee, and hip pain.
- Letting one arch flatten more than the other, which is common, creates a functional leg-length difference with every step you take.
- If your big toe joint does not bend pliably when walking, it throws off your gait. You will either take small stiff steps, or your foot will turn out (duck-footed).
- Walking with your feet turned out contributes to hip and knee pain, and is often mistaken for "flat-foot" because it shifts your weight to the inner side of your foot and presses downward on the arch.
- Turning the feet outward when walking causes and perpetuates several problems at once. Pushing off against the side of the big toe with each step exacerbates tendency to bunion and means the fascia on the bottom of the foot, the Achilles tendon, and calf muscles don't stretch as they would during normal walking. They shorten, and continue the cycle.

- When the bottom of your feet gets tight, it contributes to a condition where tissues attached to the heel irritate the heel because they pull on it too tightly with every step. This condition is called plantar fasciitis. Plantar means the bottom of your foot (that you "plant" on the ground), and fasciitis is an inflammation of the fascia, the fibrous connective tissue spanning the bottom of your foot. Untreated plantar fasciitis can lead to heel spurs. Your heel gets irritated from the pulling that, like an oyster, it grows a "pearl" of a bony spur.

Exercises for Arch and Foot Positioning

In most cases, you can control the position of your feet and arches using your own muscles. Supportive inserts are not needed.

- Check to see if you allow the arches of your feet to sag and flatten downward toward the floor, a motion called pronation. Practice lifting your arch while keeping the rest of the sole of the foot on the floor. Then, let the arch flatten again to see the difference. See how the muscles work on the inside and outside of your foot and leg. Hold normal arch with your foot and leg muscles.
- Look in the mirror to see if your feet point inward or outward. Practice walking with your feet and knees facing straight ahead.
- When walking and jogging, land softly on the heel first, then roll through to the toes. Toe-walking and running shifts body weight more on your joints rather than the muscles. Sprinters run more up on the toes, but they are not running for their health, they do it for speed gains. If you are running to stay healthy, do it in more healthful ways. Step lightly, and use muscles to decelerate to come down lightly. Good shock absorption uses your muscles and burns more calories than hard walking habits.

> Think of your feet as the front-end alignment of your car.
>
> The tires are your feet and can have posture problems in three directions—caster, camber, and of course, toe.
>
> If your tires are crooked, they will wear. It does not fix the problem to stop driving. Instead, you check why they are crooked and fix that. The same easy solution follows for bad knee and foot posture—learn to hold your knees and feet using your muscles, not letting them sway and slump.

Exercises for Preventing Falls and Ankle Sprains

Retraining balance and knowledge of positioning, called proprioception, is more successful than high-top shoes, taping, orthotics, and bracing in preventing falls and ankle sprains.

Sense organs all over your body pick up and send information about what is happening to your body. These sense organs are called proprioceptors. *Proprio* means "self," and the word root *ceptors* refers to "receiving information." Proprioceptors tell you about yourself. The most abundant proprioceptors in your body are structures called muscle spindles. Spindles lie embedded in your muscles.

When maintaining balance, you make thousands of minor adjustments all day without thinking about it, while sitting, standing, and walking. If you start to trip forward, for example, the spindles in your back and the back of your legs stretch. The spindles signal your spine to send a return message to your muscles to contract. They also tell your muscles how much to contract. With this information, your muscles know to return you to an upright position, but no further. The muscle stretch-contraction loop is called the myotatic reflex, or stretch reflex.

A sudden overstretch activates sensory nerves in your muscle spindles. The sensory nerve carries a message to your spinal cord about how much and how fast your muscle stretched. Your nervous system sends a signal back to tell your muscle not to stretch so much. Your spindles send a sensory message up your neural chain of command, triggering a motor message back down to contract the muscle. This process is important to train your legs and ankles to work to hold you in proper position. Training this system helps prevent falling, or spraining your ankle.

In an inversion sprain, the bottom of your foot turns toward the other leg and your ankle bends too much, overstretching or tearing the outer connective ligaments. Inversion is the most common source of sprains. The receptors become damaged and lose their ability to tell if you are about to sprain our ankle again. This receptor damage is a common reason for repeat sprains—not retraining balance and proprioception. Various therapy programs concentrate on strengthening the ankles. High rates of repeat sprains have led some medicine groups to conclude that strengthening will not help, and only bracing will stabilize a previously sprained ankle. Preventing sprains requires something else—training the receptors that tell you if you are about to invert. Without it, the ankle does not send signals to your leg muscles to prevent you from turning it. With proprioception training, you learn how to sense ankle position and balance to keep it from inverting. Allowing inversion when stepping up or down is surprisingly common, even in people who exercise frequently.

Using easy positioning and proprioception training, you can train your ankles to sense when they are rolling too far outward (foot inversion), and send signals to your

Weak or injured ankles do not have normal "knowledge" and control of balance. They cannot correct for a sudden slip quickly enough. Instead of righting you, these weak, slow, overstretched, and "unaware" ankles let you fall.

You need balance exercises, good motor-control exercises, and real strengtheners more than high-top shoes, supportive wraps, and ankle stretches.

ankle, foot, and leg muscles to straighten your ankle and prevent the sprain. This approach works well, even with damaged and overstretched ankle ligaments, and is key to rehabilitating and preventing recurring sprains.

Wearing supportive shoes, an air cast, splints, taping, and elastic bands to brace injured ankles are common practices that can perpetuate weak, unstable ankles because these devices prevent sense of balance and positioning. Wearing these devices to support non-injured ankles for hiking and walking can be counterproductive, because balance is diminished when wearing an ankle brace.

Proprioception exercises are simple. Do these exercises in a safe area.

Drill #1:

- Stand up. Keep both feet facing straight ahead, not turned out.
- Rise up on tiptoe. Notice if you allow your weight to teeter over the small toes, tilting feet and ankles outward. This poor positioning lacks the stabilization that allows your ankle to turn in the outward direction that allows sprains. You don't want this bad positioning to occur any time you are walking, hiking, jumping, dancing, or moving.
- Shift your body weight over your big toe and second toe. Don't let ankles sag inward or outward. Hold ankles neutral.
- Stand up on tiptoe with straight, good positioning as long as you can. You can practice this position on the phone, or when doing dishes or laundry. Make sure you use it in real-life activities whenever standing on your toes to reach and lift.
- Walk on tiptoe, using the stable positioning, not teetering outward to the small toes.

Drill #2:

- Stand on one foot. Keep neutral arch, not letting your arch flatten
- Stand on one foot with eyes closed. Without visual cues, balance is more highly challenged.

Drill #3:

- Work up to rising to toe and lowering on just one foot without letting your weight shift to the small toes.
- Work up to careful jumps, first coming down on both feet, then on one foot. Each time, land with your weight centered over your big and second toe, not turning your ankle outward, then roll gently down until the whole foot is one the floor.

Use stabilization each time you step up or down stairs, curbs, or any uneven surface. With this practice, you can train your ankles to hold stable, healthy position with each foot-fall, reducing risk of sprains, and increasing health and strength of the ankle.

Physical therapy settings may work on proprioception rehabilitation on a balance board or other balancing device. You can make your own stability challenges by standing and practicing different sports movements on a board over a small rock, or a variety of inventive household items like cans, books, and pillows. Lifestyle balance training is covered in Chapter 8.

Ankle exercises should not be limited to "spelling the alphabet" in the air with the foot and using resistance bands. A high incidence of repeat sprains occurs in people following only range of motion and strengthening. The missing link is balance and proprioception training. Balance and proprioception training also strengthens feet in a functional and more effective way than isolated strengthening exercises.

Exercises for Foot and Ankle Strengthening

The previous positioning and balance exercises strengthen feet and ankles functionally, meaning in the way you use your feet in daily life. Some prescribed strengthening exercises, such as walking with feet pointing outward or inward, will strengthen, but not in a functional way. Others can strengthen the components. A few follow. Then, you need to use the strength to walk and move in healthful ways.

- Loop a short rubber tube or bungee cord (without the hook) around both feet. Roll the outside edges of your feet outward and upward, and hold. Repeat. Gradually increase the number you can do and the thickness of the band.
- With the same tube, keep your heels together and point your toes away from each other, resisted by the tube. Hold and repeat.
- Repeatedly press the outside of your ankle upward against a wall, as if you are resisting an ankle sprain (which is what you are doing) and hold for 10 counts. Repeat at different angles.

- Get a towel and any 5- to 10-pound weight, even a big book. Set the weight on the towel, and your bare foot next to it. Pivot on your heel to slide the towel with your toes. Do both directions, pivoting inward and outward (Figure 9-6).
- Pull a weighted towel (or whatever is handy) toward you by scrunching it with your toes.
- Walk back and forth on only your heels. Step lightly, not hard on the heels
- Pick up things with your toes while balancing on the other foot. Bend at the hip to lift the object to your hand.

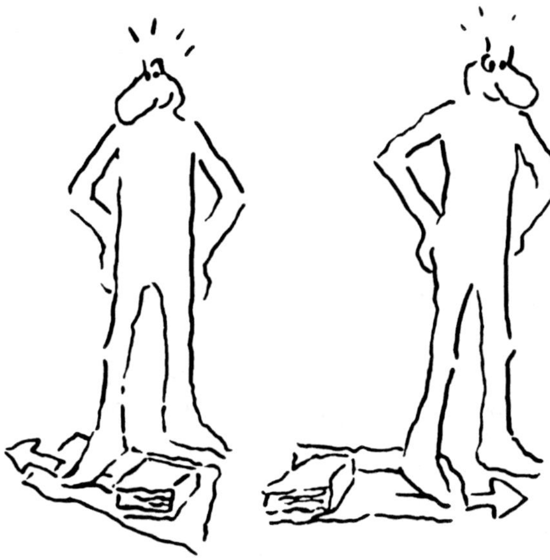

Figure 9-6. You can strengthen the feet, but then you need to use good foot and ankle mechanics during all movement to stop pain and injury.

Strengthening your feet and ankles will not change the bad positioning that creates tightness of the fascia and injury. You need to apply the strength with good positioning and balance exercises.

Swimming

Swimming can increase strength, endurance, and cardiovascular function. Swimming does not use every muscle, as often thought, but is excellent exercise for the upper and lower body. It is a myth that swimming does not burn fat or does not provide as much exercise as land-based activity because heart rate is lower in the water. If you only swish around, you won't get enough exercise to burn much fat or strengthen to a high degree. More vigorous swimming will burn calories and fat, like other active exercise. Taking a stroke mechanics clinic to improve your swimming stroke can increase your enjoyment, the distance you can swim, and teach you to swim more comfortably and safely for your joints.

- Poor stroke mechanics can create shoulder and neck pain.
- Bad stretches can hurt shoulders (refer to Chapter 6).
- Keeping the body level when lifting arms in the front crawl instead of using a side body-rolling technique will overrotate the arm when lifting it out of the water, and crane the neck for each breath.
- Allowing the lower back to overarch like a hammock instead of holding a straight profile with neutral spine decreases streamline and increases lower-back pain.

Good Swimming

- Keep neutral spine to prevent overarching during front strokes. (Refer to Chapter 7 to see how to readjust to neutral spine.)
- Use a smooth body roll for the front crawl, as if you have a pole from head to feet. With a good body roll, you can lift your arms from the water to each side safely and smoothly, the shoulder does not exceed normal motion, and you can breathe comfortably to either side without lifting your head forward.
- Try arm-only and leg-only work and swimming with fins for variety and additional leg workouts as part of your routine.
- Have your stroke checked by a good stroke-mechanics specialist or coach to be able to do more of a workout and reduce chance of mechanical injuries.
- Dry your toes after swimming to avoid athlete's foot. Wear clean, dry socks. Powder your feet before dressing, if needed, with baking soda. Don't put damp feet into socks. Don't keep toes moist and pressed together in tight shoes.
- Dry your ears to prevent swimmer's ear. Don't use cotton swabs or other devices to remove the protective earwax that keeps germs out. Earplugs do not keep much water out of your ears, and in fact, usually keep water in. You don't need to keep water out. Sloshing water helps remove debris and germs. Ear plugs prevent this normal removal process. Pressing a phone to an ear can create a moist environment, allowing swimmer's ear. You don't no need to stop swimming to prevent or treat swimmer's ear.
- Don't drink large quantities of water or other fluids before long cold swims. The greater volume has been linked to cases of pulmonary edema in scuba divers and open water racers and swimmers.

- Avoid bad stretches, such as lifting arms upward behind your body.
- Don't round your upper body when swimming in the front crawl. The forward position created by the rounded shoulder will compress the rotator cuff each time you lift the arm to the side.

Leg Lifts

Leg lifts do not make the hips or abdomen smaller. You cannot remove fat from an area by exercising that area. Moreover, exercising "for body parts" does not result in even, natural-looking, whole-body fitness. You will look better, without having "difficult body areas," if you do real lifestyle movement (refer to Chapter 8) outside a gym. Leg lifts are sometimes prescribed as part of back- or knee-strengthening programs, and then done in ways that are not healthful for the back or knees.

Side Leg Lifts

Leg lifts lying on your side to work the gluteus medius muscle do little for the muscle, even with an ankle weight, unless you are debilitated from sedentary living or injury. Your leg is too light to give the resistance you need for strengthening. It is a small muscle, so it easily "burns," but that doesn't mean it is working the way you need it. A side leg lift while lying down is not a "functional" movement exercise. In other words, it is not a movement that you use for your daily life or for sports or recreational activities. Side leg lifts lying on your side are not usually an effective use of exercise time.

Back Leg Lifts

Leg lifting to the back done on hands and knees is sometimes called the "bird-dog" exercise, or "donkey kick" when done with the back knee bent. From a hands-and-knee position, one leg is lifted to the back, and sometimes with one arm to the front. When done resting on the knees, back leg lifts do little for the back and leg muscles, is hard on the knee, and is prone to the same overarched poor lower-spine positioning that perpetuates back pain. The bad habit of lifting the leg by pivoting at the lower back is the same bad habit that contributes to lower-back pain when walking and running. The leg should lift from the joint where the leg meets the hip, not by arching from the lower spine. Back leg lifts should be used to retrain leg movement habits without arching the lower back.

Front Leg Lifts

Leg lifts to the front are usually not a good abdominal-muscle exercise. They use other muscles more than the abdominal muscles, and they promote and practice a bent-forward position at the hip. Front leg lifts contribute to tight front hip and all the problems of forward bending. The front hip muscles are usually already tight and short, and do not need bad postural reinforcement to be tighter and shorter.

Healthier Leg Lifting

Side. To work the muscle on the side of your hip functionally, stand to exercise. When you raise your right leg to the side while standing, the gluteus medius on the side of your left hip must work to keep your hip stable. If not, it drops down like the walk of a runway model. That jolts the hip with each step, and grinds structures into each other. It is one interesting and often missed cause of hip pain. You need strong medius muscles for posture stabilization while walking, going up and down stairs, running, and any time you need to shift your weight from one leg to the other. Balance on one leg and use the resistance of a band, the wall, or the foot of a partner who is standing to do the same exercise. Practice not letting the other hip drop downward.

Another fun side hip strengthener that trains stabilization is to hold a push-up position, then turn to the side, raising one hand in the air. Raise the top leg in the air and lower many times. If you hold your body straight without sagging while doing these side leg lifts, your hip muscles on both sides must work hard

Front. Substitute the abdominal exercises covered in Chapter 7 instead of leg lifts to the front.

Back. Leg lifts to the back while lying flat are described in Chapter 21 on back pain. Lie facedown with your chin on your hands. Lift one or both legs up slowly with a straight knee, hold, and then lower. This action of prone (facedown) hip extension benefits your lower back and posterior hip (gluteal) muscles. Don't lift so high that it hurts.

For back leg lifts from a hands-and-knees position, if you let the lower back arch, the pivot is the lower spine, not the leg and hip muscles. Don't arch your back. Tuck hips under to make your spine flat and straight across your back. It will immediately feel like more work, since you are no longer just swinging from your lower back, but using the back hip and leg muscles instead. Watch yourself in a mirror. Use only your leg and gluteal muscles.

Once you learn the hip tuck to stop overarching, then get off your hands and knees and do back leg lifts from a push-up position. Hold a "plank" face down on hands and feet. Lift one leg upward, not allowing the lower back to arch. You will immediately feel the exercise shift to your abdominal and leg muscles when you tuck the hip.

Push-Ups and Planks

Push-ups can be an excellent abdominal exercise, if done without arching the lower back. Use push-ups instead of crunches for functional core training. Although principle movers for the push-up are biceps, triceps, and pectoral muscles, if you use back and abdominal muscles to prevent overarching the lower spine, you will train core and legs. Push-ups are a good exercise to maintain ability to get up off the floor, more important with every passing year.

Even if you don't do complete push-ups, holding the push-up position, called the plank, is a good functional exercise for most of your body if done with a straight neck and back. If you can't hold a plank for more than a few seconds, then it is no wonder your posture sags and your back hurts.

A sagging inward curve to the lower back is not the normal curve; it is too much curve. Doing a push-up or holding a plank with a sagging (overarched, hyperlordotic) lower spine "hammocks" body weight onto your spine joints called facets, adding to lower-back pain, and does not use your core muscles. It is counterproductive as an exercise. For push-ups and planks:

- Don't let your hips stick upward or droop downward. This position trains your posture muscles the way you need them for real life.
- Tuck your hip under so to straighten your back, as if starting a "crunch." When you do this exercise correctly, you will immediately feel the effort shift to your abdominal muscles.
- Hold your body as straight as you would if you were standing up.
- Keep your head up.
- Don't lock your elbows; keep them slightly bent. Although it makes the exercise easier to shift weight to locked elbow joints, it is better to strengthen your arms instead.
- Don't flop your weight on your wrists. Distribute the weight across your entire hand and use forearm muscles. Press with hand and fingers to reduce wrist compression and shift weight to surrounding muscles.

> The push-up uses so many muscles that, if you are pressed for time and have to choose just a few exercises to work as much of your body as possible, do push-ups.

The push-up is a bench press upside-down, using your body weight for resistance. Push-ups use the same motion and prime mover muscles as the bench press, but have different training effects. In the bench press, your hands move freely, while your shoulders remain a fixed axis. In the push-up, your hands stay fixed against the floor. Your elbows and shoulders rotate around them. The forces in each joint are different in the two situations. The adaptations are close, but separate. Push-ups won't improve your bench press as much as doing bench presses.

To Get Started. For someone severely debilitated, start with holding a plank. If that hold is too much, begin building up to regular push-ups by standing up, leaning against a wall, and pushing away. Do not allow the hip to sink in toward the wall. Work up to a lower starting position, such as the arm of a couch. Then, move to the floor, holding a plank, and follow by trying regular push-ups.

To Progress. When push-ups become easy (or possible), prop your feet up on a box, then on a chair or other sturdy support, and then work up to putting your feet up on a wall (Figure 8-4) to do decline (head-down) push-ups. Lie flat with your face down and press upward without lifting the upper body first. Hold a tucked neutral spine, lifting the entire body flat at once.

When Push-Ups Are No Longer Enough. To increase resistance during push-ups and head-down push-ups, put weights on your back, or have a friend actively resist your push-ups, or eventually even sit on you while you keep correct posture and prevent your back from sagging downward under their weight.

Wrist Exercises

Strengthening wrists is important. In daily life, you need to open jars, prepare food, and do actions using the hands without hurting your wrists. Putting wrists in a splint or "supportive glove" weakens then and does not fix the source of wrist pain. Your wrists need movement and strength to stop pain and injury.

Resisting weight with your wrists strengthens the bones. The wrist is one of three major sites of osteoporosis and needs healthful weight-resisting activities. Healthy wrist bending is needed for weight lifting, push-ups, holding a plank position, handstands (Figure 8-4), and other activities that weight your arms. Putting weight on the bent wrist strengthens your wrists and arms. The idea is to not shift all the weight to the bent wrist joint. When putting weight on a bent wrist:

- Distribute weight over your entire hand and fingers. For example, when holding a push-up position, press with your fingers and flat hand, don't let the fingers curl, putting all weight on the heel of the hand.
- Use forearm muscles to prevent the wrist from pinching back under all the weight.
- Keep your weight and the effort on your muscles, not just passively compressing the wrist joints.

Use healthful positioning and muscle use to prevent wrist pain, and bend the wrist without compression when cutting food, using a keyboard or data-entry device, driving, gardening, opening jars, wringing wet clothes or towels, and all the fun exercises you do. Confining the wrist to a splint does not stop the source of the problem, and it is not healthful in the long run. Wrists need movement and loading to keep the joint healthy, the muscles strong, and the bones dense.

Wrist and Ankle Weights

Swimmers, boxers, and martial artists may use hand, wrist, or ankle weights to add to their workouts. When swimming, you want to increase your ability to pull backward in an S-shaped curve. When punching, you want the power of your punch to go forward. Using hand weights for boxing or swimming weighs your arms downward. That approach preferentially builds muscles and neural pathways that raise your arm upward to resist the downward pull, which is not what you want.

Ankle weights for kicking while swimming have similar problems. They throw off your streamline, meaning they throw off your body positioning so that you are no longer horizontal, which reduces your efficiency. Incorrect swimming posture, in turn, makes poor swimming habits by building the wrong neuromuscular patterns. Tying weights on is also not the safest thing to do in the water.

A more direct way to improve swimming or punching ability, is to increase resistance against your forward progress, not weigh your arms or legs down so that you build patterns that lift upward.

- Use resistance like tethers, drag suits, and other devices designed to resist your forward progress.
- For punching skills, use pulleys, or bands that pull your arm directly opposite from the direction you want to develop your punch.
- If you are punching forward, use a band that hold your arm to the back.
- If punching diagonally upward, move the band so that it pulls your arm diagonally downward.

Healthier Exercise

Neck. Don't press the neck forward, or roll in circles. Use upper-back extension exercise and daily movement with the chin in.

Military Press, Shoulder Press, and Overhead Lifting. Prevent forward head that damages rotator cuff when reaching upward. Prevent lower back from increasing in arch. Hold neutral spine.

Squats. Squats can be excellent for general health, strengthening, and many sports. Keep weights off your neck. Keep both heels down. Keep knees over feet, not forward. Keep knees from swaying inward or drooping forward. Keep neutral spine, not rounding forward or overarching the lower back.

Leg Machines. Look for machines where you push the weight with the bottom of your feet, over those where you sit swinging the weight upward at your ankle. Don't round or overarch your back as you press or lower.

Lunges. Stand in place with both feet facing forward, not turned. Lower straight down. Keep your front knee over the heel, not forward or inward. Keep your hands off your front knee.

Step Aerobics and Stairs. When stepping up, keep the heel down that is stepping up. Don't let the knee sway inward or slide forward over the foot. When stepping down, use shock absorption to land lightly. Bend the knee upon landing.

Feet and Ankles. Training positioning and balance prevents flattened arches, plantar fasciitis, and sprains more effectively than strengthening, high-top shoes, shoe inserts, and elastic wraps.

Sense of Balance. Train balance daily for functional daily life and safety.

Swimming. Use body rolling for the front crawl for speed and healthful neck and shoulder positioning. Don't overarch your lower back. Keep neutral spine for streamline. Don't crane your neck by jutting the chin forward, or keeping the head low so that you have to crane to get a breath. Keep slight forward facing head position by stretching the upper body instead of craning the neck backward at one joint.

Push-Ups and Planks. Uses many upper-body and torso-stabilization muscles if done with neutral spine—don't let your lower back sag downward into an arch.

Wrists. Wrists need strengthening and positioning retraining to prevent injury, not restricting movement in a splint. When resting weight on a bent wrist, distribute weight over the entire hand, using finger and forearm muscles, instead of compressing all weight on the joint.

Avoid Artificial Gym Exercises That Only Work "Sides" and "Parts"

Many of the most common gym exercises work body parts of muscle groups. Isolating parts is not how you move in real life. Machines can get you started, and are an easy way to make an organized progression of exercises in a short period of time, but they leave out real, functional, practical movement skills.

Choose Good Exercises

Your daily life can be more exercise than a gym if you use your body properly and use your muscles, instead of letting your posture sag, walking heavy, and bending incorrectly.

Improve your health and fitness by choosing good exercises for the hour you are in the gym, and using good postural and daily-life habits for all the rest of your day. Have fun.

Resources for More Information

Healthy Martial Arts
Dr. Jolie Bookspan
ISBN 0-9721214-4-7
www.DrBookspan.com/books

10

Soreness, Overuse, and Misuse

A good laugh and a long sleep are the best cures in the doctor's book.

—Irish proverb

Doing more physical activity than usual can be fun, productive, healthy, and mood boosting. When soreness results in your muscles, it usually means you moved and exerted your muscles more or differently than usual, which is often a good thing. Soreness in joints should not occur, and usually means you need to retrain injurious joint positioning, as discussed in the chapters on stretching (Chapter 6), abdominal muscles (Chapter 7), good and bad exercise (Chapter 9), and back pain (Chapters 20 and 21).

Muscle Soreness

Anyone can be sore after activity, even trained athletes. Soreness usually begins the day after activity, so it is called delayed onset muscle soreness (DOMS). Several complicated theories explain the mechanisms and consequences of DOMS. In brief, unaccustomed mechanical stress leads to a cascade of events, including changes to the proteins in your muscle fibers and an inflammatory response. You are stiff, sore, and weak for one to three days. As long as the soreness is in the muscles, not joints, soreness isn't usually dangerous, and it eases quickly.

Soreness Creams

Various muscle rubs and creams contain ingredients to mask soreness, or provide a feeling of heat or cooling. It is better not to rely on these preparations, and, instead, prevent joint soreness with good body mechanics, and treat muscle soreness with heat and stretching. Some pain rubs contain toxic ingredients, such as turpentine oil and camphor. Many use methyl salicylate to dilate blood vessels to bring blood to the area and redden the skin. Methyl salicylate is an oil of wintergreen (betula oil). Salicylate poisoning is not rare or unknown.

People becoming sick from medicated rubs and oils accounts for "48% of acute salicylate poisoning cases treated in the general medical ward of the Prince of Wales Hospital" in Hong Kong (Chan TY. *Vet Hum Toxicol.* 1996 Apr;38(2):133-4). A study comparing severe salicylate poisoning from aspirin and topical oils found that the oils pose "the threat of severe, rapid-onset salicylate poisoning" because of the concentrated form and lipid solubility of the methyl salicylate in the rubs (Chan TY. *Postgrad Med J.* 1996 Feb;72(844):109-12). A New York teen cross-country runner is reported to have died in June 2007, after using large quantities of a muscle soreness rub over many days. According to various news stories, the medical examiner concluded she died after using too much Bengay® cream containing methyl salicylate.

Aloe for Cuts

For cuts and small wounds, you can use fresh aloe vera to help cell repair. Straight from the plant, it is cheaper and probably more effective than bottled. If the aloe leaf is small, just cut an end and squeeze out the gel. Apply to cuts and small wounds. Rub the gel and inside of the peel on your face, hands, and hair for healthy skin and shiny hair. The gel dries without stickiness. For large thick stalks, cut a one- or two- inch section, and remove the side spines. Peel the skin and scoop the cool gel. Be careful cutting the slippery insides. When eaten, aloe is said to be anti-inflammatory and to help move slow digestion. Add a chunk of aloe gel when making your own healthy fitness water and sports shakes (refer to the recipes in Chapter 16). Ethnic markets may be good sources of cut leaves, or you can grow your own plants.

Misuse and Poor Positioning Causing Injury

Soreness in the muscles is common and normal after energetic activity. Muscle soreness does not just occur in out-of-shape people. However, your joints should not be sore after exercise.

If your joints (not muscles) are sore after activity, it may be misuse, rather than overuse. You may be using body mechanics that put joints in positions that grind or rub. You may be shifting weight off your muscles onto your joints to make the exercise easier. Most repetitive movements should not overload the joints, when using good muscle mechanics to take up the load.

If you experience tenderness in small joints following the use of video games and small electronics, check yourself to see if you're using an overly tight grip on input devices and tensing your muscles in the hands and upper body. Larger areas may be sore from virtual sports simulation games. Check for joint positioning and muscle use during movement. For example, in a virtual tennis game, power the arm swing using forward motion from the torso instead of merely swinging from the shoulder and elbow, and don't increase the inward curve of the lower back to raise your arm (refer to Chapter 7).

Your joints should not be sore, hot, or swollen after any activity. Joint injury is unhealthful in itself, and can alter how you walk and stand, which can eventually stress previously healthy structures into new injuries. (Refer to Chapter 6 on stretching, Chapter 9, and Chapters 20 and 21 on back and neck pain.)

Overdoing

With any unaccustomed exercise, you can overdo, even with activity that seems mild to a more conditioned exerciser. Mild to moderate overdoing usually should not present major problems. Have fun doing new fun things, and go home destressed, exhilarated, and tired. Chronically overdoing anything, with strain, mental stress, not eating healthful food, eating junk food, and too little rest can be unhealthful overdoing.

Up to a point, regular physical exercise enhances health, athletic ability, and feelings of energy. Findings from mental health research indicate positive mood change, increased intellectual function, and improved self-concept. Overdoing in unhealthful conditions reverses the situation. Athletic ability, energy, physical health, and state of mind suffer. "Fatigue," Napoleon observed, "makes cowards of us all."

Studies of immune function show a trend where exercise helps immune function, but intense overtraining can suppress the immune system. Most of the changes so far identified are small, variable, and temporary. It is still not known if these changes increase your risk of recurrent infection or other diseases during periods of extreme ultra-training. Diminished physical performance sometimes drives frustrated exercisers to push harder to offset the decline. The overtraining cycle of fatigue, depression, and overdoing continues.

Preventing Overdoing

How do you know if you're overdoing it? According to basketball coach Dean Smith: "If you make every game a life-and-death proposition, you're going to have problems. For one thing, you'll be dead a lot."

Check which aspect you overdo. Is your intensity level all right, but you're not getting enough rest? Is it more a problem of improper use than overuse? Is it poor eating habits? Eating refined sugar and flour, high fructose corn syrup, soda, junk food, fried food, and foods with artificial sweeteners and coloring will detract from your health and top capacity, even if the foods are sold as sports or health food. Do you smoke, drink alcohol too often, or take drugs? If you are still tired and unhappy doing appropriate and safe activity, consider changing the kind of exercise you do. Try a different activity that you like.

Train in Cycles. Adequate rest is needed for physical improvement. Alternating days of hard exercise and active rest by doing a different activity is called exercise cycling and periodization.

Get in Shape. Improving fitness increases the variety of activities you can do without injury. Occasional activity will not provide the fitness needed. Be regularly active. Have fun doing a variety of regular lifestyle and recreational activities to increase your physical capacity.

Warm Up. Warm-up, just as it sounds, means raising your body temperature. Warm-up is not stretching, arm waving, or rising up and down on tiptoe. Those activities do not raise body temperature. Once warm, move through the range of motion of your activity, repeating each time closer to full speed and range. (Refer to Chapter 5 on warm-ups.)

Enjoy Yourself. Do you enjoy the exercise you do? A point to consider is: are you happy? Some disciplined people concentrate only on the results, forgetting that a painful journey isn't always necessary. Change the activity so that you enjoy yourself. Find aspects of the exercise that you like. Incorporate rest periods. Performance should improve. If you enjoy obsessing, go ahead and obsess. Identify and modify aspects that injure your body, social life, or happiness. Then, if overdoing is really for you, then just overdo it. Remember to reassess periodically. Get outside and enjoy the day sometimes. Go to a nice clean comedy show and laugh. It is good exercise.

> *Avoid errors in technique. It's estimated that about two-thirds of all injuries come from training errors.*
>
> —Dr. Stanley L. James, University of Oregon, 1997 meeting of the American College of Sports Medicine

Fixing Injury and Soreness

First Aid for Injury

The first letters of the words *rest, ice, compression*, and *elevation* spell RICE, the acronym for standard treatment of many acute injuries. RICE is for injury, not muscle soreness. Ice can reduce pain and swelling. You can make a nice cool slush bag by freezing a mixture of one-third rubbing alcohol with two-thirds water in a ziplock bag. Bags of frozen vegetables are another easy source of pliant ice packs (then, have a nice vegetable meal for good nutrition to help you heal). Compression with various elastic and non-elastic wraps reduces swelling in limb injuries. Make sure not to restrict circulation into or out of the area with overly tight compression dressings. Elevation means raising the injured part above the level of your heart, not simply propping it on a low chair. Rest includes proper activity to rehab the injured area and bring blood flow to help heal the area, and exercise for the health of the rest of you. Rest doesn't mean stopping all movement, or getting out of shape so that you injure yourself trying to get back into shape. It does not mean letting the rest of your body suffer the health losses of stopping exercise. Lack of movement is generally unhealthy, slows healing, and increases risk of deep vein thrombosis. Exercise at levels below what it takes to reproduce pain. Keeping active is necessary to stay healthy so that you can heal.

Does Hyperbaric Oxygen Treatment Work for Injuries and Soreness?

Some athletes and private citizens are using high-pressure oxygen treatments, believing it will get them in shape or help speed injury healing. Like other specific medicines, hyperbaric oxygen helps some things and not others, and can have side effects. What is hyperbaric oxygen treatment, and what is the basis for its use?

"Hyper-" means more or above. "Baro-" comes from a Greek word meaning weight or pressure. Some words that use this word root are barometer, an instrument measuring atmospheric pressure, and bariatrician, which is a physician who manages obesity. Hyperbaric oxygen treatment consists of breathing 100 percent oxygen while inside a dry treatment chamber that is pumped to a pressure higher than you are breathing now. Hyperbaric oxygen treatment does several things, including bringing additional oxygen to a deprived area, increasing the body's white cell ability to fight problem-infected wounds, and reducing inflammation by constricting blood vessels and preventing white cells from sticking to the blood vessel lining. These actions allow healing of certain problem wounds, and help prevent spread of infection and damage to adjacent non-involved tissue.

Hyperbaric oxygen treatment can be life- or limb-saving for a sick patient with decompression sickness or air embolism from a scuba-diving accident, carbon monoxide poisoning, gangrene, necrotizing fasciitis (flesh-eating bacteria), radiation necrosis, problem wounds that do not heal because they have a poor blood supply (i.e., hypoxic), and certain infections of problem wounds.

Debates continue about whether hyperbaric chamber treatment can help athletes or muscle injuries. Sprains and delayed-onset soreness are not injuries where low oxygen prevents cells from doing their job to fight infection and rebuild. For non-geriatric athletes, most sports injuries should not be hypoxic, which is an area of low oxygen. Often, the opposite problem occurs. For example, an area that is hot and swollen may have plenty of oxygen and blood supply. Adding more oxygen would not make it heal faster. With the normal oxygen level in regular injuries, you also do not increase antibacterial action. Elevating oxygen levels doesn't turn normal cells into super cells.

The idea that there may be other effects of injury that are not from low oxygen has led to more research on sprains and muscle injury. Dr. Kazuyoshi Yagishita and colleagues at the Tokyo Medical and Dental University looked at 20 patients who sustained muscle injury during sports, who were admitted to the Tokyo hospital within seven days after injury. The patients received hour-long hyperbaric treatments for one to seven sessions. Patients were tested before and after each treatment for pain at rest and with motion, subjective evaluation of edema, muscle stiffness, and leg volume. All parameters slightly improved with treatment. They concluded that, in this study, in patients with muscle injury, hyperbaric treatment was effective. Further study is needed to assess healing acceleration and its intermediate and long-term results. Chronic exposure to hyperbaric oxygen has side effects including vision changes, and should not be casually used for regular treatments by people hoping for gains in sports or general health.

Stretch for Soreness

Stretching helps relieve delayed-onset soreness. Warm up gently, then gently stretch the affected muscles. Warmth while (safely) stretching sore muscles in a hot bath or shower helps.

Heat for Soreness

Most muscle soreness is not an injury. It will go away by itself. It is a good sign that you are out having a good time and are living, and were exercising enough to have effects. Rub the sore areas. Stretch. A helpful prescription is a hot bath.

What to Do

Muscles Not Joints. Don't be afraid of muscle soreness—it means you're working. Joints should not hurt. Don't injure yourself.

Identify Problems. Are you doing healthful movement? Are you eating junk food and too much simple sugar? Do you get enough sleep? Do you like the exercise you do?

Avoid Misuse. Is it overuse or misuse? Bad gait? Poor lifting technique? Bad exercises?

Train in Cycles. Vary exercise. Do functional exercise rather than isolating "muscle groups" or "body parts." Get enough rest.

Get in Shape. Improving physical condition increases the variety of activities you can do without soreness and injury.

Warm Up. Raise your body temperature. It is not stretching, arm waving, or rising up and down on tiptoe.

Enjoy Yourself. Make your program one that satisfies your soul along with your body.

Keep Moving. You need regular movement for the health to heal injury and regular movement to prevent and sooth soreness.

Heat. Rub sore areas. Take a nice hot bath.

11

Getting Out of Shape, and How to Avoid It

We can now prove that large numbers of Americans are dying from sitting on their behinds.

—Bruce B. Dan

You may not be an exerciser—or you may have been active, then went on vacation, or got busy with work or family. You may have worked hard to be in shape at one time, but gave it up. You may have had an accident or illness and were told to reduce activity, or forced into reduced activity by surgery and debilitating medical treatments. After a layoff from exercise, your problems are more serious and far-reaching than just gaining some weight.

Loss of strength, endurance, balance, speed, coordination, flexibility, even blood volume and bone density make packages feel heavier, shelves harder to reach, stairs more difficult or even dangerous from loss of balance, and daily tasks more tiring What can you do?

How to Get Out of Shape

Following weeks of weightless space flight, astronauts come home with less muscle, blood volume, and bone than they left with. After only a day or two in bed with flu, you get up weak and dizzy even though you're not sick anymore. The principle of "use it or lose it" is technically called "reversibility." Physical performance gains made through exercise reverse with inactivity. The deterioration of your physical condition is called deconditioning.

Periods of inactivity often follow injury or illness. Deconditioning may begin locally, as in a limb in a cast, and quickly become a global problem of whole body inactivity. An immobilized limb dramatically decreases in size, strength, and endurance. Bed rest, being restricted in activity, or using a wheelchair too readily severely reduces the mechanical stresses your entire body needs not just for athletic ability but for health itself. Complete rest so effectively diminished bodily health you that aviation scientists use it to study the huge physical decrements following zero gravity in space flight.

What Goes Bad?

Deconditioning seriously affects the functional state of your entire body. Strength, cardiovascular capacity, blood, mental skills, and even your bones and immune system suffer. Treating an injury in one area with restricted activity can harm many other areas.

Muscle. Without use, muscles decrease strength, endurance, and size, and lose blood vessel and nerve associations. They become less able to extract and use oxygen to do work, not only because your entire body's oxygen-carrying and delivery system declines, but for chemical reasons of their own.

In-shape muscle is able to burn more fat as fuel than out-of-shape muscle, which uses more carbohydrate. Deconditioned muscles lose intracellular fluid, stored carbohydrate, and contractile protein, contributing to loss of muscle tone. Your body gets soft and weak. Daily life becomes harder, and chance of injury increases. Eating extra protein will not stop muscle-protein loss. Only exercise does that. When muscles decondition, you may not look as good, feel as good, exercise as much, or do as much around the house or in life.

Cardiovascular. A deconditioned cardiovascular system can't process, deliver, or burn enough oxygen to do intense exercise because several of its components go to seed with inactivity. The total amount of blood your heart pumps per minute decreases, probably from an overall decrease in blood volume in the initial weeks of detraining. You lose oxygen-carrying molecules called hemoglobin.

The size and contractile force of your heart diminishes. The maximum rate your heart can beat doesn't change, yet it has to beat faster and work harder to do the same work you could easily do when you were in better shape. More lactic acid builds up than if you weren't deconditioned. Cardiovascular deconditioning even lowers your ability to regulate body temperature in the heat and cold. Without regular cardiovascular exercise, you become more prone to weight gain, and serious disease and disability.

Bone. After your mid- to late-forties, you usually begin losing bone if you don't exercise, no matter how much calcium you eat. To maintain mineral density, bones need the mechanical stress of muscles pulling on them. Lack of regular weight-resistive activity is a major risk factor for osteoporosis. Activity restriction at all ages, particularly in an elder, is a serious oversight in health care.

Body Composition. Changes in body composition over time without exercise include higher body fat percentage and less lean muscle, even with no change in weight.

Cholesterol. One of several reasons regular exercise decreases risk of coronary artery disease is a favorable change in blood cholesterol. High-density lipoprotein cholesterol (HDL), popularly called good cholesterol, increases. "Bad cholesterol," or low-density lipoprotein (LDL), can decrease.

One study of male runners accustomed to 30 to 40 miles per week found detraining of only two to three weeks resulted in a 12 percent reduction in their aerobic capacity and a 7.7 percent reduction in good cholesterol. For more on good and bad cholesterol, refer to Chapter 28.

Immune Function. Your immune system needs regular exercise. Without regular exercise, it loses a large stimulus to make and move immune cells and products around your body. You become more prone to many disease and illnesses, and have reduced healing time.

Memory and Coordination. Physical skills not used dull and fade from active memory. Both memory and specific skills, like hand-eye coordination and fine motor coordination, involve physical and chemical connections that require practice to stay sharp.

Flexibility. Inactivity, not exercise, reduces flexibility. Joints tighten and your range of motion diminishes for normal, daily activities. You become more likely to lean back when reaching upward, for example, adding back strain because of a still shoulder, bend incorrectly because your hip and legs are too stiff to bend in healthful position that prevents back pain, and crane your neck forward because your upper back is too stiff to straighten.

Balance. You quickly lose sense of balance when you are inactive. Your risk of slips, falls, sprains, and injury soars. You may do less due to of fear of falling. A negative cycle of doing less and losing more balance develops.

Reaction Time. The time it takes you to mobilize a response to something is another skill that you can improve with training and lose with lack of use. Reaction time, coupled with good judgment, allows you to react well in dangerous situations like oncoming traffic and falling objects.

How Long Does It Take?

Even brief detraining periods remarkably reduce physical ability. After only days to weeks of stopping exercise, your capacity for exercise decreases. After longer periods of weeks to months, you can suffer serious losses. Gains made from an active summer can disappear over a winter indoors.

The more drastic your inactivity, the greater and more rapid your losses. Complete bed rest for a week can decrease your capacity to use oxygen, your strength, hemoglobin count, and blood volume by up to 7 percent. It would take several weeks to deteriorate to the same extent without bed rest even if you didn't exercise.

Does It Hurt?

Deconditioning isn't physically painful, at first. Great harm comes from the fact that getting out of shape is more serious than just gaining a little weight.

Capacity for routine walking, lifting, and carrying dwindles. You slowly weaken, and as a result you do less and push it less. Your sense of balance dwindles. In turn, you decondition further. A negative cycle self-perpetuates. Risk of cardiovascular disease, falls, back pain, obesity, musculotendinous strains, and certain cancers may increase. For these reasons, you could say getting out of shape hurts a great deal. The global physical decline not only hinders specific sport activities, but activities of daily living, and many aspects of health. It is a major cause of death in populations after hip fracture.

In older people, deconditioning often continues to the point of severe and even dangerous weakness. Getting out of chairs and ordinary daily activities become too much. A serious handicap results, not from aging, but from preventable and reversible deconditioning.

Several studies of exercise for populations debilitated by what we formerly called "aging" found dramatic reversals after simple weight lifting and activity programs. These people no longer needed canes or wheelchairs, they decreased medications they took for high blood pressure, arthritis, or diabetes, and they went back to unaided daily activities.

How to Prevent Getting Out of Shape

Maintain Activities. If you must take time off from exercise, try cutting back, not out. You can hold on to physical fitness, even with less frequency of exercise, if you maintain the intensity. According to some studies, decreasing from three regular days of exercise to two days can preserve oxygen-carrying capacity. Substituting one day for three will not prevent, but can reduce several consequences of detraining.

Avoid Secondary Losses From Medical Rest. In many instances, the original illness or injury is worsened through the physical degeneration resulting from bed rest. Sometimes, irreversible problems develop. Treatments for many illnesses and injuries have been found more effective when they involve early ambulation and active physical rehabilitation, although often this recommendation is not observed or appreciated enough to make sure it is carried out. Don't allow medical care to make you unhealthy.

Get Active, Stay Active. Stay as active as you can all year, every year. If you are sedentary, find some kind of regular activity you enjoy and get started. The older you get, the more beneficial exercise, including weight lifting, becomes. Exercise counteracts physical declines of aging.

Prevent Debilitating Losses

Inactivity is a debilitating condition. Restricting your activity and mobility, either by choice or after accident or illness, can cause problems more serious than just gaining a little weight. Inactivity sabotages your cardiovascular condition, strength, endurance, bone health, blood-fat status, body composition, and joint range of motion. In a short time, these decrements can become the functional equivalent of aging many years.

Serious problems can result from a vicious cycle of deconditioning, weakness, and poor health. This cycle is easily preventable. Get up now, stretch your arms overhead, breathe deeply, and safely do something active, brisk, and fun.

Resources for More Information

The Fitness Fixer
www.healthline.com/blogs
Regular online health column of all aspects of keeping exercise healthy, fun, and effective

12

Exercise Gimmicks

The actress Billie Burke was dining in a restaurant where a man at the next table was obviously suffering from a bad cold.

"I can see you're very uncomfortable," she volunteered. "So, I'll tell you what to do for it: drink lots of orange juice and take lots of aspirin. When you get to bed, cover yourself with as many blankets as you can find. Sweat the cold out. Believe me, I know what I'm talking about. I am Billie Burke of Hollywood."

The man smiled and introduced himself in return: "Thank you. I am Dr. Mayo of the Mayo Clinic."

It seems to be common for exercises to be taught, and health and fitness products promoted, by Hollywood stars and fitness personalities. Many humorous and wrong ideas and statements become commonly accepted.

> "Lose fat while you sleep by drinking miracle liquid, not available in stores."
>
> "Watch TV while motorized stomach vibrator burns more calories than 500 sit-ups a day."
>
> "Shrink your waist with secret device known for years to scuba divers."

Regarding the first claim, everyone burns fat when they're asleep. When they're awake, too. Metabolizing stored fat is part of your around-the-clock energy production for body functions, whether you drink "miracle liquid" or not. (Refer to Chapter 4 for more on fat burning, and Chapter 14 for more on how potions get sold by carefully worded, but false, claims.)

The second advertisement compares the relative number of calories burned in a longer time frame to a shorter one. In two hours sitting in front of the television, you would burn more calories than during the theoretical 15 to 30 minutes it would take to do the sit-ups, with or without a vibrator strapped to your abdomen. That rate is just your normal metabolism at work.

Claims of Continued Fat Burning

Some products claim to give a workout so intense that you burn fat for hours after you finish. You burn fat 24 hours a day as part of being alive. It is also the case that during vigorous exercise, you increase your metabolism to meet your energy needs. It slows when you stop exercising, but takes a while to return to your resting values, sometimes up to a day. Any product can truthfully claim to produce increased calorie burning after a workout. A nice run, swim, or weight-lifting session will do the same.

Aerobic Benefits by Increasing Heart Rate

Many activities like to promote themselves as beneficial for your cardiovascular system. Not everything that increases heart rate or blood flow gives you aerobic benefit. For example, it is sometimes stated that the yoga position of standing on the head or inclining head-down on a tilt or inversion table improves circulation and oxygenation to the head, and therefore confers aerobic benefit, or that a specific stretch that is difficult to hold and raises heart rate therefore gives aerobic benefit. These practices do not improve aerobic conditioning.

Aerobic exercise is more than increasing blood flow and heart rate. Many things increase heart rate—for example, fear—without having anything to do with cardiovascular improvement. Increased heart rate from stage fright, for instance, is termed *neurogenic*, meaning it is produced as a nervous system effect, not *cardiogenic*, a cardiovascular system effect. Just moving the legs of a person lying in bed raises heart rate. It is a neurogenic increase, as that seems to be the body's way of preparing for exercise. Taking a long, hot shower or sitting in a hot tub increases heart rate because the blood vessels in your skin open up to try to dump the extra heat from your body. The vasodilation lowers your blood pressure, and your heart usually must speed up to keep enough blood pumping around. No large aerobic benefit results from overheating. Even massage has sometimes been promoted as beneficial to the cardiovascular system on the basis of increasing blood flow. It doesn't improve aerobic fitness level. It doesn't mean that massage is not helpful, just that it doesn't increase your cardiovascular capacity. True aerobic benefit comes from a collection of effects that you can get only through long-duration exercise, at least at moderate intensity, repeated regularly over time.

Ab Isolators

Several products on the market claim to better isolate your abdominal muscles, and to therefore somehow give you the same abdomen as pictured on the package. The true way to get a trim, well-defined abdomen is to lower your body fat through long-term exercise, eat healthful meals on a regular basis, and do exercises to improve the size and shape of the abdominal muscles in a healthful way (Chapter 7), whether you use an "isolator" or not. An isolating device does nothing you cannot do without the device. For instance, the advertising for one device claims to hold your feet and legs in the specific position required for crunches. You can do the same yourself without the device. In addition, crunches and other forward spine-flexing exercises are not healthful exercise, promote forward-bending posture, and are not the way your abdominal muscles work in daily life when you are standing and going about your day.

Other various devices on the market add resistance to the abdominal exercises. More resistance increases the muscle-unit activation you require to do the exercise, the same as carrying extra packages adds more weight to your arms. There is nothing secret or scientific about doing more work to get more results.

Dr. Steven Fleck, sport physiologist formerly with the U.S. Olympic Training Center, reminds us: "The value of these devices is their novelty. If they get you to exercise areas that you wouldn't normally exercise, they might pay for themselves." Remember that the fine print on the packaging mentions that these products need to be combined with healthy eating and regular exercise. However, more important to remember is that forward-bending exercise is not a functional abdominal exercise, and is often counterproductive for health and function, whether in yoga, Pilates, a fitness class, or using a machine.

Secret Scuba Device

What is the secret scuba device at the beginning of this chapter? Neoprene. Neoprene bands are sold to wear around the waist and thighs. They shrink the areas, but it has nothing to do with weight loss or sweat loss. It temporarily compresses the area, just as when you take off your socks and notice a ringed dent around your leg where the elastic compressed your leg. You return to normal circumference soon enough. It is healthier, more economical, and longer lasting to just get in shape.

13

Get Started

A man ought to have a doctor's prescription to be allowed to use a golf cart.

—Paul Dudley White

Lifetime Activity

You don't have to go to a gym to get exercise. You don't have to do push-ups or jumping jacks, or run. You can develop fitness through an active lifestyle. Being active for fun, and for things you have to do anyway, is the concept of lifetime activity.

Your daily activities become more active in a natural way, instead of a sedentary life that has to be made up for by going to a gym. Improve your concept of exercise from a mandatory session with strange rules about heart rates, intensities, and minimum calories to burn, into a daily-life-exercise playground—yard work, shopping, cleaning, or painting. Lift properly all day. That's work? Good. Stand and sit without slouching in unhealthful ways. Make opportunities to move and burn calories as part of your normal day. You could burn a few hundred extra calories a day. You might lose two pounds a month without doing any special exercises or diet. That difference may not sound like much, but it is a clothing size every three or so months, and about 20 pounds by next year. Add specific movement skills outside the gym for more exercise for more fitness. (Refer to Chapter 8).

Goal-Specific Exercise

Activities to choose depend on what you what to achieve. For a sedentary beginner to increase aerobic capacity, a three-times-a-week aerobic effort is a good starting place. For disease reduction, three 10-minute walks a day can reduce your risk of early death by disease by 60 percent, according to the Cooper Institute for Aerobics Research in Dallas. For fat reduction, use both cardiovascular sessions and weight lifting. Different fad fitness groups have debated which system burns more fat for weight loss, with each group claiming the other's exercise system is not necessary. Both cardiovascular exercise and weight lifting are needed for health, and for improving life abilities.

Body fat is not removed in single bouts of any exercise. Small calorie expenditures multiply over time. A 150-calorie walk per day can translate into close to 15 pounds lost in a year.

Start Daily Fun

A key to getting fitter is finding activities you love to do, and making your daily routines more active in general. Some people want the same routine each day; others need variety. Rather than think of fitness as intentional isolated exercise at set periods for specific body parts, enjoy an active life. Enjoy yourself. Following are some ideas:

- Do you like to go dancing? Find a club for a fun cardiovascular session. Drink water and whole juices instead of soda and alcohol through the night.
- Walk or bike to the market, carry bags home, and help put away groceries. It is both aerobic and muscular endurance, and depending on weight of the bags, some strength work, too.
- Try bicycling for errands or scenery for aerobic endurance and muscular endurance of the legs. Maybe commute by bike or walk or jog instead of driving. It can be quicker and cheaper than driving and paying for parking.
- Try bicycling or walking for grocery shopping instead of driving.
- Take nature walks.
- Plant a garden.
- Vacuum the house.
- Lift right for everything you need to bend and reach. Bend your knees properly, and it will strengthen them. You'll burn twice the calories or more with each bend—all day, every day.

- Wash your car by hand, and have fun getting your helpers or yourself soapy.
- Take a walk, and feed a few expired parking meters for strangers.
- Instead of only swimming laps, play in the water with beach balls, floats, and kickboards.
- If you hate jogging, play Frisbee®, tag, catch, soccer, or badminton instead. It may be less exercise or more than jogging (depending on how you do it), and it is a way to get started and have fun.
- Race the elevator or escalator.
- Take stairs, and walk up hills.
- Help your local club or group with chores.
- Instead of the golf cart, walk.
- Use a push mower instead of a power mower, or a walk-behind mower instead of a ride-around mower.
- Don't use a remote control. Walk away from the television to stretch instead. Stretch on the floor while watching something uplifting.
- Give a friend a piggyback ride.
- Play with children.
- Be a hero, and carry things for people.
- Take housebound neighbors' dogs for walks and romps.
- Carry groceries with your arms and good positioning rather than using a cart.
- When you eat, take time to really taste your food. Turn down seconds. Breathe. Smile. Help clean up. Keep your shoulders back. Enjoy the roof over your head. That process is healthy eating as a lifestyle.

Healthy Getting Started: What Not to Do

Don't Believe Gimmicks. People flock to outrageous weight-loss regimens, programs, gizmos, and outright hoaxes. Why are starvation, dehydration, stomach stapling, unhealthy fad diets, vibrating machines, and amphetamines considered acceptable, while normal daily movement and exercise are avoided as extreme? Avoid unhealthy gimmicks in favor of a healthy lifestyle. Healthy exercising is detailed in Part I of this book.

Don't Fad Diet. Fad diets restrict your nutrition, are usually not healthy, and don't keep the weight off in the long run. Remember that many so-called diets are just gimmicks. Just because something is called a diet doesn't mean it is a weight-loss diet or a healthful way to live.

Don't Restrict Water. Water is not fat. Losing water weight has no effect on fat loss. You need enough water to be healthy. You don't need too much water, but don't restrict water in hopes of losing water weight. Dehydration lowers exercise capacity and your ability to thermoregulate. For those who eat when they're not hungry, a glass of water is a helpful substitute.

Don't Lose Weight Too Quickly. Diets that promise large rapid losses usually do most of it through water loss, which is not fat loss. Don't spend money and fix your beliefs on them. Losing weight too rapidly can sometimes be tough on your heart, doesn't give your skin a chance to adjust to the new size without sagging, and is believed to promote loss of bone density. Avoid losing weight too quickly unless your physician has determined that the benefits outweigh the risks.

Don't Believe Claims of Spot Reducing. The idea of spot reducing is to lose fat from a specified area by repetitive movement of that area. If that were true, then the people selling spot-reducing devices would have thin mouths from all their talking, typists would have skinny hands, and bicycle riders would have skinny legs. If you want to lose fat, then burn more calories than you eat. Include exercise to do it in healthful ways that keep you mobile and fit. Find a variety of exercise that you enjoy such as walking, running, biking, cross-country skiing, rowing, weight lifting, gymnastics, dancing, swimming, and active work occupations.

Remember Error of Measurement. Don't believe health-club personnel who measure your body fat with calipers at intervals and state that you have lost 2 percent fat, or 5 percent fat, or other small percent since starting their program. The error of body fat measurement inherent in caliper testing is too high to compare specific percentages over time. A 2 percent loss measured on calipers could just as easily be a 1 percent gain. Go more by the fit of your clothing. (Refer to Chapter 25.)

Don't Stress. Driving hurriedly in a stressed manner to get to a gym or exercise class or personal training appointment to do little artificial "reps" and "sets" is not fitness as a lifestyle. Stressing to get to yoga class, then becoming upset when someone's cell phone goes off during class is not peace and focus. Do happy, real-life activities and eat healthful meals without overeating. Stop searching for peace. Make your own home and body your peace. It matters more nowhere else. No gimmicks, CDs, gurus, DVDs, special equipment, mats, Zen cushions, or any other thing that collects dust. Be good. Do good. Be happy.

- Don't believe gimmicks.
- Don't fad diet.
- Don't eat high-sugar, high-calorie unhealthful foods because they are "fat-free" or high-calorie food with bad fats because they are labeled "low-carbohydrate."
- Don't restrict water.
- Don't lose weight quickly.
- Don't believe claims of spot reducing.
- Don't fixate on artificial measurements.
- Don't stress. Healthy peaceful happy mind and body need to be trained together.

Healthy Getting Started: What to Do

Everyone, whether thin or heavy needs to exercise and have good nutrition to be in good shape.

Eat More Filling Food. Eat less high-calorie food. Studies at Tufts University found that low-calorie but physically "heavy" food like cantaloupe can make you feel fuller than an airy donut.

Not all calories are the same. When you eat 100 calories of complex carbohydrate, your body burns 25 calories just to digest the carbohydrate. When you eat 100 calories of fat, your body burns three calories to process it.

Exercise. Exercise is the necessary to healthful fat loss. Exercise doesn't only mean going to the gym. Find a few regular activities that you enjoy, that fit your lifestyle, which you can build into your ordinary day.

Reclaim Built-In Exercise (Fitness as a Lifestyle). Many activities of daily living are built-in exercise. (Refer to Chapter 8.) Exercising in a gym is a substitute for having an active lifestyle. Even if you prefer to drive to a health club, and take the elevator to an exercise class, reclaim healthful movement the rest of the day, instead of going back to injurious positioning when lifting, walking, reaching, bending, and sitting.

Lift Weights. Weightlifting to keep bones and muscles strong is important to health. Remember that lifting your body weight is lifting weights. Bend properly. Get up from your chair often, and see if you can easily get up without your hands, then back down. Get up and down from the floor.

Have Fun. Be active in real life with things you love to do. Be creative.

Be Happy. Be happy. Why not?

- Eat less. Try more vegetables. Fruit makes good desserts.
- Try heavier, low-calorie foods. They fill you more than physically lighter, higher calorie foods.
- Get more exercise.
- Find all the things that you can do in a day to be more active without going to a gym.
- Use your brain. Don't get sucked in by hype and sales.
- Lift weights. Weight lifting strengthens bones and muscles. Lift children (safely). Use your body weight for weight lifting by bending properly.
- Stand up straight. It burns more calories than slouching and prevents common body aches.
- Get fun activity every day. Do things you used to love. Enjoy being active.
- Be happy. It's healthy.

Start Lifestyle Nutrition Mindset

The following tips will get you started with developing a lifestyle nutrition mindset. Refer to the healthy-nutrition chapters in Part II for additional recommendations.

- Everyone benefits by good examples and support. Be a support system to someone else. Start children early on knowing that cookies, ice cream, candy, and cake are not healthful food, and are not synonymous with love, their birthday, holidays, or parties. Teaching them to avoid bad habits is a better love. You can start them on the habit of not routinely putting harmful things in their body. Remember that automobile coolant tastes sweet, and animals and babies who find and drink it can be seriously harmed, even killed. It tastes sweet, but it is not good for you. You can teach a similar concept about sweet tasting junk food, soda, and harmful drugs to children and yourself. If you don't believe that junk food is unnecessary and unhealthful, that is fine. Make sure to understand that increased body weight and risk of disease is no longer a mystery to ascribe to genetics or metabolism.

- Don't smoke, drink soda (diet soda is also unhealthful) eat junk food (even if it has marketing words like "organic" on the label), or undo the health benefits of fruit and vegetables by adding cream, sugar, and cornstarch (refer to Part II).
- Are you feeding your body more when it doesn't need it while starving your mind and your spirit? Develop beautiful activities that fill you.
- Add up all the money you no longer will spend on cigarettes, fast food, and junk food, which take a healthy body and give it health problems. Add the money for prescriptions and treatments for the pain and jitters you were causing yourself with the bad habits. With all you save, you can feed a village and still take a vacation.

Some Lifestyle Exercises

Light Exercise:	Moderate Exercise:	Vigorous Exercise:
Less than 200 calories an hour	250 to 450 calories an hour	More than 450 calories an hour
Walking or strolling around 2 miles per hour	Fast walking around 3 to 4 miles per hour	Fast walking up a hill, or with a load
Golfing with a cart	Golfing carrying clubs	Racquet sports
Home care, like vacuuming	House cleaning	Moving furniture
Mowing the lawn with a riding mower	Mowing the lawn with a power mower	Mowing the lawn with a push mower

Your Fit Life

Instead of thinking you have to lose weight first to try things, or fix knee or back pain first before you can exercise, use healthful positioning to stop joint pain as described throughout this book. You may find that you can exercise for the first time without injury. Make daily life active and fun, and you never have to go to a gym if you don't want to. Don't spend on pills and gadgets to have a healthy, fitter life. Find activities you like to do anyway, and make them a part of your daily life. Find things that you like, or used to like, that would make your life better if added back into your day. Sit down and plan them. Then, get up and do them. Enjoy.

Part II

NUTRITION

How strange a creature is man, who will at times go to such extremes to preserve his life, only to shorten it at the dinner table.

– William H. Gordon

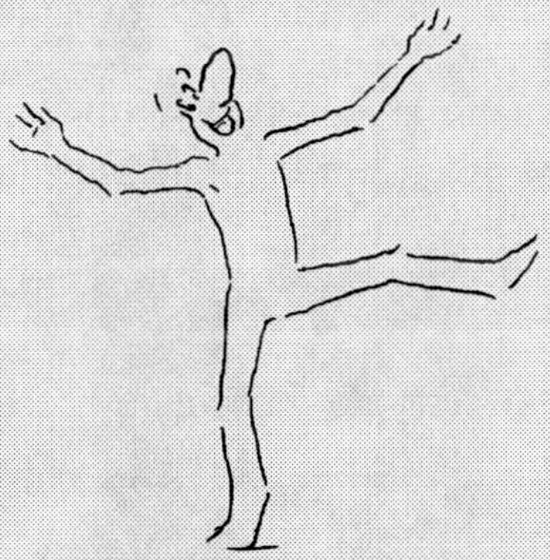

14

Nutrition Myths

You believe easily that which you hope for earnestly.

—Terence (Greek-born Roman playwright, second century B.C.E.)

Nothing is so firmly believed as that which we least know.

—Michel de Montaigne (16th-century French essayist)

If you heard of a nutrient that your body requires to transmit nervous-system signals, manufacture sex hormones, and is a precursor of the bile that handles ingested fats, would you want lots of it in your blood stream?

It's cholesterol.

Would you pay a lot for a substance your brain can't do without to process decisions and retain memory?

It's sugar.

Do you avoid a common practice using a chemical that constricts brain blood vessels, reducing cerebral blood flow?

It's breathing oxygen.

Descriptions in isolation can mislead, which is how nutrition myths begin. Ordinary food items become income producers to the slick packager. Nutrition myths are no exception. This chapter explores just a few.

The "Isolated Aspect" Myth

Oxygen, in high concentrations, is toxic to every life form on the planet. If you breathe high levels for long periods, you will suffer ill effects. You don't avoid breathing oxygen in the air around you. You use it for other characteristics in its favor, like staying alive. In similar ways, vitamin and food-supplement advertisements divert your focus to and from isolated aspects of their product. They concentrate on problems occurring only from excesses or deficiencies, or on only one effect of the substance, usually exaggerated.

Claims

- A powdered bodybuilding supplement for weight lifters and athletes advertises that it is insulinogenic. The suffix "-gen" comes from a Greek word meaning "producing." In other words, it encourages insulin production. The advertising states that insulin is instrumental in getting the building blocks of protein into your muscle cells, and since this product is insulinogenic, it therefore builds muscle. Wouldn't that be great?
- Another product uses the opposite property of insulin for marketing. A popular high-protein diet promotes the idea that you must avoid non-protein foods because they stimulate insulin. Since another property of insulin is to promote fat storage, these people say to eat only high-protein, non-insulin-stimulating foods, to be in a fat-burning "zone."

Critical Reading

- Insulin has several functions. It transports amino acids into your cells for protein synthesis. It also activates enzymes, which stimulate fat cells to synthesize and store fat. That process is part of how you digest food. The function of insulin to store fat is left out of advertising for insulinogenic muscle-building supplements. They tell you only about storing protein. The function of insulin to help store protein is left out of promotions for fad diets that limit carbohydrate.
- Two opposite, seriously unhealthful practices are centered around isolated beliefs about insulin. Certain body-builders illegally inject insulin trying to build muscle and create a look of thinner skin because they believe insulin will build muscle. At the same time, a growing subpopulation of people with insulin-dependent diabetes skip or reduce prescribed injected amounts, believing it will reduce body fat, a practice popularly called "diabulemia."

- Almost all food is insulinogenic. Every time food enters the non-diabetic bloodstream, it stimulates insulin release. Nothing is particularly special about a specific "insulinogenic" muscle-building product. It is food.
- Claims for high-protein diets are misleading and potentially unhealthy. High-protein diets (and other diets) "work" to produce weight loss when they are low-calorie, not because of any insulin-stimulating or suppressing quality.
- Some diets are centered around the insulin-producing quality of food. They rate foods according to their ability to raise blood sugar, called the glycemic index. They avoid high-index foods and stress lower index foods. It is an important and healthful practice to limit junk fat and sugar and eating too much of any food that raises blood sugar and insulin levels frequently. In a few cases, helpful foods are restricted for having a high index, such as carrots, while milk products produce high insulin responses even with a low glycemic index. In general, it is unhealthy to have high and continual insulin responses from constant eating of any food, particularly junk fat and sugar. Use common sense and healthful control to eat smaller portions of more healthful food. Don't rely on artificial products or unhealthful practices, or get bogged down counting numbers and grams and zones. Eat less. Relax.

The "More The Merrier" Myth

Most of your brain is water. Almost no one would expect to get more brain by drinking more water. (I say "almost no one" with great optimism.) If you eat an extra amount of something, your body doesn't always use it to do what you hope. The most flagrant examples involve protein and calcium supplements.

By themselves, protein and calcium won't grow muscles or strengthen bones. Your body continually "turns over" the protein in muscle fibers, calcium in bone cells, and fat in fat cells. It uses some for body function, recycles some, and takes small amounts of incoming material from food for rebuilding. The constant breakdown and resynthesis is called modeling. Modeling doesn't grab extra protein or calcium and add it on to you. It takes what it needs to keep you the same as before and discards the rest, unless you give your body a reason to make you different than before. That reason is resistance exercise, which includes weight lifting and pushing and pulling against resistance. Resistance exercise will make your body add more protein to your muscles, and calcium to your bones. By itself, eating a food will not. For more on calcium and your bones, see Chapter 22.

Given normal functions of vitamins in your body, a common assumption is that taking more vitamins must do more of that process. The B vitamins, for example, work as coenzymes. Coenzymes help an enzyme do its enzyme job. The enzyme/coenzyme interdependence is like a lock-and-key relationship. Only one key fits one companion lock. Taking more of a vitamin when your body is not making more of the corresponding enzyme will have no effect; from three wheels you can still make only one bicycle. Taking the companion enzyme in pill form will not help because eating the pills destroys the enzymes, as described in the "No Digestion" myth.

A precursor of bile, a fluid that handles fat digestion, is cholesterol. However, if you eat more cholesterol, your body will still not digest more fat. Your body uses what cholesterol it needs and dumps the rest back into circulation. Too much cholesterol can create unhealthy effects.

The "More Can't Hurt" Myth

Claim

- Protein builds muscles; therefore, more protein must build more muscle, and after all, more can't hurt.

Critical Reading

- Extra protein doesn't build extra muscle unless plenty of resistance exercise tells your body that the muscle is needed.
- Even then, your body can use only so much, regardless of how much you exercise.
- Past that amount, extra protein can be harmful.

Problems of Too Much Protein. Extra protein is not stored; it goes several routes. One is through your excretory system, taking water with it to produce urea. With excessive protein intake, you can dehydrate yourself a bit. Another exit route for excess protein is conversion to fat, which can't be turned back to protein later. Another problem with too much protein is that it increases calcium loss through the urine. In other words, eating too much protein makes you "pee" out calcium. Epidemiologic studies point to excess protein, particularly animal protein, as contributing to osteoporosis.

What about high-protein diets that claim you need extra protein to get you into a fat-burning zone? It turns out that if you follow their meal plans, the meals are low-calorie, and for that reason, you lose weight. It does not have anything to do with extra protein, or insulin, or zones. Problems occur because the meals are also low-complex carbohydrate meaning decreased intake of important nutritional components needed for health. You need energy to carry out daily activities, and to exercise for weight loss and health. Chapter 18 covers how much protein you may need.

Problems of Too Much Iron. A high blood-iron level is also frequently thought to be a good thing. It is not always true. Iron is essential to your health in several roles. Iron is also involved in certain harmful reactions in your body, involving special molecules called free radicals. (More on free radicals can be found in the glossary, and the following sections on the "No Digestion" myth and "Reverse Reasoning" myth.) Free radicals can sometimes be destructive in your body, which is their job. People with high iron levels have been found to develop high rates of heart disease, possibly from high amounts of free radicals generated through too much iron.

Although women are frequently labeled as at a disadvantage for tendency to lower iron levels than men, it seems that may be an advantage. Populations with lower-than-average iron levels have been found to have lower-than-average incidence of heart disease. Iron supplements are also constipating. It is now a common recommendation that people should not supplement iron without high need and physician supervision.

Problems of Too Much Water. Even drinking water can be overdone. Extreme prolonged exercise in the heat with no food or fluid replacement other than large amounts of water, or drinking extreme quantities of plain water, for example in a hazing ritual, can cause a problem called water intoxication. You dilute yourself too much. Seizures, even deaths have resulted.

More is not always better. Philosopher Allen Ross Anderson capsulized maximalist thinking: "We should have our minds open, but not so open that our brains fall out."

The "No Digestion" Myth

More is not always better. Sometimes, more becomes nothing at all. Some health-food stores sell pills containing enzymes. The claims are that your body needs these enzymes for various functions, so if you eat a supply of these enzymes in their pills, you will get more of the benefits. This claim does not work.

Enzymes do not pass into your bloodstream after eating them. They cannot pass through your intestinal wall except by breaking down into constituent parts. This process destroys them as enzymes.

Broken-down enzymes will not automatically reassemble on the other side of your intestine, so eating enzymes will not raise your body levels of enzymes. Your body makes all the enzymes you need out of the ordinary food you eat. Eating enzymes by themselves, except those that aid digestion (like lactase to digest dairy products), is useless and expensive.

An interesting example is superoxide dismutase (SOD). SOD is an enzyme. It is one of several antioxidants your body makes to counter effects of free radicals. Free radicals have an unpaired electron, so they go around trying to get another electron by taking one from other molecules in your body. Free radicals particularly target fatty acids and proteins, harming them in the process of stealing their electrons. Then, the fatty acids and proteins become free radicals themselves, and go around grabbing electrons from other molecules, like a destructive game of tag. Your body has several built-in systems for removing radicals, but can get overwhelmed by too many free radicals, which can then go unchecked in their damage.

Eating SOD in pill form won't protect against free-radical damage or other oxidative stress in your body. If eaten, SOD, like any other enzyme, is destroyed in your intestine by digestion.

As is often the case with sham cures offered in pill form, research studies seem to back up the claims. Studies do show that SOD reduces free-radical formation. None of these studies involved eating the SOD, but injecting it into laboratory animals under specific conditions. More on free radicals, oxygen toxicity, and antioxidants can be found in the "Reverse Reasoning" myth.

The "Stimulants and Sugar Water Are Health Food" Myth

Sales are high of sports products advertised as "giving energy." Technically, the potential energy in food is measured in units called calories. "High-energy snack" is a euphemism for "high-calorie food" or, in other words, "fattening food." Even though fat is stored energy, an obese person will not automatically be energetic. An increasing number of sports and "health food" contains stimulants such as caffeine, ginseng, ma huang, or other substances.

Sugar helps delay fatigue if used during long endurance events where you can't stop to eat. For regular use, simple sugar is not health food, even though sold in "energy" and sports food. Simple sugars raise insulin levels, which drop soon after. Constant insulin production and circulation is not healthy. Complex carbohydrate mixed with a small amount of protein is often a better choice for nutrition for energy. You can do this with a piece of fruit and some raw nuts, like almonds or walnuts. For healthy energy, instead of relying on special energy foods, get good nutrition, keep your emotional health strong through practice (Chapter 2), and get regular exercise. (Refer to Chapter 17 on ergogenic aids.)

The "Need It Now" Myth

Some sport-food advertising implies that since vitamins and minerals are removed from your system by sporting activities, that you need their specific foods that have those nutrients. General recreational exercise does not sufficiently deplete any nutrients to affect athletic ability or health. For that reason, after a one-hour hike or game of tennis, you don't need to replace specific vitamins or minerals immediately. Your next good meal will cover you. It is unnecessary to take extra vitamins or minerals ahead of time to offset any loss predicted during your exercise. You don't lose enough to affect performance or fatigue level. Regular healthy eating and hydration assures you don't start your day in an already depleted state. Moreover, your daily requirements of most nutrients typically balance out over days. Minute-to-minute deficits don't matter as much.

Claim

- A common claim is that you are in danger of B12 deficiency if you don't eat red meat every day, or often, to replenish amounts you use each day.

Critical Reading

- Vitamin B12 is stored in your liver in enormous quantities, sufficient for years.

The "Reverse Reasoning" Myth

In this myth, if a deficit causes a weakness, then a surplus will bring strength. However, just as the right glasses prescription corrects vision, getting too strong a correction will not make you see better yet.

Vitamin E is a nutritional example. In experiments with rats years ago, researchers removed all Vitamin E from the rats' food. The rats became bald and sterile. Restoring Vitamin E restored the rats' hair and fertility. Marketing and advertising people used those results to launch campaigns to sell Vitamin E with claims of giving you hair and virility. Vitamin E does not do that for humans with adequate nutrition. (But bald, sterile rats, take note.)

Claims

- Vitamin A is often promoted as: "Needed for good night vision."
- High-calorie foods are often labeled as: "Giving you energy."
- Special powdered mixtures are advertised as: "Providing all the nutrients contained in healthy spinal discs," or containing "All the nutrients crucial to healthy hair."
- Free radicals are known to be involved in the various damage to the body caused by their oxidative nature. Vitamins C and E are known antioxidant agents against the oxidative free-radical activity. People often take extra Vitamins C and E on the presumption that it will reduce their risk of the various damaging effects of free radicals.

Critical Reading

- Vitamin A deficiency reduces ability to see in dim light. No amount of carrots or vitamin supplements will make adequately nourished eyes see better.
- Calorie deficiency makes you tired. Eating extra calories will not make you energetic. It will make you fat.
- Potions containing the nutrients or component substances of your back and hair don't fix your bad back or grow hair. They are regular food. Countless products line the shelves, stating they are for skin, nerves, strength, fingernails, or whatever—all just glamorized food. Your body needs specific nutrients to do its job, but eating more of them won't increase the processes.
- Vitamin E is lipid (fat) soluble and protects cell membranes, which have a major lipid component. Vitamin C is a water-soluble antioxidant, having protective effects in blood and the fluid inside and outside of cells. Vitamins E and C work together in their free radical inactivation work. The way Vitamin E inactivates radicals is to accept the extra electron that makes the molecules radical and reactive. When Vitamin E takes that extra electron, it becomes radical itself. Vitamin C then takes the extra electron from E to restore Vitamin E. Vitamin C is special in that it can accept this extra burden without injury to itself or surrounding molecules.

  You need a minimum amount of these vitamins to do their jobs. It is true that many people, particularly those on a typical meat-eating Western diet, may not get enough Vitamins E and C, and many other disease fighting anti-oxidants which are found in vegetables and fruits. Taking more of Vitamins E and C than you need has not been shown to increase their usual effects on radicals in the body. If you are vitamin deficient, they may help, but not if you are vitamin sufficient. Taking too much in isolated vitamin supplements may be injurious.

  Free radicals are not all bad. Some perform critical functions in your body, such as muscle contraction and immune response. You may not want to push your resting levels down, even if it were possible to do so by eating antioxidants. If you got rid of the radicals stored in special cells in your body that fight infection, you would be at risk of catastrophic infections.

The "I Can Eat Anything I Want as Long as It Is Low-Fat (or Low-Carbohydrate)" Myth

Are you eating low-fat or low-carbohydrate diets and still not losing weight? Despite the claims about needing to eat fat for "zones" or fat burning, or that carbohydrates make you fat, it is the number of calories you eat of those "low-fat" foods compared to how much your lifestyle burns the calories. Low-fat cakes, cookies, and candies can easily be high-calorie and full of sugar.

A sack of sugar is nonfat, and a 1,000-calorie block of fat is sugar-free. Keep your common sense about you. Several hundred extra calories a day of "non-fat" or "low-carbohydrate food" will store as fat.

The "I Eat Right" Myth

An average person sits down to an evening meal of steak or burgers; potato mashed with butter, salt, and milk; coffee with cream and sugar; and a small side of buttered vegetables; then has ice cream and/or cake for dessert. A good dinner of protein for muscles, calcium for bones, and energy for exercise? No. The U.S. Department of Agriculture recently surveyed American dietary habits. The findings? Many Americans who think they eat healthy don't at all. The sample dinner is typical of three times too much fat, saturated fat, cholesterol, and salt; double the needed protein; too much simple sugar; insufficient fiber, vitamins, or complex carbohydrates; and not enough water. This kind of eating is increasingly associated with heart and vascular disease, vitamin deficiency, dehydration, calcium loss, high blood pressure, and some cancers.

The "Healthy Eating Is Awful" Myth

Why should low-fat, vegetable-based meals be called drastic, while cardiac-bypass surgery, stroke, and colon cancer are considered normal? It is good news, not bad. Good meals need no secret energy foods and no special supplements. They can be good tasting and healthy in many ways and are cheaper than special health and sports foods. Good things to eat, and how to prepare them quickly, inexpensively is covered in Chapter 18.

15

Healthy Digestion

Kitchen physic is the best physic.

—Jonathan Swift

Gas and Mystery Bloating

Modern commercial sports and "health" products commonly contain products that produce a swollen, uncomfortable gastrointestinal tract. Sometimes, without knowing the cause stems from products used, concern of disease may lead to uncomfortable, time-consuming, and often risky medical testing, unhealthful prescription medicine, and occasionally needless surgery.

Dairy. Dairy products—including milk, cheese, yogurt, and protein supplements made with whey—are a common source of gas. Use vegetable protein and calcium sources, which have several healthier characteristics (refer to Chapter 21).

Soy. Protein supplements and sports bars and drinks made with unfermented soy cause much gas. High amounts of unfermented soy are not as healthful as initially thought. The estrogenic effects contribute to estrogen-sensitive problems, from fibroids, breast, and ovarian cysts in women, to migraine in both women and men. Unfermented soy is increasingly recommended to be limited. (For more on soy, refer to Chapter 17.)

Sweeteners. Sweeteners like sorbitol and corn syrup produce painful gas. They are found in drinks, candies, many protein supplements, "health" foods, and dietetic foods.

Wheat Gluten. People with sensitivity to wheat protein, a condition called celiac, or sprue, have painful gastrointestinal symptoms after eating wheat and related products. Effects also extend to mood, bones, and joints. Celiac is an often overlooked contributor to osteoporosis. Glutin sensitivity can be determined by blood testing. Chapter 22 provides more information on celiac.

What Does Fiber Do?

Soluble fiber helps digestion and has been found to lower high blood cholesterol (refer to Chapter 28). Insoluble fiber reduces the risk of colon disease, hemorrhoids, and overeating, and keeps digestion regular and moving more quickly and easily. Insoluble fiber is named because it doesn't dissolve in water. Good amounts of insoluble fiber are found in brown rice, seeds, carrots, cucumbers, zucchini, bulgur, whole-grain, bran, celery, and tomatoes. The National Academy of Sciences has recommended phasing out the terms "soluble" and "insoluble." Many fruits and vegetables have both types of fiber.

Concerns about "blocking" digestion through eating more fiber can be addressed by looking at the rest of your eating patterns for unhealthy foods that slow digestion, getting enough water, getting fiber from food, not supplements, and getting regular exercise that moves the legs and whole body, such as most aerobic-system exercise. Exercise is highly important in keeping digestion comfortable and moving.

Diet, Exercise, and Colon Cancer

A prospective study published in the Journal of the American Medical Association in 2007 found that colorectal cancer survival after initial cancer treatment depended greatly on dietary habits. Participants who are more red and processed meats, sweets, and refined grains were more likely to have a recurrence or die. Those participants who ate more fruit, vegetables, whole grains, and less red and processed meats and refined foods were less likely to have a recurrence and more likely to survive. Researchers in India, found that a vegetarian diet started early in life was associated with reduced risk of colorectal cancer. Colorectal cancer risk was inversely related to both vegetarian diet and body mass index. The term "inversely related" means that the higher one factor is, the less high or likely the other. Body mass index is a measure of how much you weigh relative to how tall you are (refer to Chapter 25).

Regular exercise lowers incidence of colon cancer in both men and women. Regular moderate exercise increases survival rate of colon-cancer patients. Exercise is also found to reduce risk of new tumors in people who survive cancer the first time.

Why Stomach Acid?

Needed for Digestion. You need stomach acid for food digestion. Pain, reflux, and constant burping are often a sign of low acid, not high acid. Taking antacid medicines is often the opposite of what is needed to stop these symptoms

Fights Gastrointestinal Germs. Stomach acid is necessary to kill unhealthy germs and food-borne infection. Low stomach acid allows infectious organisms to grow in your system. Taking acid-reducing medicines is a known risk factor for traveler's diarrhea and other gastrointestinal illnesses.

Fights Ulcer-Producing Bacteria. You need enough stomach acid to kill the bacteria associated with ulcers. Although acid suppression is commonly used to treat ulcers, the resulting lack of stomach acid encourages overcolonization of the bacteria *Helicobacter pylori*. *H. pylori* is not all bad, and has important functions in your system. However, in some circumstances, it is associated with promoting ulcers. Using acid suppression with *H. pylori* colonization present has been linked in some studies with development of atrophic gastritis, one step in the progression to gastric cancer.

Antibiotics Hurt Good Bugs in Your Gastrointestinal Tract

Antibiotics reduce the gastrointestinal tract's "good bugs" along with the bad. The good bugs manufacture several compounds that you need for health and good nutrition. Without the beneficial flora that normally live in your GI tract, normal nutritional and disease-fighting products in your body are not made.

An example is antibiotic-associated *Clostridium difficile* (*C. difficile*) colitis, an infection of the colon that occurs primarily among patients exposed to antibiotics. More than three million *C. difficile* infections occur in hospitals in the U.S. each year. It is estimated that more than 20,000 *C. difficile* infections occur each year in the U.S. outside the hospital.

Time-Honored Food as Medicine

One effective remedy to stop gastrointestinal illness and pain, historically used in many societies, is eating fermented food. The use of "probiotics," which are beneficial bacteria and yeasts, dates back thousands of years. People in ancient civilizations, from Mongolian nomads to Babylonian royalty, drank soured milk, and Asiatics ate fermented beans and vegetables. Russian and Mongolian military troops campaigning across vast distances ate sauerkraut, which is fermented cabbage, to prevent scurvy and diarrhea. Sauerkraut is a version of kimchi, Korean fermented cabbage, that was brought to the Teutonics with the Mongols and other wandering tribesmen who had contact with the Far East. Modern major studies support that probiotics prevent and reduce duration of acute diarrhea in adults and children.

Cabbage may be an accepted antibacterial for stomach ulcers, now known associated with the gastrointestinal bacteria *Helicobacter pylori*. Clinical trials indicate that some types of probiotics also help control several diseases, such as ulcerative colitis, reflux, and irritable bowel.

Fermented vegetables like kimchi are nutritious in themselves, plus produce nutrients that beneficial lactobacteria need to thrive and produce antibacterial action. Two top foods for promoting beneficial bacteria and inhibiting unhealthy bacteria are cabbage and onions. Broccoli sprouts have been found to specifically reduce *Helicobacter pylori*. Seasoning food with raw crushed garlic and fresh ginger root may inhibit strains of *Helicobacter*, *E. coli*, *Staphylococcus*, and *Streptococcus*, without harming beneficial digestive bacteria.

Several spices have bacteria-inhibiting properties: garlic, allspice, and oregano have been found to have action against "bad" bacteria, followed by thyme, cinnamon, tarragon, and cumin. Capsicum, such as chilies and other hot peppers, have moderate antimicrobial action. White and black pepper, ginger, anise seed, celery seed, and lemon and lime juice follow in effectiveness. Researchers at the University of Kansas found garlic, cloves, cinnamon, oregano, and sage kill *E. coli*. Research in Mexico has found the spice oregano to be more effective than prescription drugs against Giardia.

Studies show that extracts of cocoa (not candy chocolate, but the cocoa it is made from) can prevent the *Helicobacter pylori* associated with stomach ulcers, and disease-causing strains of E. coli.

In addition to antibacterial properties, many foods have been long used against fungal and worm infestations. The World Health Organization recommends crushed garlic, curry, and cloves for their specific anti-worm properties, confirmed in studies.

In Russia, a lacto-fermented beverage called *kvass* has long been made from old rye bread. It tastes like beer, but it is not alcoholic and can be purchased in modern supermarkets packaged like soda. *Kvass* was used by peasants, military, and even the Czars. Another kvass made from beets was made during war times and taken during travel to protect against infections. Ancient Iraqis and Egyptians made similar drinks from bread. Fungus and yeast-fermented teas have long been used throughout Russia, China, Japan, Poland, Bulgaria, Germany, and Southeast Asia (called *chainyi grib* in Russia, *kombucha* in Asia, and elsewhere as *teeschwamm* or *teewass*, *wunderpilz*, *cajnij*, *fungus japonicus*, and *hongo*, which means, simply, "mushroom.") The drinks are not made of mushrooms, but the fermenting culture forms a mushroom-like mass.

Australian aborigines lacto-fermented grains and legumes to make a bubbly, sour drink that modern Australians call "wholegrain." South American Native Indians fermented several drinks they say prevent digestive problems including diarrhea. In Africa, lacto-fermented *munkoyo* was made from millet or sorghum (sorghum beer) and given to babies to stop infection and diarrhea. Missionaries (and others) suppressed *munkoyo* in favor of commercial soft drinks.

What to Do—Simple and Inexpensive Food

For serious cases of gastrointestinal trouble, seek medical attention to determine what is wrong. Most of the time, several things may lessen, prevent, and alleviate ordinary discomfort.

Instead of antacids for stomach pain, it is healthier and often as effective or more effective to eat cabbage and fresh sauerkraut, and drink cabbage juice, or apple cider vinegar diluted in a little water. Squeeze lemons and limes on fruit and vegetables, and add to drinks and blender shakes. Add balsamic vinegar to salads. Soothe an uncomfortable stomach with fresh ginger. For gas, season food with cardamom, coriander, fennel, or cumin, or just chew the seeds. For traveler's diarrhea, try kimchi, tempeh, vinegar water, and sauerkraut. Avoid overuse of antibiotics. Instead of soda, try kvass.

Eat fermented vegetables like fresh pickle (fermented, not vinegar cucumbers), sauerkraut (fermented cabbage), fermented chutney, tempeh, oncham, and kimchi. Season with spices like garlic and curry. Look for fermented food with live cultures. Many products kill the cultures through heating, processing, and packaging. Use fresh-made sauerkraut, not pasteurized or canned. The packaging process deliberately removes helpful nutrients and living cultures created through fermentation so that the lids don't blow off. There are "quick" sauerkrauts made with vinegar. The vinegar is fermented, but the cabbage isn't. To get real fermented cabbage, check the label for sauerkraut made from cabbage, water, spices, and salt. Although probiotics are often packaged in expensive and overconcentrated supplements, you can have the benefits from inexpensive, simple, normal food.

What to Do—Simple and Inexpensive Containers

An interesting problem is becoming known among group camping expeditions. Traveler's diarrhea is turning out to be frequently a result of the dishwashing techniques in hiking camps and expedition kitchens. It has become a point of debate in hiking groups, how much bleach to use to disinfect camp dishes, flatware, and pots. Some say the bleach is not healthy for the streams where the dishwater is discarded. Others say bleach needs to be used to stop germs from spreading, for camper gastrointestinal health.

One solution is not to use dishes. Wrap food in leaves like banana, spinach, grape leaves, chards, and other greens for cooking, and to use for sturdy plates and napkins. The leaves pack lighter and flatter than dishes, with no washing needed. Make pronged vegetable roasters from long, narrow stems and branches. Cut lengths into simple spoons, spatulas, and chopsticks. Return them to the earth when finished. Don't destroy living trees, and keep your impact low. It is healthier for you and the camping areas.

Exercise for Good Digestion

Exercising right after eating delays stomach emptying. Eating large, fatty meals right before exercise seems to be related to upset stomach and decreased ability during exercise. Regular exercise speeds small and large intestine activity, helping move chronic slow digestion. Stay hydrated to help prevent nausea from dehydration during hard exercise.

Medicines and Stomach Pain

Several commonly prescribed medicines, for example, drugs for anxiety, blood pressure, and even gastrointestinal illness, are known to cause upset stomach. Common prescriptions for joint and muscle pain can lead to serious stomach erosions. Further prescriptions to reduce acid production or accumulation may be taken trying to counter this problem. These medicines reduce calcium absorption and are known to increase bone fracture and osteoporosis risk. Use the information throughout this book to stop the common causes of many conditions to avoid the need for medicines. Medicines often do not address the cause and cause more problems of their own in an unhealthful and expensive cascade of problems.

Simple Good Digestion

Get exercise, and eat fruit and vegetables for fiber, and a sensible amount of fermented food. Real food can work more effectively, more quickly and without the health problems caused by pills and supplements. Choose good food for a simpler life and better health.

Instead of Antacids for Burping and Digestive Upset

- Drink a little apple cider vinegar in water, and sprinkle balsamic vinegar, wine vinegar, or other vinegar that you prefer in your food.
- Clinical trials indicate that the "good" yeasts and bacteria called probiotics in fermented food like real fermented sauerkraut and kimchi help control diseases, such as reflux, ulcerative colitis, and irritable bowel.
- Cabbage has been found in studies to be an effective antibacterial for stomach ulcers associated with *Helicobacter pylori*.
- Use ginger root to sooth stomach pain, rather than medicines.

Stopping and Relieving Gas

- Stop eating dairy, unfermented soy, and sweeteners like sorbitol and corn syrup.
- Season food with cardamom, coriander, fennel, or cumin.
- Do exercise that moves the legs to help mobilize digestion.

Stopping Bad G.I. Bugs

- For traveler's diarrhea, try kimchi, tempeh, vinegar, and sauerkraut.
- Broccoli sprouts have been found to specifically control *H. pylori*.
- It is established in scientific studies in standard Western medicine that several spices have bacteria-inhibiting properties. Seasoning food with raw crushed garlic, onions, and fresh ginger root may inhibit strains of *Helicobacter*, *E. coli*, *Staphylococcus*, and *Streptococcus*, without harming beneficial digestive bacteria.
- Garlic, allspice, and oregano have been found to have action against "bad" bacteria, followed by thyme, cinnamon, tarragon, and cumin.
- Capsicum, such as chilies and other hot peppers, have moderate antimicrobial action. White and black pepper, ginger, anise seed, celery seed, and lemon and lime juice follow.
- Researchers at the University of Kansas found garlic, cloves, cinnamon, oregano, and sage kill *E. coli*.

16

Sports Drinks

The greatest mistake a man can make is to sacrifice health for any other advantage.

—Arthur Schopenhauer

Health food makes me sick.

—Calvin Trillin

Dehydration reduces your capacity for exercise and your tolerance to heat. Various advertisements for commercial sports drinks claim they prevent dehydration better than water. Is that so? Sports-drink ads may state they replace electrolytes. What are electrolytes, and why and when do you need them? What else may be in these drinks? Are some of these drinks even healthful?

What Are Sports Drinks?

You lose water and salts in normal processes all day. You also burn carbohydrate for energy. You need to replace what you lose. Even though you can normally do so with regular healthful meals, commercial replacement drinks of all kinds have become a multi-billion-dollar industry. Just as worrisome, even if sugar water will extend endurance, it is increasingly recognized as junk food, and not healthful for the long term.

A major 2007 study by the World Cancer Research Fund made 10 recommendations for reducing risk of cancer, including getting exercise every day and drinking water rather than sugary drinks. Trendy sports and energy drinks add cost, plastic-bottle litter, and sometimes dyes, synthetic isolated vitamins, and questionable sweeteners. Increasingly, they contain stimulant compounds such as caffeine, guarana, ginseng, ephedra or ma huang, and others, discussed in Chapter 17. Use of stimulating compounds is linked to sleeplessness and increased nervousness and anxiety, and can become habit-forming. Drinks containing dyes, sweeteners, and stimulants are not a healthy choice for adults, and even less so for children and teens. Instead, you can easily make healthy whole-food sports drinks and vitamin water yourself for pennies. Recipes are provided later in this chapter.

You Get Thirsty Two Ways

One way you get thirsty is when you are low on water, called hypovolemic thirst. If you replace only water, your body sees that you have more fluid relative to electrolytes, because you have also lost electrolytes. Your body responds by "peeing" out some water to balance things. You may still be a bit low on water because of this response, even after drinking water, which is why it helps to get water from eating a piece of fruit. You replace a variety of needs through a whole food.

The second way you get thirsty is when you have a high-electrolyte blood content, regardless of your body's total water volume. This condition is called osmotic thirst. It is why salty things make you thirsty, even when you are drinking, and why bars serve salty finger food—to keep you drinking. Small amounts of sodium in electrolyte drinks stimulate your osmotic thirst, and then help you retain what you drink. It is why people drink more of these beverages than plain water, whether they need it or not.

What Is an Electrolyte?

An electrolyte is a substance that, when you dissolve it in liquid, becomes electrically conductive. Why does your body need an electric current? To transmit every signal for all the thousands of functions that nerves control to keep you alive, moving, and thinking, and to maintain an electrical potential across the membrane of every cell in your body, so that the cells can do their jobs.

No current flows through pure water. Dissolving even a trace of electrolytes in water makes water conductive. Electrolytes that are put into a liquid break up into ions. Ions are atoms or molecules with at least one or more fewer electrons than normal, giving them a positive or negative electric charge. Table salt, for example, becomes the positively charged sodium ion, and the negatively charged chloride ion. Both elements are principle ions in your body. In physiology, the ions themselves are called electrolytes. Salt itself is not an electrolyte, but in liquid it becomes the ions that are electrolytes.

> Flashlights run on current passed by electrons through wire. Your body runs on current passed by ions through nerves.

The difference between current in electronic equipment and in your body is that electronic signals race through wire, passed by electrons, at up to half the speed of light, while in your body, nerve signals move through ions, thousands of times more slowly. Current in electronics uses electrons to pass the charge. The electrons themselves don't move far, but pass the charge along from one electron to the next like toppling dominoes. In your body, nerve signals move along dissolved ions. Like electrons, the ions themselves don't move far in the nerve, but propagate the signal by positive and negative ions switching places on either side of the nerve membrane. That exchange makes neighboring positive and negative ions want to switch places too, in a continuing action called the action potential, until the signal is passed along the nerve. Then, the nerve ending uses a transmitter chemical to jump to the next nerve to start the signal traveling again, until the message is delivered.

Why Replace Electrolytes?

Losing some electrolytes through sweat is a good thing, to an extent. If you lost only water, your blood would become too concentrated with electrolytes. Even though you lose electrolytes, your body regulates the loss so you don't lose too much. When you sweat, you lose proportionately more water than minerals, leaving your blood slightly more concentrated than normal, or hypertonic. You can lose a substantial amount of electrolytes with prolonged sweating, creating a need for replacement. Without replacement, your electrolyte and fluid levels fall too low, and your ability to exercise decreases.

With extreme electrolyte loss during long exercise, and only water to drink without food to supply other nutrients, you may abnormally dilute your body fluids and cells, a condition called water intoxication. Effects range from weakness to convulsion and occasionally death. Water intoxication is also called hyponatremia (high-poe-nay-TREE'-me-uh), meaning low sodium in the blood. Cases are usually reported in hikers and distance runners who drink only large amounts of water and eat no food. Occasionally, serious cases of hyponatremia occur in infants swallowing pool water during parent-baby swimming lessons.

Your Body Regulates Electrolytes

You eat varying amounts of electrolytes in your food and drink, and lose varying amounts with exercise and daily activity. Your body ordinarily keeps levels of everything within narrow ranges, no matter how much you vary input and output.

Your body restricts electrolyte loss when your supply is low, and gets rid of excess when you eat or drink too much. When you are inactive, the major exit avenue for surplus electrolytes is urine and feces. When you are active and start sweating more, your body restricts the amount of electrolytes that exit with sweat, and secretes a hormone called aldosterone (al-DOHS'-tur-own) into your bloodstream to help your kidneys retain more sodium.

Most people in Western society eat many times more salt than their bodies require, sometimes in astounding quantities in fast foods, before they even pick up the saltshaker. When you eat more salt than you need, your body retains water to dilute the salt, and aldosterone secretion drops, encouraging your kidneys to excrete the excess.

"Salt-sensitive" people with high blood pressure need to restrict salt to allow them to lose the extra water that salt retains. Their blood pressure increases with salt intake. For the rest of the population, your kidneys tightly regulate your output to get rid of excess electrolytes and water, or hang on to them, depending on what you need at the time.

> Many people in Western society eat far more salt than they need.

When Should You Replace Electrolytes?

Except for extreme endurance activities, you usually eat and drink more than enough electrolytes with your regular meals to keep you going. Ordinary recreational exercise does not deplete electrolytes enough to affect athletic ability or health. For that reason, after a one-hour bout of exercise, you don't ordinarily need to replace electrolytes immediately. It is also unnecessary to take extra electrolytes ahead of time to offset any loss predicted during your short bout of exercise. You don't lose enough to affect performance or cause fatigue. Unless you are in endurance races, or work long hours in hot environments with limited chance to eat and drink fluids other than water, health problems from electrolyte loss are unlikely.

Consider Long-Term Effects

Commercial electrolytes drinks often contain refined sugar and other ingredients that are not healthful over the long term. Salt and sugar drinks can be helpful for specific uses: if a person is dangerously ill from a dehydrating disease such as cholera or dysentery, is suffering dehydration from prolonged vomiting, or has serious heat illness from lack of blood sugar and salt. For healthy athletes who are exercising, replacing blood sugar and salt helps performance and helps prevent heat injury. However, habitually consuming refined sugar is not healthful over the long term. Dyes and stimulants are linked with negative effect on emotional control. Isolated vitamins may also negatively affect health. Simple drinks you can make yourself using ordinary, whole, healthful food are a better choice.

How To Make Your Own Sports Drinks

You don't no need to purchase commercial drinks. You can make your own healthier drink of various kinds, quickly and more cheaply. To make simple vitamin water:

- Put clean water in a blender
- Add a few grapes with the skin and seeds, and blend well.

Grape skins and seeds have been found to contain cancer-fighting and other disease-fighting compounds. Think of the money you save by not buying expensive grape seed oil products.

For a different light flavor, squeeze in fresh lemon. It helps keep the container cleaner, too. If you like tea, put a tea bag in the container. No need for hot water. To make different flavors, try a few strawberries with the green tops, watermelon with the seeds, or some raw sweet red pepper to make a variety of light, vitamin-water drinks.

"Energy drinks," also called loader drinks, are different purpose and recipe from fitness water. They have more carbohydrate content than vitamin water, and sometimes added protein. To get started making your own, throw the following ingredients in a blender or other mixer:

- Clean water
- Peeled banana
- Peeled orange with the seeds
- Some of the well-washed orange peel
- Raw walnuts or other favorite
- Some cooked brown rice left from a meal
- Sweeten with raisins or a prune softened in clean water and optional molasses. Adds many minerals.
- Cinnamon powder to level blood sugar

Considerations for Sports Drinks

- You need to replace lost water and nutrients if you do endurance events lasting more than an hour or so, like marathons and triathlons.
- Consuming some food and water helps if you exercise in the heat for long periods.
- You do not need commercial or special sports-drink products. You can make your own from ordinary food and water.
- Be aware that commercial drinks promising energy may contain stimulant compounds. Habitual use can produce dependence, emotional change, sleeplessness, and unsafe interactions with common prescription and other drugs. Other common effects include feeling nervous with the consumption of the drinks and unwell without it.

Tips:

- For the day of the event, you can substitute tea for the water.
- Experiment with amounts to get preferred consistency
- If you want a chocolate shake, add a scoop of unsweetened cocoa powder (unsweetened non-alkalized baking cocoa). People with migraine can leave out the cocoa.
- Don't junk it up with milk, sugar, artificial sweeteners, commercial sports powders.
- If you use a juicer, put the solids and pulp back in, or you will be drinking sugar water and throwing away the point and the nutrition.
- Try different fruit—persimmons, mangosteen, pineapple, melon, berries, or your favorite. Raw red beets are an overlooked sweet fitness food good in shakes.
- For flavors, add a small slice of unpeeled ginger root or washed mint leaves.
- Experiment, and have fun.

Healthier Containers

Commercially bottled fitness water and drinks may not be healthful, from the drink inside to the container they come in. Plastic containers may leach chemicals into the drink they hold, and the bottling, transport, and disposal all seriously weaken environmental fitness—and ultimately your own. The plastic water bottle manufacturing process requires 1.5 million barrels of crude oil a year. Bottling and shipping water produced more than 2.5 million tons of carbon dioxide in 2006.

When you carry your homemade fitness drinks and water with you, use safe, non-plastic bottles. Instead of spending money on bottled water, get a water filter for your tap water. Research demonstrates that the water supply increasingly contains medical drugs excreted by the users and other chemicals that constitute a "body burden" of compounds with potential health effects.

Healthier Sports and Energy Drink Choices

Your health benefits from good hydration. During extended intense exercise, you can replace needed electrolyte, carbohydrate, and protein with ordinary food or simple homemade drinks. Commercial sports drinks are not a magic energy food, and often contain unhealthful ingredients. You can easily make your own healthier sports drinks. Don't worry that you must eat engineered commercial products or you can't win. You can win better in the long run without them.

Why You Get Dehydrated From Drinking Seawater

Sea-going birds, such as penguins, seagulls, petrels, and albatross, can drink seawater. Special glands in their heads excrete excess salt. Humans have no salt-excreting glands, yet you have to get rid of the extra salt in seawater because the amount is just too much for your system. Your blood is not similar in composition to seawater (contrary to popular belief). Your blood is several times more dilute. If your blood were like seawater, you could safely drink seawater, which is not the case. In the process of excreting the excess salt in salt water, the human kidney draws water from the body's supply, a process so dehydrating that if seawater were the only fluid replacement available, you could die of thirst faster by drinking seawater than if you didn't. Human inability to drink seawater for fluid replacement is reflected in Samuel Taylor Coleridge's Rime of the Ancient Mariner: "Water, water everywhere, nor any drop to drink."

17

Ergogenic Aids—Performance-Enhancement Food and Drugs

Fillet of a fenny snake,
In the cauldron boil and bake;
Eye of newt and toe of frog,
Wool of bat and tongue of dog,
Adder's fork and blind-worm's sting,
Lizard's leg and owlet's wing,
For a charm of powerful trouble,
Like a hell-broth boil and bubble.

—Second Witch: Macbeth, Act IV, Scene I

A miracle drug is any drug that will do what the label says it will do.

—Eric Hodgins

The search for a personal edge that you can eat is a common one. Hundreds of years ago, Aztec warriors ate the hearts of fearless enemies, believing it would increase their own bravery. To prepare for battle, the Inca Indians chewed coca leaves, and Berserkers ate muscaria mushrooms, which made them seem and act wild. Norsemen drank the milk of Arctic reindeer in heat. In the Middle Ages, Dervishes whirled longer using coffee. Sigmund Freud used cocaine. Today, South American Indians know chewing coca leaves reduces hunger and fatigue. In the Middle East, *khat* leaves are chewed for similar effect. Betel nuts are chewed in Asia and the South Pacific Islands, and the kola nut in the Sudan. Some people take diet pills, eat protein supplements, use steroids, drink coffee, or try preparations with labels promising everything from muscle growth to energetic hair.

What Is an Ergogenic Aid?

Substances and practices that help physical performance are sometimes called ergogenic aids. An *erg* is a unit of work. The word "energy" contains the erg root and means the ability to do work. The suffix "*-gen*" means "producing" or "generating." Putting them together forms the word "ergogenic" and refers to things used and, not incidentally, believed to enhance physical performance. Not everything claiming to be ergogenic is really ergogenic.

Some ergogenic aids are psychological, such as mental rehearsal, confidence training, and good-luck charms. Some are physical, such as hard exercise, lifting weights, or training at altitude. Nutritional ergogenic aids include an assortment of drugs, supplements, and food concoctions. Some are hokum—many products on the market claiming to be ergogenic have no ergogenic properties. Others work well enough to be banned by athletic associations and Olympic committees. Certain products work, but are unhealthful or addictive.

Why Do People Use Ergogenic Aids?

Would you pay to eat a product called "This Won't Work," or would you prefer "Beautiful Body For Certain"? Many products are sold through clever advertising and false hope. Product names are not required by law to do what they imply, allowing ads to combine suggestive words like *power*, *energy*, *natural*, *super*, *organic*, *health*, and *mega* on their labels. Who could think a vitamin named Ener-B® didn't have anything to do with feeling energetic? Ads targeting the serious bodybuilder market suggest anabolic steroid capability with names incorporating word segments like *ana*, *testo*, and *bolic*, even if they do not have those components. Product promotions may include quotes from flawed studies in obscure or faux journals. The Food and Drug Administration (FDA) does not currently require testing these products for proof of efficacy. An athlete may work and slave, eat low fat, train diligently, but then attribute all gains to a capsule or pill, and go on to promote the product through testimonials.

Another reason people use certain substances is that some of the potions work to various degrees. Cardiac relaxants can improve aim in target shooting. Stimulants boost speed and endurance. Other substances increase muscle mass.

Many stimulant preparations are sold as "natural" and "herbal," which does not mean they are harmless or non-addictive. Cocaine and nicotine, for example, are naturally occurring plant substances. Do not buy stimulants thinking they will have no problems because they are labeled "natural." Herbal medicines are not necessarily safer or more natural than any other pill or medicine. Dependence on Eastern medicine is no different than dependence on Western pills. Check to see if you are relying on products instead of making healthy lifestyle changes. You could have energy, weight loss, and increased physical abilities by exercising more, eating better, and stopping smoking, without spending on dubious pills.

"Natural" and "herbal" do not mean harmless or non-addictive.

Methylxanthene Stimulants

Coffee. "Black as hell, strong as death, sweet as love," according to a Turkish proverb. Few who drink coffee or cola drinks consider themselves drug users. These drinks contain caffeine, the most commonly used stimulant drug in the world. Other people shun caffeine, and instead take "natural" stimulant herbs. Caffeine is no less "natural" than any health food herb. They can all have the same unwanted effects.

The effect of caffeine after eating berries and seeds containing it was probably discovered in the Stone Age. It has been widely used ever since. Caffeine can extend endurance, and it is banned in high concentrations by the International Olympic Committee for that reason. A big rage for caffeine as an ergogenic aid may have begun in 1978 when exercise physiologist David Costil, told *Runner's World* magazine that caffeine could improve marathon times. According to Professor of Medicine Randy Eichner, "This led to long coffee lines at big marathons, followed by long potty lines."

How caffeine helps is still studied and debated. Caffeine is thought to help endurance by directly stimulating your central nervous system, decreasing your perception of effort, helping your body save some fuel called glycogen, and possibly improving your use of fat as fuel. More recently, caffeine is thought to help short-term activity (so brief that your body has no time to use either glycogen or fat) possibly by increasing recruitment of more of your muscle fibers and/or directly increasing their resistance to fatigue. Coffee itself may have antioxidant properties.

Reactions to caffeine vary and may change throughout your lifetime. Effects may be partly genetically based, and partly due to how much you eat with it, time of day, how much you are accustomed to, and other interactions. For most people, nervousness, increased urine production, and heartbeat irregularities begin after one cup, and increase with dosage, with increasing tendency to irregular heart rhythms from caffeine as you get older. Many commercially sold preparations claiming energy effects from herbs contain caffeine or caffeine-like substances.

The body becomes accustomed to regular caffeine intake. Regular drinkers frequently experience withdrawal symptoms of headache, irritability, and weariness as soon as missing even a single expected dose. If you are a coffee drinker, try to keep use low to moderate.

Theobromine. Cocoa, gotukola nut, and several other foodstuffs contain theobromine, among other substances. Theobromine stimulates the nervous system, opens airways, and increases heart rate, but less intensely than caffeine. Theobromine is used in certain medicines and advertised in some supplements promising energy. Eating real unsweetened cocoa is a healthful source of theobromine and several healthful antioxidants and other compounds. Dark chocolate has more theobromine than lighter chocolate, with flavonoids and phenolics, which are plant substances that are good for the heart. Candy and chocolate product manufacturers may use a process called dutching to remove flavonols, polyphenols, and other healthful compounds in cocoa, because of their bitter taste, and often add fat and sugar, which are harmful to the heart and arteries. Instead of buying cocoa made into unhealthful chocolate candy, look for powdered unsweetened, non-alkalized (non-dutched) cocoa or unsweetened baking squares. It can be found easily in the grocery baking section. Add to blender drinks, baking, and desserts. (Refer to recipes in Chapters 18 and 19.) For some people who get a kind of vascular headache called migraine, chocolate may trigger the headache. They do better not to eat chocolate.

Sympathomimetic Stimulants

Part of your nervous system increases heart rate and constricts blood vessels, getting you "ready to go." That part of your nervous system is called the sympathetic nervous system. Substances with properties that mimic your sympathetic nervous system are called sympathomimetic (sim-path-oh-my-MET'-ik). Three examples are amphetamines, cocaine, and ma huang. (Not everything that is a central nervous system stimulant is sympathomimetic, for example, caffeine and nicotine). People use sympathomimetics because they inhibit fatigue and appetite. Overstimulation and addiction are common, resulting in various effects that are not healthy. Many products sold as "health" and energy food have stimulant compounds that have unhealthful, even dangerous effects, especially when combined with other stimulating compounds, coffee, many prescription medicines, cold medicines, and various performance-enhancing substances.

Amphetamines. Amphetamines are addictive stimulants. Amphetamines became popular as "pep pills," athletic enhancers, anti-depressants, and diet pills because they mask tiredness, sadness, and hunger. Amphetamines were given to military forces during World War II to delay fatigue, even mixed with chocolate, called "flier's chocolate" and "tanker's chocolate." A large post-war health epidemic followed. Methamphetamine, or meth, is an amphetamine prone to abuse and addiction. A large population, including young children, has become addicted from wide use in medical prescriptions. Dangerous effects have been dismissed as "side effects."

Amphetamine users may experience abnormally high or irregular heart rates, raised blood pressure, and sometimes mental states resembling paranoid schizophrenia. Abdominal cramps, incoordination, dizziness, dry mouth, nausea, and vomiting may accompany initial use. Some people experience unusual effects on their blood cells. Stimulants like amphetamines, ephedra, and Ritalin® raise risk of heart trouble. Amphetamines constrict the arterioles of the skin (small, end branches of skin arteries), increasing risk of overheating. Deaths in endurance competitions in the heat have been connected to amphetamine use.

Amphetamines usually addict their user physically and psychologically. Abusers can gradually increase their doses from 10 to 1,000 times to retain the initial effects. Withdrawal brings uncomfortable rebound symptoms of hunger and weakness. Users are prone to unhealthful actions to procure more amphetamines to stop the withdrawal pain.

For solving problems in concentration and mood, amphetamines are not a healthy practice. For weight control, diet pills undermine sound nutrition and allow the user to ignore the requirement of exercise in fat reduction, predisposing the user to serious health consequences. Newer diet pills replacing the older amphetamine types still require extreme caution. Moreover, after two to three weeks, diet pills begin losing effectiveness.

What is an effective substitute for amphetamine drugs? Exercise. Exercise increases feelings of energy and happiness, and offsets food calories for weight control.

Cocaine. Cocaine enhances physical performance, with an unhealthy price. Cocaine is sympathomimetic. Your nerve endings release nerve transmission chemicals called catecholamines across a space, called a synapse, to the next nerve ending. After they have done their job to transmit their signal, you have to get the catecholamine back out of the synapse so it doesn't keep signaling and signaling. Several normal mechanisms accomplish that task, including gathering the catecholamine back up into storage areas in the nerve endings, ready for more signaling at another time. Cocaine blocks this re-uptake, prolonging the effects of released catecholamines. For this reason, you get so much signaling with cocaine—lots of it. Signaling in some areas of your brain feels good.

As with other central-nervous-system stimulants, the extra signaling increases heart rate and muscle contraction, allowing more physical work, and making you feel "geared up" to do that work. Signaling to your heart and blood vessels, from the catecholamine called norepinephrine, raises blood pressure and increases abnormal heartbeats. Too much of this signaling to the heart can cause a sudden, sometimes fatal, heart attack. Surviving that situation, the problem with not taking up your catecholamines again for reuse means that you can run out. Running out of your catecholamine stores leads to severe depression (the cocaine crash).

Many health foods and herbal remedies sold as "pick-me-ups," athletic enhancers, and weight-loss aids contain various central nervous system stimulants.

Ma Huang. Ma huang is an herb that has direct nervous-system effects. Many potions sold over the counter claiming energy and weight loss contain ma huang: Hydroxycut®, Yellow Jacket®, Xenadrine®, Optidrene®, EnerGel®, Diet Pep®, and Up Your Gas®. Some have Asian-sounding names to somehow lend authenticity, like Chi Power and Jade Energy. The products contain one or more of the several forms of ephedrine, a stimulant compound that comes from the ephedra plant.

Ma huang is sympathomimetic—it mimics activation of your sympathetic nervous system, mostly by urging your nervous system to release the chemicals noradrenaline and adrenaline from your nerve endings. One effect is to open airways and decrease secretions, so ephedrine is used in allergy and asthma medications. In doses common in over-the-counter "health" and diet products, ma huang affects your body like an amphetamine (to a smaller degree). It can have serious side effects of raised heart rate and blood pressure, erratic heart rhythms, and chest pain, plus any of several nervous system effects like insomnia, tremors, anxiety, or seizures, depending on dose. When mixed with caffeine, cold medicines, alcohol, and certain medicines, it can create seriously unhealthful effects.

An advisory panel of experts convened by the U.S. Food and Drug Administration in 1996 reviewed reports of more than 600 health problems thought to be associated with ephedrine since 1993, including 17 deaths from overstimulation of the heart. The panel generally concluded that the amount of ma huang in products should be far smaller. Investigators from New England Medical Center looked at 926 reports of problems associated with ephedrine. They reported 14 sudden deaths, 13 strokes, two mini-strokes, nine heart attacks, and six cases of rapid heartbeats. Thirty-eight of the people had no history of heart trouble.

Many people take ma huang thinking it is somehow safer or more natural than caffeine, but caffeine is as naturally occurring as ma huang, as is the nicotine in tobacco. All have negative side effects in large doses. Ma huang is advertised as "used medicinally in China for over 5,000 years." That claim doesn't mean it is healthy or safe.

Opium was used medicinally, too. If you think you need stimulant drugs, look at your health habits and determine why you can't function without them. For weight loss or to increase energy, it is safer and quicker to just go out and exercise.

Other Stimulants

Ginseng. Herbal energy potions claiming that they are caffeine-free does not necessarily mean they are free of side effects or are healthy for you. Ginseng is an example. Because of ginseng's stimulant effects, it is popularly used for a variety of health problems and for a general "pick-me-up." Ginseng is used in pills, teas, sodas, candies, and drinks. Ginseng can affect glucose metabolism and raise heart rate and blood pressure. If you overmedicate yourself with ginseng, you can wind up with diarrhea, nervousness, skin rashes, and insomnia. Most symptoms will disappear when use is reduced or discontinued. It doesn't mean ginseng is bad; just that it is not harmless. It has effects, which is why people take it.

Most of the biological effects of ginseng come from ginsenosides. Investigations have found that content varies greatly, with some ginseng preparations containing no ginsenosides at all. Laws do not require uniformity or even labeling to identify content.

As with other stimulant use, take a look at your health habits to find out why you want stimulants. Taking them can produce a vicious cycle of dependence and fatigue without them, and a cycle of being too stimulated to sleep well at night, creating daytime fatigue. Poor eating habits, too much simple sugar, not enough exercise, and too much time spent indoors contribute to general malaise. Don't use stimulants to combat poor habits. Use healthy ways to give you energy. Herb stimulants are drugs the same as any other potions and pills.

Steroids and Steroid Substitutes

Anabolic Steroids. The word "anabolic" means promoting tissue growth. Not all steroids are anabolic. The anti-inflammatories cortisone and prednisone are steroids, and they are not anabolic. They do not stimulate growth. Neither does Vitamin D, another steroid that is not an anabolic steroid.

Anabolic steroids are controlled substances. They are prescription oral and/or injectable drugs that have anabolic and masculinizing or androgenic effects. They are often used to fatten cattle to enhance market price. A large problem of steroid use exists in school-age and older athletes wanting physical gains at any price. A large black market exists for prescription medical and veterinary anabolic steroids. Adverse physical and emotional side effects of anabolic steroids include high blood pressure, elevated "bad" cholesterol (LDL), liver and kidney damage, greater risk of heart and vascular disease, and volatile, aggressive, and recklessly uncontrolled behaviors. Long-term use reduces your own body's production of male hormones. Male genitalia can shrink. Some steroids increase female hormones, causing men's breasts to grow. Users trying to avoid these side effects add use of anti-estrogen drugs, which have their own side effects. Users may not be aware that their personality is changing. Side effects are common and incompatible with physical and emotional health. Don't let your ego get in the way of your health. You can be a bigger, more powerful person by giving the money spent on self-indulgent drug use to the poor and being a role model for honest exercise. Exercise increases your body's production of anabolic hormones without the side effects. Decreases in normal body levels with aging can be offset by healthy fun exercise.

Growth Hormone. Growth hormone is naturally made in the pituitary gland of your brain. It does several things, including stimulating protein to make muscle. Injections of synthetic growth hormone are used by bodybuilders and athletes hoping for strength and size increase and by actors and models hoping to look more muscular and lean. Some cosmetic procedure doctors promote it as a drug against various signs of aging. Growth hormone use is not yet detectable by drug testing. The American College of Sports Medicine (ACSM) strongly advises against supplemental growth hormone for athletic enhancement because of ethical and physical problems.

In children, one function of growth hormone is to stimulate bone lengthening. When the pituitary doesn't produce enough, children don't grow enough, causing one form of dwarfism. Occasionally, with too much hormone, a child can grow to a giant. An adult taking growth hormone after bone maturation will not increase long bone length, so cannot get taller. Instead the forehead, hands, feet, and jaw may elongate.

Human growth hormone for medical use was originally extracted from the human pituitary glands of cadavers and abbreviated "hGH." By 1985, concerns about transmitting incurable fatal brain diseases like Creutzfeldt-Jakob Disease led to replacing pituitary-derived hGH with synthetic growth hormone. The injectable form is not human growth hormone (made from humans), but synthetic, which has a different name.

Human growth hormone (hGH) is no longer used in medicine or sport doping. Instead, biosynthetic human growth hormone is used, called recombinant human growth hormone (rhGH), somatropin, somatotropin, or somatotrophin (somatotrophs are the pituitary cells where the human form is made). Even if products are marked "HGH" they would contain no growth hormone (and you would not want them to). The underground market of performance-enhancing drugs is known for having many fake (counterfeit) drugs for sale, including fake growth hormone.

Growth hormone "doping" is expensive, and must be done for a long time before results occur. For bigger results, some bodybuilders and athletes combine, or "stack," growth hormones with anabolic steroids (body-building hormones). Some users add the dangerous practice of injecting insulin in combination with growth hormone (and/or steroids) for bigger muscles, more veins showing, and the appearance of exceptionally thin skin, looking as if shrink-wrapped over the muscle (believed a desirable look by some people). Insulin doping can cause serious, long-term illnesses.

Problems from growth hormone doping can include joint pain, wrist pain, carpal-tunnel syndrome, joint swelling, facial swelling, facial elongation, and increased blood pressure. Using large doses can decrease thyroid function and increase risk of diabetes. Sadly, users may think these effects are signs of aging, so they take more growth hormone believing it will stop this "aging." If the user already has cancer, it can increase growth of the tumor.

Growth hormone is naturally produced in your body throughout your life. Older people produce less growth hormone, but they still produce it. Some advertising for GH tries to persuade its targets that older people are somehow at a disadvantage without a lot. Remember that older people (above the age range of puberty) need less because they are not growing, although they still need enough for strength and tissue repair. Aging alone is not what makes you not have enough growth hormone. Four main factors reduce your body's growth-hormone levels:

- Lack of exercise. Without exercise, your muscles, bones, and other tissues have no reason to rebuild; you aren't using them, after all.
- High blood sugar from dietary sources (e.g., eating too much, eating too often, eating without enough exercise to use the blood sugar, and eating junk food)
- Too much growth hormone. Your body reduces its growth hormone levels if it already has too much. Growth hormone stimulates your liver and other tissues to secrete "insulin-like growth factor-I" (IGF-I), which is the real factor behind most of the effects of growth hormone. Having high blood levels of IGF-I decreases secretion of growth hormone as a normal regulatory function.
- Ongoing dosage with anti-inflammatory and immune-suppressive medicines called glucocorticoids (such as prednisone, dexamethasone, and hydrocortisone). People taking these medicines for injuries and pain should keep in mind that ongoing dosage can lead to osteoporosis, muscle weakness, delayed wound healing, and increased infection risk.

How do you get more natural growth hormone in healthy amounts without side effects? Three main agents stimulate GH secretion in your body:

- *Exercise.* Getting exercise in healthful ways, described throughout this book, boosts GH at all ages.
- *Deep sleep.* With good exercise, you will sleep well at night, too.
- *Low levels of sugar in your blood.* It is shown that both high fat and high refined-sugar diets increase blood sugar. It is not rocket science to eat less junk and more fruit and vegetables to be healthier and to lower high blood sugar.

Taking supplemental GH in adults may irreversibly increase growth of the jaw, forehead, hands, and feet, even in cases where it does not increase strength. It may also increase risk of diabetes, high blood pressure, and heart problems.

Compounds supposedly having GH-releasing potential sell briskly in health-food stores and gyms. Ornithine and sapogenin are two growth hormone hopefuls that fall short. Ornithine is often packaged in 250 mg capsules, although the effective dose is far higher. Sapogens are derived from plants found in desert regions. Your body will excrete them without making any GH. If you want results similar to taking growth hormone, but in a natural, safe, and inexpensive manner without side effects, vigorous exercise does that.

Anabolic Activators, Multipacs, and Enhancers. Packs of food elements are usually labeled with the suggestive name "anabolic." They have no special muscle-building abilities, and contain nothing that is not available in regular food. They are not anabolic steroids or steroid substitutes, except by name, and no law currently prevents anyone from selling you potions called steroid substitutes, even if they have no anabolic steroid effect. The name "steroid substitute" means only that advertisers would like you to buy their products instead of steroids, not necessarily that the product works like steroids do. The use of the word "anabolic" could technically mean that, since some of these supplements have so many calories, they do promote tissue growth—of fat—the same way any other high-calorie food does.

"Women's" Sports Supplements

A large and unfortunate industry exists of convincing people they need to spend money on separate sports and health supplements for women. Estrogenic, or estrogen-promoting supplements are easily overconsumed and are increasingly documented to contribute to estrogen-dependent tumors such as fibroids, cystic ovary, breast cysts, and endometriosis.

A partial list of estrogenic products includes unfermented soy, primrose oil, damiana, chasteberry, kudzu, black cohosh, St. John's Wort, dong quai, pennyroyal, flax seeds, burdock root. More are absorbed through the skin in lotions and oils containing lavender, clary sage, high amounts of tea-tree oil, and from hair products and shampoos with hormone containing placenta and estrogen or its precursors.

Hundreds of thousands of women annually have needless, serious, and painful surgery for conditions they might alleviate by avoiding overloading on estrogenic foods and the numerous "women's" supplements sold in "health-" food stores.

Protein

The most common belief about protein supplementation is that eating more protein will build bigger muscles. It won't. Consider the following: Protein enters into thousands of body functions besides muscle assembly. Eating more protein will not automatically increase all those functions. Protein builds skin, enters into the reactions that create the pigment in your skin, and is a building block for the smooth muscle in your blood vessels. Extra protein doesn't grow you more skin, make you turn brown, or make your blood vessels more muscular.

> Protein has many functions in your body besides growing muscles. Eating more protein does not increase any of those functions in speed or amount. For example, protein is involved in pigmenting your skin, but eating extra protein does not darken your skin.

Do You Need More Protein When Active? Studies find that for a brief time after beginning an exercise program, your body's protein balance falls, then restores to previous levels. Your need to increase protein (over the recommended minimum) may be brief and mild. Most people routinely eat more protein than the required recommended daily allowance (RDA). Because of all they already eat, any increased intake in meals or supplements is often unnecessary.

> A high-protein meat dinner can keep you from sleeping well. Get legume- and vegetable-based protein meals throughout the day, and most of your protein at breakfast and lunch.

You can't store protein the way you can store fat and, to a lesser extent, carbohydrate. Whenever you eat more protein than you need on any given day, most will convert to fat, and you will excrete the rest, a process requiring water. In high amounts, dietary protein contributes to dehydration and loss of calcium.

For the average inactive person, the minimum RDA for protein is 0.8 grams for every kilogram of body weight. A kilogram is about 2.2 pounds, making your minimum requirement less than half a gram of protein for every pound you weigh. Protein requirement for a 180-pound (82 kilogram) person varies around 65 grams per day, or about 2 ounces. A 130-pound person (59 kilograms) meets minimum requirements with less than 50 grams.

An active athlete may need at least 1 gram per kilogram of body weight. Muscle magazines often state that you need a gram of protein or more per pound of body weight. This amount does not seem to be the case, and has not been shown to have any effect on muscle building. Strength athletes usually need less protein than endurance athletes. Endurance athletes need a bit more protein, as they burn more calories. Muscle requires little protein for growth. For active people, carbohydrate supplementation seems to be more important and contributes more to muscle building.

You need a certain amount of protein every day. You may need more than that amount when you are active. The average person already eats more protein than required and so has no need to supplement.

Not All Protein Sources Are Healthful. Check supplement protein powders for fillers, dyes, sweeteners, thickeners, and hidden stimulants to give a false good feeling or weight loss in unhealthful manner. Dairy and whey products have many of the unhealthful components of dairy, listed in the chapter on osteoporosis, compounded by drying, processing, and concentrating them. Products with soy are usually unfermented soy. Unfermented soy contains enzyme inhibitors (which block digestion), goitrogens (which inhibit thyroid function), phytic acid (which blocks minerals like zinc and calcium), and estrogen-promoting compounds. Anyone with a tendency toward estrogen-dependent tumors or cancer, fibroids, cystic ovary or breast, or endometriosis should avoid unfermented soy. In general, vegetable, non-soy sources of protein from real whole food are best.

In a study published in the *European Journal of Clinical Nutrition* (November 29, 2006), researchers found that eating diets of low carbohydrate and high protein was associated with "increased mortality and risk of cancer." Another study, published in the *American Journal of Clinical Nutrition* (December 2006), concluded that a low-protein diet may protect against certain cancers. Lead author Dr. Luigi Fontana stated that if people ate more whole grains, beans, fruits, and vegetables and far fewer animal products, they would be healthier. Research published in 2007 from the University of Leeds found that those with the highest intake of red meat, the equivalent to one portion a day (more than 57 grams), run a 56 percent greater risk of breast cancer than those who eat none. Women who eat the most processed meat, such as bacon, sausages, ham, or pies, run a 64 percent greater risk of breast cancer than those women who eat none. Large studies in England and Germany found a 40 percent lower risk of many kinds of cancer in vegetarians, both men and women, compared to meat eaters.

Good quality protein is available without meat, dairy, or supplement powders. Try beans, peas, lentils, sesame seeds, oats, brown rice, nuts, chickpeas, muesli, seaweed, kelp, brewers yeast, hummus, tahini, and spirulina. These foods have protein, antioxidants, many nutrients, and fiber.

It is not true that you need to carefully mix specific foods in each meal to get complete proteins from vegetables, grains, and legumes. Proteins combine on their own in the body over the day of eating a variety. It is another food myth that you must avoid eating protein with starch (carbohydrate), or not eat one food group in combination with others. Nutrients usually work better together.

You can build much strength and muscle without eating any supplements or high protein diets. Save your money. Just do honest exercise in healthy ways.

Carbohydrate

Carbohydrate provides energy for activities. Carbohydrate is so important that your body stores it, mostly in your muscles and liver in a form called glycogen. The larger your stores, the longer you can exercise before you fatigue, depending on your physical fitness. You increase your body carbohydrate stores when you exercise regularly and eat regular meals with (healthful) carbohydrate.

Many commercial energy bars, mixes, and drinks are little more than unhealthful candy, with refined sugar, fillers, dyes, hydrolyzed proteins, unhealthy fats, and some synthetic vitamins. Eating them does not make you healthy just because they have the words "natural," "healthy," "vitamins," or "exercise" on the label. You would get more vitamins and health from eating a pear and some walnuts. Any product that contains high fructose corn syrup is not something you need to eat. Processed packaged sports supplement foods cost far more than the ingredients, and you can get healthier ingredients at a lower cost, and just as easily to make your own without commercial sports powders, bars, drinks, and other preparations.

Because athletes exercising at high intensities for long periods can delay fatigue and therefore work longer and harder with added carbohydrates, misunderstandings result. Taking carbohydrate drinks and preparations will not transform you into a better athlete. Your ability to do submaximal exercise like recreational running, swimming, biking, dancing, walking, skating, and so on, does not improve from any particular food or drink. Moreover, drinking sugar water is not fitness or health.

Carbohydrate Loader and Replacement Drinks. Carbohydrate loader drinks have a higher carbohydrate content than regular electrolyte-replacer drinks for intense, long-duration exercise.

"Energy food" technically means it has calories. Extra calories alone will not enable you to build muscle or win a race. Carbohydrate loader drinks are not magic energy elixirs. They won't give you a performance edge if taken before or during exercise much shorter than an hour or so, like an aerobics class, a half hour to an hour of cycling, skiing, or basketball, or even a 6- to 10-kilometer jog. Athletes generally have enough of their own stored carbohydrate, called glycogen, to last about an hour to 90 minutes.

Carbohydrate replacement drinks have a higher carbohydrate content than the loader drinks. Long, intense exercise depletes glycogen, an important fuel. You need to replace glycogen soon after exercise. If you don't, your body can't make enough glycogen to replace the loss. Your muscle and liver reserves remain low even days later, limiting further exercise ability.

The first 30 minutes after hard exercise are crucial to the major restocking. Your muscles can restore more total carbohydrate if you begin to eat or drink carbohydrates within 30 minutes after hard exercise. The next two hours are the second important stage. You benefit by eating complex carbohydrate food such as fruit, sweet potato, or a homemade drink recipe as soon after exercise as you can.

An example of homemade sports drink:

- Make healthier, less expensive sports drinks by putting an apple, banana, grapes, or other fruit, with nuts, (an optional sweet pepper), and clean water in a blender, grinder, food processor, mixer, or just mash them in a bowl.
- Add any combination of unsweetened cocoa powder, cinnamon, cloves, ginger root, sesame seeds, and healthy items for flavor.
- More sports-drink recipes can be found in Chapter 16.

In general, no commercial processed "sports food," no matter how engineered or marketed as effective for training, will give you the health of healthful real food. Whole foods, for example, a simple apple with the skin contain combinations of nutritional and disease fighting chemicals that are not available in supplements. Many nutrients need to work in the original food containing other components that make each part work better. Some do not work, or have even been found to increase health risks when concentrated in vitamin and mineral supplements. Good nutrition all year will give more benefit than eating special foods for an event, race, or hike.

Drinks With "Buzz"

Packaged "health" and "sports" drinks may contain stimulants of many kinds: ginseng, ma huang, guarana, ephedra, caffeine and its variants, and others. These products are advertised as "energy" drinks. Check the label. You don't need them to exercise or lose weight. A cycle starts of needing the product to avoid feeling weary and headachy. Nervousness, anxiety, inability to concentrate by day and sleep at night, and irregular heart beats can occur. Mixing these products with energy pills, diet pills, coffee and espresso, and other pills and medicines, can produce effects even more serious.

Users with uncomfortable effects may add over-the-counter or prescription medicines to try to stop those effects. That approach is not health. The practice of regularly taking stimulant drinks and products is a foolhardy one to become accustomed to, building cycles of inability to focus, exercise, or feel well without them, and varying degrees of agitation with them, sleep difficulties, and various cardiovascular risks.

> If amphetamines and cigarettes were discovered today, they would probably be in stores advertised as "wonder energy enhancers" and "natural" diet aids. Remember that they once were promoted that way with devastating health effects. Compare that when spending money on other commercial products for "energy."

Creatine

Chapter 4 explains how you use a molecule called ATP to fuel short, hard activity. As quickly as you use ATP, you rebuild it for more activity using creatine phosphate that you store, mostly in your muscles. You can't store much, only enough for 8 to 10 seconds of intense activity, like a 100-meter dash. When you run low, you shift to another energy system at lower intensity. The hope of supplemental creatine to fuel intense short efforts is behind sales of creatine as a supplement.

Creatine monohydrate is a synthetic of the creatine phosphate you make in your body. Not everyone can absorb it, which may be why some people find results using it and others don't. Advice to eat lots of steak and pork, which contain creatine, doesn't work (for you or the pig). Once you cook meat, the creatine denatures (changes permanently), so you can't use it. Harming your arteries with high-meat meals won't help athletic ability either. You don't need to eat creatine directly because your body makes what you need from balanced meals, including vegetarian meals. Ergogenic effect of creatine supplementation seems to be counteracted by caffeine. One thing known to work well is to get in better shape. Good aerobic ability increases your ability to store the creatine that you make and use it to rebuild your energy stores.

Even after years of inquiry, the USDA issued an advisory statement saying more is unknown than known about creatine side effects over the long term, and that adverse effects may result on your kidneys and liver.

Androstenedione (Andro)

"Andro" is another expensive "health-food store" supplement. You make it in your own body out of DHEA. People buy it because androstenedione breaks down to testosterone, a male hormone. However, another hormone that androstenedione makes is estrogen. Body chemistry is more complicated than "andro makes muscles because it makes testosterone." Your body is smart. If it has too much of a substance, it will try to reduce the excess. Andro supplements can increase urinary levels—not because more hormone is in your body, but because your body is getting rid of the extra. Sometimes your body will stop producing its own testosterone if it intakes too much, making you more deficient than when you started. Sometimes andro supplements have other elements not on the label that can cause a positive drug test for banned substances.

Reports from gyms and androstenedione manufacturers state that andro always greatly helps athletic ability. Carefully done studies in real labs don't always find that it increases lean body mass, strength, or testosterone levels in healthy adult men. Some studies show increased strength, but only the same amount of strength as a control group who also exercised hard but didn't supplement with andro. Great changes into a muscular athlete don't happen from pills alone. Although andro is available over the counter, its use is banned by athletic bodies because of harmful side effects and ethical issues.

Vitamins

Many people regard vitamins as ergogenic aids. No scientific evidence supports vitamin supplementation as ergogenic. Unless you have a nutritional deficiency, increasing your intake will not improve physical ability.

Vitamins have no calories, so by definition they furnish no energy. Vitamins are often advertised as giving energy, even labeled with suggestive names like "Ener-B." Unless your fatigue relates to a deficiency, they will not make you energetic.

> Vitamin B12 has been called the least likely vitamin to affect sport performance and the most likely to be abused for nonexistent ergogenic effects.

Taking too many vitamins can be unhealthy. Some vitamins are fat-soluble. With repeated overdosing, they can accumulate in your body to toxic levels. Other vitamins are water-soluble and you excrete them, but can still have side effects with long-term overdose. Vitamins do not work in isolation. Studies find unhealthful effects of taking vitamin supplements, with some studies showing increased risk of cancer. It is better to get vitamins from whole foods where they exist along with many other compounds they need to work with that cannot be isolated into pills

Minerals

Like vitamins, minerals have no calories and no known ergogenic effects. Deficiencies may result in weaknesses, but taking amounts above your needs will not improve your physical fitness. Even so, many have been advertised with claims of ergogenic effects.

Boron is one of several minerals misrepresented as an ergogenic aid. A widely misquoted study found low dietary boron decreased testosterone in postmenopausal women. Levels rose when the deficiency was corrected. From that misquoted study came claims of boron as helpful to athletes to increase their testosterone levels, with "studies" seeming to back up those claims. Although problems stem from nutrient deficiency, no evidence suggests that extra boron elevates testosterone. Large doses are toxic. Boron is an ultra-trace mineral. You need only tiny amounts and can get them from fruits, vegetables, nuts, and legumes.

Chromium (including chromium picolinate) and vanadium are ultra-trace minerals in the diet that have been advertised as ergogenic. If a deficiency exists, the benefit of supplementation is to correct the deficiency. No good evidence suggests that they alter your body composition or enhance athletic ability to any extent that it matters to most exercisers.

Carnitine

The excitement over carnitine began when the Italian soccer team won a title while taking carnitine. The team did many other things besides taking carnitine, such as train at high levels. No specific evidence shows that carnitine had anything to do with their season outcome, yet such advertising sells many bottles of carnitine.

Your body makes its own carnitine and distributes it to many of your body's cells. Primarily, it works to carry unoxidized fatty acids. These acids have a D form and an L form. Those initials just tell how the molecule rotates—to the right (dextro-, or D-rotatory) or left (levo-rotatory, or L form.) Eating too much of the D form of carnitine in supplements can make you lose the L form. In this case, supplementation can be harmful.

It is difficult to become carnitine deficient through training. No good evidence suggests that taking carnitine in any of its forms does much that can be considered helpful, but we do not have enough evidence to reject it completely. Some studies show minor gains. For the small gains and big price, the average exerciser can gains as much and more through regular exercise.

Carnosine

Carnosine a compound made of amino acids. It is thought to have antioxidant properties. Some claims suggest that vegetarians might not get enough carnosine, as it is found only in meat. You manufacture carnosine in your own body. It is not an essential nutrient, meaning you don't need to eat it to have enough. Your body makes more antioxidants when you exercise.

Carbohydrate Injection

Korean speed skaters were reported to have been experimenting with glycogen injections directly into thigh muscle. For elite athletes, it is not known if it can be used or beneficial. The answer for regular exercisers is that it is completely unnecessary.

Fluid Retention

Fluid retention has been examined as an ergogenic aid. The theory is that muscle leverage favorably changes as the muscle swells with extra water. You can increase your total body water in several ways—carbohydrate loading increases the water your muscles can hold, eating salt retains more water, and anabolic steroids swell you with water, before they have a chance to exert any androgenic effect.

But should you count on fluid retention to help you in sports or exercise? Most people don't drink enough water, which is a common, and hidden, cause of fatigue. Getting enough water is a good idea and can make you feel better by itself. As far as dosing on extra water, the effect would be small, if any. Your body will usually regulate things so that any excess is quickly eliminated.

Water

For exercise, you need enough water to distribute to your skin for cooling and your muscles for working. Without enough to go around, you may overheat or not work at strong capacity. People overdo carrying water with them for minor exercise in air-conditioned gyms. If you are so dry that you cannot get through an hour of ordinary exercise without a bottle in your hand, you may have started out underhydrated.

Expensive bottled water is not always better or cleaner than tap water. Plastic bottles create a substantial problem of litter and waste in manufacture, transport, and disposal, harming the fitness of the environment. Chapter 16 provides ideas on making your own fitness water and drinks, and using filtered tap water in your own healthful, non-disposable containers.

Despite various fad-diet advice that extra large quantities of water must be consumed every day, or that large quantities of water will somehow remove substances, vaguely labeled "toxins," these claims have no solid support. Drinking enough good, clean water is important, healthy, and can help control appetite. Drink more water in the heat. Eating fruit and vegetables supplies water in healthy form. Drinking too much water will not make you healthier. Too much water, like many other things, is not good. Claims that you must drink eight glasses of water per day have little basis.

Avoid the Hype

Masses of products crowding store shelves claim to fix this and cure that. Product sales have risen to billions of dollars annually. Products seem dazzling, but much is hype and many produce unhealthful effects. More dollars follow on pills and products for problems that result, then more medicines when ill effects result in turn. Stop the cycle, and save time, money, and unhappiness. If it is not healthy, it is not health care.

What Will Give You an Advantage?

Regular good nutrition, good hydration, and regular exercise (not supplements) give true athletic advantage. What can you do?

- Eat a healthful breakfast. Include real raw fruit and nuts rather than toast and jam or processed cereal.
- Do not eat fast food or junk food.
- Know the difference between simple sugars and complex carbohydrates. Eat complex carbohydrates for the vitamins, nutrients, and energy-giving fuel you need for activity.
- Get enough protein early in the day. Don't have a coffee and Danish for breakfast and a salad for lunch. Get protein from vegetables and nuts, throughout the day. You'll sleep better without a high-protein dinner at night.
- Rest is a greatly ignored ergogenic aid. Get enough sleep, and enjoy your life.
- Exercise for fun and health.
- Drink water instead of commercial sports drinks or store-bought juice.
- Make your own juice with the pulp by putting your favorite fruit with clean water in a blender or mixer or get exercise by mashing it by hand.
- Make your own sports drinks instead of drinking sugar water in plastic bottles.
- Cut back (or out) on stimulants. Vicious cycles of dependence build. Stop unhealthy food, drink, and life habits that sap energy.
- Get outdoors in the sunshine (or the rain or snow) safely every day.
- Add up all the money you save on supplements. You will have enough to give to the poor and take a vacation.
- Be good to your mind and your body—a neglected personal-enhancing device.

Resources for More Information

Healthy Martial Arts
Dr. Jolie Bookspan
www.DrBookspan.com/books
A large resource on training all aspects of physical and mental fitness for any athlete in any sport.

18

Healthy Eating

To avoid sickness, eat less; to prolong life, worry less.

—Chu Hui Weng

Eating nutrition-poor food is common. Sometimes, unhealthy foods are the only offerings at restaurants, movies, ball games, theme parks, and public events. Unhealthy eating is so easy to do, and so well-accepted as normal, that it often goes unnoticed as a major factor in fatigue, extra pounds, and some of the most common Western diseases, such as cardiovascular disease, diverticulitis, high blood pressure, and diabetes. Many people turn to vitamins, supplements, drinks with stimulant compounds, and various medicines, both over-the-counter and prescription, hoping these will fix their low energy or poor health, without ever looking at the unhealthy daily eating habits behind their problem.

This chapter looks at a few common eating habits that lead to weight gain, fatigue, and health problems. It gives ideas for more healthful food habits, some myths of healthful and unhealthful eating, and how simple, good-tasting choices can improve your health.

Eating Backward in Quantity

Healthy eaters have smaller evening meals than their breakfasts and lunches. If you eat backward in quantity, you do the opposite—eat little or nothing for breakfast, have unhealthful lunch, candy and packaged snack foods during the day, then a large meal at night and a snack or two later on. The results are often fatigue during and after work, cravings, crankiness, and extra pounds.

You don't need to have a huge, sugary breakfast to "have energy for the day," particularly if you sit at a desk. You do need a meal of some healthful foods for the work you do. You may feel fatigued when you don't eat enough at the beginning and middle of the day. Your body does not only burn fat if you skip eating breakfast or don't eat carbohydrate. Your body also turns to protein stores when dietary carbohydrate is low. You need healthful sources of carbohydrate energy to work, do physical activity, and get around enough to enjoy life. Sugary snacks are unhealthful sources, high-calorie, and may contribute to mood swings and food craving. Large high-protein and high-fat meals at night add more calories, protein, and fat when you need less. After eating too much, too late, you are less likely to sleep well, and more likely to wake to use the bathroom. Junk food and "health-food" products that have sugar substitutes like sorbitol can make you uncomfortably gassy. Some products that are labeled "low carbohydrate" are high in unhealthy trans-fat and hydrogenated fat. Many products labeled "low fat" or "no fat" have much junk refined sugar. Junk fats and sugars damage your health over the long term.

Eating Backward in Quality

The second way you may eat backward concerns what you eat. You may have a good-sized breakfast, but filled with sugar and fat. Backward meals may be high in fat, protein, and simple sugar, but have little of an important nutrient—complex carbohydrate. Eating backward in quality, as with quantity, often results in fatigue, poor nutrition, and increased risk of various diseases. Several studies of a "Mediterranean" style of eating, which is high in fruit, vegetables, and nuts, and low in dairy foods and red meat, show greatly reduced numbers of deaths from cancer and cardiovascular disease. A study of thousands of Chinese women looked at what is called the "meat-sweet" diet. Half the participants followed a "Western" pattern of eating beef and lamb, pork, poultry, organ meats, saltwater fish, shrimp, candy, desserts, bread, and milk. The other half followed a traditional daily diet of vegetables, sprouts, tofu, fresh-water fish, and beans. The postmenopausal women in the Western "meat-sweet" eating group of the study had a 60 percent greater risk of estrogen-receptor-positive (ER+) breast cancer than women eating the traditional vegetable diet.

A day of backward meals may be no breakfast, or a breakfast of coffee or tea, pastry or donuts, or eggs and sausage, and then a sugary snack at a midmorning coffee break because of low energy. Lunch may be fast food or restaurant food—high fat and high protein, but low complex carbohydrate. Additional eating for the day includes another afternoon sugary/fatty donut, Danish, or cookie snack because you are hungry for sugar; a fast-food snack of fat and simple sugar; a large, meat-based, high-fat dinner with high-fat ice cream, cake, or pie for dessert; and a sugary snack (or more) of cookies, potato chips, and other unhealthful food later that night to calm low blood sugar from earlier candy snacks.

Why Do People Eat Backward?

One reason for bad eating habits is the U.S. Department of Agriculture's recommendation of meat and dairy "groups" for daily consumption. Of the old "four food groups," two were meat and dairy. Modern Western diets often include meat and dairy every day, sometimes every meal. The human body is not designed to handle it. Meat is not only protein. Bacon, for example, can have roughly 80 percent of its calories from fat. Many meats are over 50 percent fat. A number of studies have been done to look at the connection between meat and dairy eating and developing cancer. Meat has no fiber and nutrients that are protective. Meat contains animal protein and saturated fat. Carcinogenic compounds may form during processing and cooking. The high fat content of meat and other animal products increases hormone production, increasing the risk of hormone-related cancers such as breast and prostate cancer.

On April 9, 1991, the Physician's Committee for Responsible Medicine released a statement that a diet based on the old four food groups will not ensure adequate nutrition, and promotes disease. This information was not new. A 1978 study showed that only 9 of 17 minimum daily-required amounts of needed nutrients were met by meals based on the old four food groups. The 1977–78 Nationwide Food Consumption Survey stated, "Americans who eat diets based on the four food groups consume an excessive amount of fat." It is still taking years to advance to healthier thinking about eating patterns. Later revision of food groups to various "pyramids" showing differing amounts of needed food still relied on high amounts of meat and dairy.

Another reason for backward eating habits is a belief that complex carbohydrates are fattening food to avoid. If complex carbohydrates are confused with simple sugars, people will eat sugar thinking it is energy food.

Another reason for such habits is that often the only food available at restaurants, office buildings, ballparks, picnics, and drive-throughs is unhealthful packaged foods and popular fast foods, high fat and simple sugar, and low complex carbohydrate. Some fast-food chains offer what seems to be healthier items, but which are offset by the actual contents and preparation of the items. Food preparation can add sugar, fat, flavor enhancers, fillers, and other chemicals, and remove the skins of vegetables. The skin of red peppers, potatoes, and other vegetables is important for fiber, which helps keep blood sugar even and contains good nutrients. Check if you turn healthy vegetables into a high-blood-sugar, high-blood-fat meal.

An additional reason for such behaviors is habit. The most popular snacks of packaged chips and lunchmeats become habits at early ages. People eat these foods because they are part of their daily routines. It is a highly counterproductive custom to spoon-feed cake and ice cream to babies in arms and young children. Eating such seriously unhealthy foods will become seriously unhealthy habits throughout their lives. To rationalize it by saying that babies need some fun too would be like giving them cigarettes or street drugs. Automobile anti-freeze tastes sweet, too, but is still harmful.

> Eating candied yams, glazed vegetables, and buttered lima beans isn't "eating healthy vegetables;" it is eating too much fat and sugar—bad for your teeth, bad for your heart, bad for your skin and eyes, and bad for the rest of your body and health and general.

Misleading food labels can also contribute to bad eating habits. Food is often labeled as health food to make it sell, although it is high fat and processed sugar (for example, granola bars, sports bars, and processed "whole-grain" snack foods).

Is It Natural?

Eating high fat and high processed refined sugar and flour is a common bad nutrition habit. It is easy to do and becomes natural. The taste perception of people accustomed to sugar and fat changes to the point where food that isn't fatty and sugared doesn't taste as good to them. After an adjustment period, the same people tasting junk again often protest that the high-fat item tastes too fatty, like drinking butter, which is not all that far from truth.

Children regularly fed high-fat and highly sugared foods develop the habit of eating them. When visiting anthropologists first gave South American Indian children candy, the children spit it out as bad tasting. Although our bodies have an evolutionary survival tendency to prefer higher sugar and fat foods, foods as high in fat and sugar as we currently eat didn't exist until recently. Many modern food preferences are just habit. It is natural to wet your pants, too, but you learn control.

How to Make Bad Food Habits Into Good Ones

Eating healthy should not be some hateful thing you do at certain meals because you have to, then discard the rest of the time to go back to your "real" foods. Like exercise, healthy eating can gradually become a desirable, normal way of life.

Don't Eat Backward. Try smaller dinners. Have healthful amounts at breakfast and lunch. Healthy meals have more of the calories as complex carbohydrate, avoid saturated and trans-fat, and don't emphasize high protein.

Various Food Pyramids. The old "four food groups" have been replaced by various new food pyramids. In many of the new pyramids, a large, two-level base of food to eat most often contains fruit and vegetables. The smallest section is a sugar and fat group, to be eaten sparingly. The middle protein group includes dry beans, lentil, peas, brown rice, and nuts.

The original seven-group food pyramid had been criticized for including meat in the larger protein section of beans, and for having an entire equally sized section just for dairy. It is often argued that meat and dairy combined should be a smaller section than the others. Various newer pyramid recommendations call for vegetables and fruit as main foods, with a smaller area for grains, similar to what is sometimes called the Asian Pyramid. The new recommendations all agree on vegetables as main dishes, an important concept for changing to healthy food habits, with meat as occasional use if you eat meat. The China-Cornell-Oxford Project and many other studies have shown that Asian people who follow this traditional way of eating have among the world's lowest rates of obesity, heart disease, and cancer.

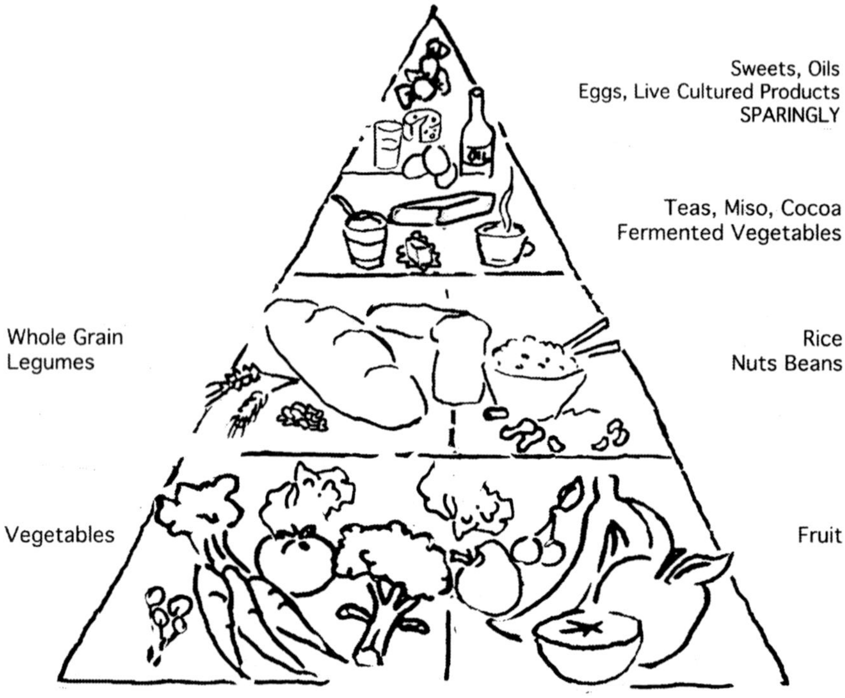

Figure 18-1. Various food pyramids replace the old four food groups and the original seven-group pyramid. Food pyramids put certain foods at the small end to emphasize they should be used only to a small extent. Main meals of vegetables and fruit form the large, supporting base. Proteins from legumes (foods like beans, lentils, and peas) and nuts, plus nutrients and protein from whole grains, brown rice, and oatmeal share the middle.

Serving Size. Eating too much is not smart, and not needed, obviously. Various food pyramids and food guides talk about serving size, but what is that? A food label may say that snack crackers have 150 calories per serving, but that serving is only a few crackers. If you eat the contents of the entire box, you consume over 1,000 calories. Too much of any food, no matter how healthful, adds up. A handful of raw nuts can be healthy. Two cups, or a small bag-full, will be about 1500 calories.

Check to see if you are eating far more than you think of unhealthful food. The following chart gives an example of the difference in eating a serving and a typical amount. You may be eating five times the amounts and calories you think.

	Official USDA Serving	Typical Restaurant Serving
Ice cream	1/2 cup	2+ cups
Typical meat dish	3 oz	6 to 16+ oz
Salad dressing	2 tbsp	6 tbsp
Slice of standard pizza	5 oz	12+ oz
Muffin	2 oz	6 to 12 oz
French fries	3 oz	8 to 16+ oz

Eat Healthful Breakfast. Trying to eat low fat by eating a refined sugar breakfast of jam and toast, or getting a pastry or toaster pastry in a hurry is not healthful eating. It can raise your cholesterol in the same way as eating fatty food. Have complex carbohydrate from fruit, healthy fat from nuts and seeds, and moderate protein to fuel the day's work and exercise. You don't have any need for an overly large breakfast (or any meal) when you sit at a desk.

Eat Healthful (Not Junk) Snacks. A common recommendation is to eat many times a day, almost continuously, to never go hungry. You don't need to constantly flood your body with food. Constant insulin "baths" are not healthy for your cells. If you eat less simple sugar and refined flour products and junk food, you will find that food cravings often stop. Try snacks like fruit, vegetables (such as sweet green and red peppers), and raw nuts for energy during the day.

Cooked Versus Raw. You don't need to eat only raw food or only cooked food. It is not true that any cooking destroys the bulk of nutrients. Processed, heat-treated, extruded, commercially-produced packaged foods and protein products greatly reduce nutritional value. Lightly cooking vegetables at home can enhance digestibility, flavor, and some nutrients. Beans, grains, and tubers need cooking. Have a variety of healthy cooked vegetables and raw fruit and nuts.

Eat Less When Not Exercising. You need fuel to work hard enough to get a good workout. Eat light, healthful food some time before exercising. If you don't tolerate a regular meal before exercise, try small snacks of fruit or homemade sports drinks. Eat less when not exercising.

Eat Smaller Dinners. Food fuels activity. Eat the bulk of your calories earlier in the day when you need energy to get things done. It is not true that you must not eat after certain hours. Calories eaten later in the day are the same calories. The reason for not eating late is because most people in developed countries have already eaten all the calories they need before then and don't need more, and that large dinners may increase trouble sleeping.

Don't Fall for Marketing Tactics on Food Labels. The sack-of-sugar example from Chapter 14 is 100 percent sugar. The 1,000-calorie block of fat is 100 percent fat. If you mix them together, the percentage of sugar and fat both drop to 50 percent but the amounts of unhealthful substances are still present. The food label for the new product may claim that is a "reduced fat" food, or that it has less carbohydrate. Another example is a vegetable. Vegetables will be mostly made of complex carbohydrate. The percentage of carbohydrate compared to fat and protein will be high. It does not mean it is high in total carbohydrates. It is still a low-calorie, healthful food. Don't lose sight of what you are really eating.

Choosing Good Food

Protein

Most people in the Western nations get more protein than they need. The extra protein does not automatically convert into muscle, even with exercise. If you stop exercising, eating extra protein will not make you keep the muscles you have. Without exercise, your muscles will shrink in size. They don't turn into fat. The cells will still stay muscle cells, just smaller ones.

Vegetables, legumes, and some grains are healthy protein sources. You don't have to carefully mix them in every dish to get the right proportions of proteins, as once thought. Have a variety, often, as you should anyway, and everything will mix itself in your system. Make vegetables your main dishes with smaller sides of grain when exercising. You will have low-fat, lower calorie, high-fiber, healthy meals with a good amount of protein. Following is a base recipe to get started:

- Choose from any combination of lentils, brown rice, barley, or couscous, for example. Cook a small amount in water or vegetable stock. They take about 30 minutes to cook.

- In the last five minutes, throw in several cups of chopped or sliced favorite vegetables, such as broccoli, spinach, mushrooms, or squash; a can of unsalted peas (or fresh peas), optional chopped raw carrots or apples to sweeten, or a few raisins or chopped dried apricots.
- Add raw or lightly sautéed onion, scallions, chives, and/or leeks.
- Season with any variety of cloves, curries, lemon pepper, ginger, or whatever you like.
- Add small sprinkles of unsalted sunflower seeds, peanuts, or almonds.

You can create enough combinations in this one example for many good-tasting, low-fat vegetable dishes full of healthy, complete protein. With any amounts left over, you can make good-tasting sandwich and wrap fillings for lunches. For example, mix with tomato sauce and spoon onto leafy greens, cheaply available in most supermarkets. It is cheaper, quicker, lower-calorie, and healthier than meat.

The World Cancer Research Fund study in 2007 concluded that, "evidence is stronger than previously realized" that eating meat, and processed meats such as ham and bacon, increases risk of colorectal cancer. The report makes 10 recommendations, including getting exercise every day, drinking water rather than sugary drinks, and eating fruit, vegetables, and fiber. Meat, dairy, and eggs contain no fiber. Vegan meals (vegetarian meals without any animal-derived products, such as dairy or eggs) can provide enough calcium to prevent osteoporosis and enough protein for exercise and health.

Protein need depends on your body weight. General estimates are to eat about 0.8 to 1.0 grams of protein for every kilogram you weigh. If you weigh 130 pounds (59 kg), get at least 47 grams of protein every day. If you weigh 150 pounds (68 kg), get at least 54 grams of protein. If you weigh 170 pounds (77 kg), get a minimum of 61 grams. If you weigh 200 pounds (90 kg), get 73 grams of protein. You can find the gram content of protein on the food labels. You don't need much more protein with heavy exercise, but you do need more carbohydrate to fuel that exercise. It is estimated that weight lifters need less protein than distance runners, for example, because the runners need more calories overall. More about protein and protein myths is covered in Chapter 14.

> Vegetables are important, healthy protein sources. Use grains more sparingly to avoid overdoing carbohydrate all day. You don't need to carefully mix certain ones to get complete protein.
>
> You can choose from a large variety of nutritious grains and legumes, such as lentils. They are quick to prepare, store easily in the cupboard in bulk, can be made delicious with healthful seasoning and herbs instead of butter or sauce, and are low cost compared to meat.

What Is Texturized Vegetable Protein? Texturized vegetable protein (TVP) is defatted, unfermented soy flour used as a meat replacement. It is better not to use unfermented soy products. Unfermented soy may promote estrogenic compounds, depress the thyroid, and inhibit mineral and protein absorption. Unfermented soy does not have the health benefits of fermented soy, which are better to use instead. Fermented examples are tempeh, miso, brewed soy sauce, and natto. Not all soy sauce is fermented. Some sham products are sold containing a caramel color to make it look like real soy sauce. TVP is not the same as HVP, hydrolyzed vegetable protein. HVP is a food additive, often with monosodium glutamate (MSG) added. MSG and HVP enhance appetite. MSG is thought to be involved in several uncomfortable symptoms, and is best avoided.

What Is Tofu? Tofu is made from soybeans. It is not fermented, but "precipitated." Various compounds are added to make the solids drop out and collect. Traditional use of tofu is to eat small amounts with a protein source so the bad effects are reduced. It is not supposed to be a protein substitute, eaten in large quantities.

What Is Seitan? Seitan is a protein food made from wheat gluten, and used as a meat substitute. Persons with Celiac disorder do better to avoid this food. Celiac is an immune response to wheat gluten and related products.

Position Statement of the American Dietetic Association:

A considerable body of scientific data suggests positive relationships between vegetarian diets and risk reduction for several chronic degenerative diseases and conditions, including obesity, coronary-artery disease, hypertension, diabetes mellitus, and some types of cancer. It is the position of the American Dietetic Association and Dietitians of Canada that well-planned vegan and other types of vegetarian diets are appropriate for all stages of the life cycle, including during pregnancy, lactation, infancy, childhood, and adolescence.

Feel encouraged. Being vegetarian or making occasional vegetarian meals does not have to involve any strange or expensive foods from specialty stores. You do not need any special pots or food-processing equipment. It is a myth that vitamin or iron supplements are automatically necessary. Plants are a good source of protein, and unlike meat, have no cholesterol and little fat. Meat, even lean cuts, often has more than the maximum amount of fat recommended by the American Heart Association. It used to be thought that plant protein was not as good as meat protein. In the modern diet, you have little chance of not getting enough of the different kinds of protein you need from vegetable sources. Nor do you need to carefully combine plant proteins, as once thought. Your body does that for you automatically, as you eat over time. Vegetables and grains are a good source of the healthful carbohydrate that fuels your body. Grocery bills can also be also far less expensive when you don't purchase meat, and don't substitute other expensive food that you do not need.

Fat

High-fat diets have been in the news as acceptable, even healthful ways to lose weight. However, the effect on the cardiovascular system is not as healthful as reported. The weight loss associated with most diets can contribute to lower blood fats; however, high-fat diets, over the long run, are being found to contribute to many serious health problems. Even a single high-fat meal has been shown to reduce lung function and increase blood fat enough to impede circulation. The American Heart Association calls for keeping dietary fat under 20 to 30 percent at most, with the majority of it as vegetable fat. Low-fat diets, when sensibly applied and not containing junk sugar instead of the unhealthful fat, lower cholesterol and have been found to not only stop advancing heart disease, but to help reverse it.

What about avoiding fat entirely? A small amount of dietary fat is needed to absorb fat-soluble vitamins like Vitamin A, and to supply two essential fatty acids (EFAs). Even if you ate only beans, vegetables, grains, and fruits, with no oil or high-fat ingredients at all, you would eat a certain amount of fat. You would have to eat only sugary junk foods to exclude all food fat, which wouldn't be healthy for several reasons, but which some people do when trying to eat "low fat." You need small amounts of specific kinds of fat in the diet for several necessary functions. Almonds and hazelnuts provide needed monounsaturated fat. Walnuts contain n-3 (omega-3) fatty acids. Eating nuts has been shown to lower serum cholesterol in non-diabetic subjects. Don't eat bacon, cream, and other unhealthful fat sources, and call it health food because you "need a little fat."

Essential Omega Fatty Acids. Your body cannot make certain specific kinds of fat. The kind you must eat to obtain are called "essential" fats. No amount of eating nonessential fat will supply or make essential fat. Essential fats are needed for certain body processes, for your heart, nervous system, and joints.

You need a small amount of two essential fatty acids (EFAs): n-6 fatty acids and n-3 fatty acids (omega-3 fatty acids)—but not too much of them. If you eat far more omega-6 than omega-3, you may produce many inflammatory compounds in the body. It is thought to relate to diseases like heart disease, arthritis, and pain syndromes. Omega-6 is found in meat, poultry, safflower oil, primrose oil, oats, corn, leafy greens, wheat, flax seeds, walnuts, soybeans, and processed food. Omega-3 is found in most plant foods. Highest amounts are in green leafy vegetables, and nuts. Eat nuts raw; high heat destroys the omega-3 benefit.

Flax Seeds, Almonds, and Walnuts. Almonds, walnuts, and other raw nuts are good tasting sources of good fat, with healthy nutrients. Add to baking, casseroles, and morning hot cereal. Use them as a butter substitute in baking. Put whole raw flax seeds

> Don't eat ice cream and cream sauce and call it "health food" because you heard "you need a little fat in your diet."
>
> You need oil in your car, too, but too much and the wrong kind will kill your engine.

in your blender or food processor or coffee grinder to mill them. You don't need to go to any specialty health-food stores. Try a nut store or market where dry goods are sold in self-measuring bulk. Most large supermarkets now carry these items, which are so common in many other parts of the world. Don't overdo flax seeds, as they promote estrogenic compounds in the body. Excess amounts can cause health problems. (Refer to Chapter 17.)

Complex Carbohydrates

They used to be called starches. It is a myth that starch, in itself, is fattening. Too many calories from any source leads to weight gain, but complex carbohydrates are healthy eating in moderation. Like fiber, which is the most complex of carbohydrates, complex carbohydrate is found only in plants. For exercise energy, try baked or steamed sweet potatoes, brown rice, lentils, beans, broccoli, fruit of all kinds, sweet peppers, and carrots.

How Much? Eat more carbohydrate from whole food before strenuous activities, and less when you are not exercising. Without exercise to use up the blood sugar, levels can rise. It is not healthy to have continually high blood-sugar spikes from bad eating habits.

What Are Phytochemicals? Besides the complex carbohydrate that fuels energy, many necessary vitamins and nutrients are only found in plant food. The word "phytochemicals" means "plant chemicals." They are compounds found only in plants that are increasingly studied as disease fighters—including cancer-fighting compounds. Find them in broccoli, spinach, tomatoes, and carrots, in fruits like apricots and cantaloupe, in nuts and seeds, in garlic, onions, cauliflower, and in almost all vegetables.

> Don't avoid fruit because you've confused healthful complex carbohydrate with simple sugar, and then eat a high-fat meal. Don't eat crackers and jelly (refined flour and sugar) because you want to eat something low-fat. Both foods can raise blood sugar and lipid to unhealthful levels. Use common sense.

Can Carbohydrates Make You Fat? "Carbo-bashing" seems to have started with a New York Times article, "Eating Pasta Makes You Fat," and the wide media coverage that followed. The concern was that emphasizing carbohydrates would exacerbate "Syndrome X" in "insulin-resistant" people, an estimated 10 to 25 percent of Americans.

"Syndrome X" is a collection of risk factors for heart disease, including high blood pressure, low "good cholesterol," high triglycerides, and obesity. "Insulin resistance" is a topic with a lot of unknowns. It seems to involve a reduced number of insulin receptors. Body cells don't know how much insulin they already have had delivered. The pancreas secretes more and more insulin, not knowing when to stop. In theory, this insulin oversecretion causes the carbohydrates to be better stored as fat.

To understand this process better:

- Carbohydrate will store as fat only if you eat too much of it, the same as any other food.
- Even "insulin-resistant" people must eat excess carbohydrate calories before the carbohydrates are stored as fat.
- Losing excess weight, increasing physical activity, and stopping junk food are far more important in controlling insulin resistance than restricting the good complex carbohydrate of fruit and vegetables.
- In most cases, insulin resistance seems to be caused by excess weight and inactivity, not the other way around.

Fettuccine Alfredo was once named "heart attack on a plate" for the high-fat, artery-clogging sauce and refined white flour. If you eat too much pasta, even low fat, you will gain weight; just like eating too much of anything.

What About Low-Carbohydrate Diets? Some weight-loss diets claim that you gain more weight eating carbohydrate than by eating fat or protein. They claim limiting carbohydrate will make you burn more fat. Neither claim seems to be the case. Weight loss may occur from limiting calories, which is good, but weight loss can be achieved by limiting unhealthy amounts of fat as well.

Several low-carbohydrate diets limit carbohydrates by lowering the carbohydrate percentage of your total intake, and raising the fat and/or protein percentage. Low-carbohydrate and high-protein or high-fat diets can eventually create health problems. Diet involves more than simply losing weight. If your long-term health is affected, the diet is not smart. Too much protein dehydrates you, is hard on your kidneys, and increases risk of osteoporosis. (Refer to Chapter 14 on nutrition and Chapter 22 on osteoporosis.) Too much fat promotes serious diseases. Many vitamins, minerals, antioxidants, and disease-fighting nutrients are found only in complex carbohydrates. Low-carbohydrate diets limit these nutrients and discourage healthy eating

Without sufficient carbohydrate, you won't have energy to do the exercise to lose weight. For athletic events, you won't have the fuel you need for high performance. You can lose weight through many unhealthful drugs and diets. For healthy weight loss, stop eating too much simple sugar in processed food and too much fat. Burn more calories through more fun movement in daily life. It is a win-win program.

> When you eat carbohydrate, have healthy, complex carbohydrates of vegetables, fruits, and legumes, not the simple sugars of candy, cake, packaged snack food, and fast foods. It is healthy to have a very low simple-sugar diet but not a very low-carbohydrate diet.

Claims of needing more fat or protein to put you into particular "zones" don't allow you enough carbohydrate to do enough exercise, and limit important nutrients from whole foods. Keep total calories to the amount you need for your healthy weight. More calories mean more weight, whether they come from fat, protein, or carbohydrate. (Refer to Chapter 14.)

White Processed Flour and White Rice. Most pastas, breads, crackers, biscuits, cakes, and other common processed foods, are made with refined white flour. The fiber and most nutrients were removed in processing. Refined white flour lacks fiber and makes problems with your blood sugar. Learn about whole grains that are healthy and good tasting.

Don't be fooled by packaged fast food calling itself whole grain. The product may include little whole grain and more simple sugar, fillers, bad fats, and other common junk-food ingredients. It may be clever marketing, calling the product a name such as "whole bread," which doesn't specify what about it is "whole."

Whole Grains. Like any hearty food, don't overdo grains. Use them more when exercising heavily. Have lighter meals on days when you don't need all the extra fuel.

Instead of packaged cereal with refined sugar and white flour, try quick oats, brown rice, millet, quinoa (KEEN-wah), or other good-tasting breakfast grains. Cook in water (or homemade rice milk, made by putting cooked brown rice in a blender with water). Spice with cinnamon, nutmeg, and fruit, instead of milk, butter and sugar (refer to recipes in Chapter 19).

Instead of white rice, you can use brown rice and wild rice, meaty-tasting lentils, and nutty barley and bulgar wheat (cracked wheat grains). Cook a small amount of these in water or healthy soup stock. Add chopped green vegetables, onions, scallions, chives, leeks, and spices. You will have a meaty-tasting casserole for a main dish. With many grains and greens, you can make interesting, healthy meals differently every day.

Instead of baking with refined white wheat flour, you can use bean flour, rice flour, rye flour, spelt, teff, barley flour, buckwheat, triticale, quinoa flour, and unsweetened carob flour, among many. Use real whole grains instead of white flours. Try non-wheat flours. Not everyone feels well after eating wheat. Celiac is an often-missed cause of joint pain, abdominal bloating, and a serious contributor to osteoporosis. Check for fresh grain, as mold can form, with various health effects. Don't overdo grains, particularly when not exercising.

Fluffy, refined white flour, soft white rice, and skinned vegetables are far from the healthy, fibrous foods that keep your entire body in shape. Eat crunchy food like raw fruit and carrots. Your gums and jaws need exercise to keep them strong and to support your teeth. Tooth loss is an early sign of thinning bones.

Fiber

Fiber used to be called roughage. Fiber is the most complex of complex carbohydrates—so complex that your digestive system can't digest it all. Fiber passes through your system with healthy effects on your lower intestinal tract, digestion in general, and can decrease the risk of diverticulitis and colon cancer.

Fiber is found only in plants, not in meat, poultry, fish, eggs, or dairy. Don't be fooled by certain packaged commercial "whole-grain" products. They may be primarily refined products with some brown coloring and a token amount of whole grain. "Multi-grain" does not mean healthy; it may only be a combination of several bleached, refined products. Some sources worry that fiber is the cause of constipation, digestive pain, and gas. However, the causes are more often unhealthful eating practices and lack of exercise, followed by piling dry food on top of poor health practices.

> White rice and white-flour noodles are part of the "an hour later you're hungry again" phenomenon—stripped of fiber and complex carbohydrate to keep your blood sugar even. Look for brown rice, vegetables, and legumes instead.

Water-soluble fiber reduces cholesterol (refer to Chapter 28). Insoluble fiber in fruit and vegetables is important to digestion and colon-cancer prevention. Both kinds of fiber are frequently found in the same fruit and vegetables. Keep the pulp in juice. The skins of many vegetables, like potatoes, can be healthy and good tasting when prepared well. Don't fry them. Look for brown rice, lentils, and whole foods. Eat apple, kiwi, pear, and potato skins (after good washing). The fiber in whole grains, brown rice, and fruit with the pulp keeps your blood sugar even. Without it, previously healthy food becomes more of a junk sugar than a healthful carbohydrate, and loses most nutrients.

The following is a quick, no-cooking recipe that is high fiber, tastes good, and has healthy protein, complex carbohydrate, and many vitamins. It makes a portable meal or snack. Throw all the following together in a bowl:

Cup or two of cooked black beans
Cup or two of corn
1 jalapeño pepper, diced
1 red onion, chopped
1 red pepper, chopped
2 tablespoons cumin powder
1 bunch fresh cilantro, chopped
salt and pepper to taste
Sprinkle of olive oil, just enough to blend ingredients.
Squeeze 1 fresh lime over the top.

Some people with celiac omit the corn. Celiac causes various discomforts after eating wheat and wheat-related products (which sometimes, but not always, includes corn).

Position Statement of the American Dietetic Association

Recommended intakes, 20 to 35 g/day for healthy adults and age plus 5 g/day for children, are not being met, because intakes of good sources of dietary fiber, fruits, vegetables, whole and high-fiber grain products and legumes are low. Consumption of dietary fibers that are viscous lowers blood-cholesterol levels and helps to normalize blood glucose and insulin levels, making these kinds of fibers part of the dietary plans to treat cardiovascular disease and type-2 diabetes. Fibers that are incompletely or slowly fermented by microflora in the large intestine promote normal laxation and are integral components of diet plans to treat constipation and prevent the development of diverticulosis and diverticulitis. A diet adequate in fiber-containing foods is also usually rich in micronutrients and nonnutritive ingredients that have additional health benefits.

Simple Sugars

A frequent argument is that complex carbohydrates must break down to the same simple sugar in the body so it is no different than eating simple sugar. However, refined, or even unrefined, simple sugars do not have the complex fiber, and variety of nutrients that work together in your body for many health issues and to keep insulin and blood-sugar levels lower, more stable, and healthier. Simple sugars raise blood sugar more than complex carbohydrates.

Save sugar for occasional, not daily use. When you stop eating sugar, you will be surprised that you crave it less. Eating simple refined sugar, common in processed foods, can make you hungry. Eating more simple sugar because you are hungry feeds the cycle.

- Don't buy bags of sugar when grocery shopping.

- In spite of the debate over whether artificial sweeteners are safe, either way they are a dubious habit. Save money and cycles of cravings by refraining from sweetening much food and drink, and get sweets from whole fruit.
- When baking, you don't need to add any sugar. Use mashed fruit. Instead of shortening, use a cooked sweet potato and ground flax seeds or walnuts. Instead of icing, mash apples (no cooking needed) for a topping as sweet as any sugar or syrup, and a better habit for the long run.

Alcohol

When estimating your daily calories, remember that alcohol adds plenty. Each 12-ounce beer is about 150 calories (light beer closer to 100). A two-ounce margarita is about 150 calories. Half a cup of hot buttered rum has 250 calories. A glass of dessert wine can go up to 350 calories. Beer nuts, pretzels, fried chips, and bar and party foods add many junk calories. A cocktail hour can run up an astounding number of forgotten calories. Alcohol is not metabolized as a carbohydrate, even though it is one, so it can't be rationalized as a "sports fuel."

More Simple Things to Try

If you are a beef-and-ale kind of eater, you don't want to be told to give that up and eat raw alfalfa. You don't have to. Simple, easy suggestions follow for making healthy eating a positive habit, not a poor-tasting thing you do because you're told you should, and quit soon after. You don't have to choose between being happy and being healthy. Be both. Happiness is part of good health. For new, healthy eating habits, start with a few of the following suggestions. Then, add others as you can and want.

- Tea and toast (or coffee and Danish) for breakfast won't fuel you and can leave you irritable, lacking energy, with unhealthful rising and falling blood-sugar events, and craving sugary food. Avoid packaged commercial breakfast cereals. They have a high amount of simple sugar and refined flour. Eat complex carbohydrates and protein from real food for breakfast. An easy regular breakfast can be nuts and fresh fruit. For a full breakfast to fuel a strenuous day, a little brown rice left from dinner, or whole oatmeal mixed with raisins or chunks of apple with a little cinnamon can make a hearty hot or cold breakfast cereal.
- Eat the skins of most foods, like apples and potatoes. The fiber makes them more nutritious and keeps blood sugar steadier.
- Try eating larger meals in the morning and afternoon, and smaller meals in the evening. Large evening meals can disturb your sleep and make you have to get up to go to the bathroom. If you can't sleep through the night, try eating earlier and less at night.

- Keep healthy snacks handy, like fruit, small amounts of raisins, or chopped fruit and raw almonds mixed together for before and after exercise. Don't eat many high-calorie snacks when not exercising.
- Avoid fad diets. They are nutritionally unsound and don't work in the long run. You don't lose fat that way, but you will lose important nutrients, water, muscle, bone, and other things you need for health and energy.
- Eat lightly before exercise. Experiment to find foods and time schedules that agree with you.
- Drink water with meals. Add a lemon for taste, Vitamin C (and other vitamins), and better digestion. Drink extra water when exercising, particularly in the heat. Don't overdo.
- Have vegetables as main dishes. If you eat meat, use as small side dishes, not the other way around. Combine different legumes, beans, and small amounts of grains with vegetables for variety, nutrition, and great taste.
- Use seasonings rather than butter or sour-cream dressings. Sauté with a small amount of oil and some balsamic or red wine vinegar instead of thick layers of butter and oil in the pan.
- If you make your own juice, keep the fruit pulp in the juice, rather than throwing it out. In blender drinks, throw in apple slices (for example) with the skins (washed). The complex carbohydrates, vitamins, and fiber in the pulp and skin help keep blood sugar stable. Without the fruit pulp, juices are little more than flavored sugar water. Constantly raising blood sugar above normal levels is not healthy.
- Don't be miserable with your new plan to eat right. Find healthy foods you love. Go over your mindset about living and eating in honest and intelligent ways.
- Good-tasting, healthier recipes are available for unhealthy foods. Take a walk to the bookstore or library for a few fun books.
- Wash commercial fruit and vegetables well to remove chemicals used against insects, foraging animals, and plant diseases. Try growing your own food without chemicals.
- Make your involvement with healthy eating a stress-free one. It makes no sense for your body and mind to be miserable in the name of health. Take a happy approach that leaves you feeling better and excited.
- Be good to yourself with good thoughts and healthful actions—possibly the most neglected healthy habit.

Refined sugar and white flour lack nutrients and fiber, and raise blood sugar and blood fat. For sweets, have fruit and a few raw nuts. Try more vegetables that you like, for the bulk of meals.

How You Eat Is Fitness as a Lifestyle

Make healthy eating an enjoyable lifestyle, not just something to try for a time then stop because you've done it (and hate it). Surround yourself with favorable environmental factors like exercise, clean water, clean air, good friends, good family interaction, and happiness. Avoid smoking, self-medicating with medicines and non-medicinal drugs, perpetually stressful situations, and too much alcohol.

When preparing food, stand straight without rounding your shoulders or jutting your chin forward. Make washing and cutting the food healthy meditative motion. Remember how lucky you are to have food. Choose good food.

Turn off the television while eating. Give thanks for having food, remembering the hardships of others. Turn down seconds. Breathe.

Resources for More Information

American Dietetic Association
www.eatright.org
216 W. Jackson Blvd.
Chicago, IL 60606-6995
1-800-877-1600

Physicians for Responsible Medicine
www.pcrm.org
P.O. Box 6322
Washington, DC 20015
202-686-2210

19

Healthy Weight-Control Habits

Eat less than you think you want; eat with your intelligence, not your stomach. Never get up from the table with an inward, silent apology for being a pig.

—Coco Chanel

Never eat more than you can lift.

—Miss Piggy

Having a necessary amount body fat is helpful for warmth, cushioning, buoyancy in the water, and health. Losing extra weight can benefit your joints, cardiovascular system, general health, and well-being. People of any weight need good nutrition and exercise habits. Good exercise and nutrition habits can become an easy, fun part of your lifestyle with attention and repetition.

You can do many things to lose weight without unhealthful fad diets or eating food you hate. It is not enough to say, "I'll lose 10 pounds by next month." You need to specify to yourself how. Get started by taking a clear look at the way you eat now, and how much activity you get.

It's Not Metabolism

Many false claims are made about metabolism. Metabolism is not the culprit with much weight gain. Are you eating more than in past years, exercising less, doing less, sitting around more, and eating junk food, snack food, fast food, and soda? That approach is not a slow metabolism from aging.

The fact that you burn fewer calories when you decrease activity can be twisted by clever product advertising as "slower metabolism." Don't fall for it. Find fun, healthy things you like to do, and start them again to get the increase in metabolic calorie burning that comes with activity.

Don't fall for pills and supplements advertised to increase metabolism and therefore promote weight loss. Some products contain stimulating compounds that increase heart rate or other functions, which is not helpful or healthy for your body. Many people feel stimulated and happy on these products, and don't notice the nervousness, anxiety, inability to focus, moodiness, difficulty falling asleep at night, and depression which also often occurs. A more serious cycle starts when people take other drugs to try to stop these symptoms—and then more drugs when the first drugs upset their stomach. Exercise will improve your mood and increase your metabolism for weight loss more safely without the negative effects of stimulants and medicines.

Eating food raises metabolism. The increase comes because your body has to do something extra: digestion. You still gain calories from the food and can gain weight if you eat more calories than you burn. Watch out for advertising that exploits the fact of the "thermogenic" (heat-producing or calorie-burning) effect of food. The effect is small compared to the calories you have eaten.

Some devices and pills claim to increase metabolism even after exercise ends. They can claim so because all exercise has that effect—with or without the device or pill. Exercise raises metabolic levels. It takes time after stopping exercise to return to resting level.

On a televised reality show reenacting an 18th-century farming community, one of the participants was removed from the show for medical reasons. His large weight loss worried the people in charge. After exhaustive medical tests, they realized that he had lost his extra weight from the exercise of the farm work and the simple, limited food. According to historical records, the man was normal weight for a farmer of his height in the 1700s.

People in many places in the world walk miles just for the privilege of digging for food and carrying heavy water pots back. That situation gives perspective on Westerners who easily eat much and exercise little, and believe only the most minor contributors to weight gain. Don't spend money on diet pills and expensive exercise devices. Put the money in a jar and go do something active instead. You will burn calories, keep your joints moving, feel better, and save enough to give to the poor with enough left for a vacation.

Change Unhealthful Eating Habits

A 2006 study in Great Britain found that exercise alone won't prevent childhood obesity. The children in one of the groups got exercise, but didn't lose weight because they were eating more calories than they burned. They still received several health benefits of exercise plus important motor skills. However, the message is that if you eat more calories than you need, it can become extra weight, of course. Changing unhealthy eating is needed, too.

More calories than you use each day results in more weight. An easy way to improve weight and health at the same time is to stop eating junk. It is called junk for a reason. Don't give children soda or diet soda any more than you would give them cigarettes. People may say, "You have to let them have a little fun," or, "If I don't let them have a little, they will want it more." Would you say the same about heroin? Antifreeze tastes sweet too, but we teach children not to drink it because it is harmful. Talk to them. Teach them a better way. Set an example of exercising strength by putting away the cookies and shakes. Don't eat the 1000-calorie bag of chips. Do fun exercise with them like catch, skipping rope, tumbling, and fun games you make yourself.

Remember that children can't wait to run away from the table to play, but are made to have the bad habit of sitting still and eating everything on their plate. Don't make them hold still when they can run. These common practices teach them to be sedentary overeaters who have too much pent-up energy to concentrate in school or sleep at night. Let them jump and play after dinner instead of sitting in front of a television. Tell them how happy you are to be together. Sing and smile together while they help you around the house. That approach is fitness and health as a lifestyle.

Some people say they don't have money to eat healthful food, yet spend the same money and more on junk food, supplements, "calming" drugs, and "energy" drinks. Put the money in a jar and exercise instead, and you can lose weight and feel calm plus feed the poor. Sports drinks with refined sugar and stimulant compounds are not healthy for everyday life or for exercise. Eat a banana instead. It is not more time consuming or difficult to steam or sauté in balsamic vinegar and spices instead of fry. It can be fun, not worrisome, to try something that will easily help your health. You don't need to buy a steamer; use any pot. Put any cut washed vegetables that you like in the pot with a small amount of water, balsamic or other cooking vinegar, and seasonings. Put the lid on and the heat will steam them in the seasoned broth. It takes not much more time than it takes to open a can of processed soup with too much salt, fillers, unhealthy fats, sweeteners, and little fiber or vitamins left after processing. The rest of this chapter tells healthy things to do instead of old counterproductive habits.

Chapter 16 tells how to make your own exercise drinks. Fitness as a lifestyle means exercising your brain and sensibilities to prepare and eat healthful food in uplifting ways for real health.

Reduce Fat and Refined Sugar

Reduce extra fat in your diet to reduce unhealthful calories so you can lose weight. Some high-fat diets that result in weight loss because of few total calories; however, it is not a healthful way to lose weight. Eating less saturated fat and trans fat reduces risk of heart disease, diabetes, and some cancers.

According to some studies, cutting back extra fat is a better way to lose weight than cutting only calories. Some of the reasoning for this idea is that your body uses fewer calories to digest fat than it does to digest carbohydrate. The human body is designed to store fat, and more easily stores it when provided directly. It does not mean to eat sugary junk food and refined white flour, which is little more than junk food. Refined flour and sugar products like toast and crackers and cookies can raise your blood fat as much as eating fatty food.

Many foods may be high fat, but because they also have so much sugar, the overall percentage of fat on the label seems low. Don't be fooled. Take a good, hard look at what you eat and where all the extra calories are coming from.

> A low fat percentage on the food label doesn't always mean the item is low in fat. It may be full of fat, but have so many calories from sugar that the proportion is low by comparison.

Make Your Own

Many common prepared "convenience" foods are just not healthy. They also cost more than making your own healthy foods. Making your own food doesn't have to take time. It often can be quicker than stopping for "convenience" foods.

- For a quick breakfast, instead of sugared cereal with milk and a toaster pastry, have fruit and some raw nuts (like walnuts and almonds). People with tree nut and peanut allergy can often eat seeds like sunflower.
- If you want cereal in a bowl, put oats in a bowl, add a few sunflower seeds, walnuts, almonds, or pumpkin seeds, and cinnamon. Pour in hot water and stir. You can add dozens of other healthy things, from homemade almond milk, to apples and bananas, to other quick grains like millet or brown rice. For simple, no-grain breakfast, put fruit pieces in a bowl with raw nuts and some cinnamon.

- For quick meals in a glass, throw water in a blender, and add any combination of hundreds of healthy foods. Add raw nuts, apple slices (with the skin), peeled orange slices, apricots, flax seeds (the blender will mill them), sesame seeds, pumpkin seeds, grapes, carrots, or blueberries. Other flavor possibilities are unsweetened vanilla bean or unsweetened powdered baking cocoa. Make as thick or thin as you like. Drink and go. Pack some in clean, safe containers to go for a lunch drink instead of soda.
- Replace commercial soda with your own. Squeeze a lemon or lime into a glass of carbonated or non-carbonated water. Throw fruit in a blender with a little water. Once blended, add seltzer to the consistency you want.
- Instead of processed peanut butter and refined sugar jelly, put fresh, raw peanuts (or other favorites, like walnuts) in a bowl and crush them for arm exercise with any kitchen pounding tool, or use a chopper, grinder, blender, coffee grinder, or other processor. Crush to powder, depending how chunky you want it. Mash in apple cubes to make moist, creamy sweet peanut butter. Spice with cinnamon if you want. In less than a minute of preparation time, you have a sweet nut butter that you can spread on fruit slices, carrots, and other good foods. Make it portable by stuffing inside raw sweet green and red peppers, in sandwich and wraps (non-grain eaters can make tasty wraps from leafy greens). Use for toppings. Vary the combinations; try almonds mashed with pears, sunflower seeds or walnuts and banana, or sesame seeds and figs. Make with a friend for healthy, social fun. Exercise your imagination for healthy food.
- Make your own sprouts. Put dry mung beans on a shallow plate and cover with water, or use any beans like small red beans, or seeds like clover. Each day or so, rinse the beans and replace the water. They will sprout in a few days. Rinse well and throw in a pan when you sauté vegetables. Season to taste. Eat them when only a few days sprouted for nuttier taste, or wait for longer growth for more vegetable taste.
- Instead of refined-sugar sports drinks, put a peeled whole cucumber into a food processor, mixer, or low-speed blender with a whole kiwi fruit. It will make a sweet, cool, slushy, green drink.
- Make your own sweet drinks by putting a red sweet pepper in any kind of food grinder, masher, or blender. Cut about an inch of fresh ginger root and add through the grinder. In about 30 seconds preparation time, you will have a sweet, cool, red, slushy drink with an exotic tang of ginger. It is healthy and good tasting.

Substitute

Substitute a lower-calorie for a higher-calorie food, and healthy food for junk. When you are about to eat foods full of refined sugar and fat, eat something better instead—an apple, a pear and some walnuts, a roasted, seasoned sweet potato without any junk sauce. Complex carbohydrates used to be called starches and were avoided. We now understand that eating sensible amounts of complex carbohydrates, rather than too much fat and simple sugar, is a key to healthier eating. Main good sources are fruit and vegetables for daily meals. Use moderate amounts of legumes like lentils and whole grains to fuel exercise. Be creative, and find things you like.

For Snacks

- For a cold treat without unhealthy junk food, mash a frozen banana with crushed raw walnuts or flax seeds. Use a food grinder, or get free exercise by mashing them yourself in a bowl. It will taste like creamy ice cream.
- Have raisins and grapes instead of candy. Not too much of these, though, since they are sugary. Brush your teeth after eating raisins. The sugar sticks to your teeth.
- Have bananas with cinnamon instead of banana cake.
- Have an apple and walnuts instead of cinnamon buns or donuts.
- Many brands of fruit-flavored yogurts contain fruit-jam, adding the equivalent of eight or nine teaspoons of sugar per cup. If you eat dairy, use or make plain yogurt, and add your own fresh fruit.
- Try chili powder and other seasonings instead of butter on air-popped popcorn. Use either multispice chili powder seasoning or the ground powder of chili peppers (e.g. chipotle or ancho). Make sure any seasoning you use does not have added sugar, MSG, or additives.
- Have dry-roasted and raw nuts like almonds and walnuts instead of roasted, honey-roasted, or salted nuts. Remember not to sit watching television eating a can of honey-roasted nuts, which can total over 1,000 calories. Don't eat many cups of nuts a day; they are not low calorie, just a healthier food than processed snack food.
- Drink juice with the pulp. Processed grape juice, for example, is a common sweetener put in factory foods to masquerade as "healthy." It is little more than sugar water. Put fruit in a blender or other mixer or grinder with clean water rather than purchase commercial juice.
- Instead of chips, pretzels, and dip at your next party, serve cut sweet peppers; grapes, strawberries, olives, and other easy finger fruit; raw nuts (not honeyed); and cubed, baked sweet potato and roasted or pan-sautéed zucchini. Use chopped hot-pepper salsa and unsweetened applesauce (easy recipe in this chapter) for dip.
- For holiday parties and Halloween giveaways, try bags of oranges and apples, notepads to write thoughts, walnuts in the shell to crack for hand strength, individual-size cans of fun clay to sculpt with, inexpensive eye-hand coordination toys, and other healthful fun treats.

- To make sweet herbal teas, try cinnamon, cloves, grated orange peel, or ginger in hot water.

For Cooking

- Bake, sauté, and steam instead of fry. You don't need to buy a steamer. Put your favorite vegetables in the bottom of any saucepan with an inch or so of water, depending on the pot size. Sprinkle balsamic vinegar, seasonings, and a small amount of olive oil over the top, and put the lid on to steam until tender.
- Put olive oil or grapeseed oil in a misting bottle to make your own non-stick spray, or wipe half a teaspoon of oil around the pan using a towel, brush, or hand.
- Use seasonings instead of butter. Seasonings have antioxidant and other healthful properties. Try packaged, ground seasonings such as curry, ginger, pepper, oregano, and others. Then, try grating fresh ginger root and turmeric using any ordinary hand-held grater. Fresh ginger and turmeric root is available in produce sections many grocery stores. Turmeric is a principle ingredient in curry, and researched for anti-cancer properties, Don't overdo turmeric; just season with it. Try fresh green mint, oregano, basil, and cilantro leaves in vegetables and soup.
- Steam and sauté using soup stock instead of oil; roast and braise in balsamic vinegar and seasonings instead of fat.
- Grind plain sea salt instead of using packaged salt, which often contains chemicals against caking, and other agents. Practice adding and using less salt to meals.
- Use aromatic foods to flavor sauces instead of butter, cream, or cheese. Aromatic foods include tomatoes, onions, garlic, mushrooms, leeks, fresh parsley, thyme, oregano, and basil. Many aromatics have been found to have high antioxidant and other health benefits.
- Refrigerate soups and stocks to separate and congeal the fat, skim it off, and use the skimmed product instead.
- Use whole grains, not white-flour pastas. Use brown and wild rice, not white rice. Don't overdo grains. They are nutrient-dense and best for days of exercise and exertion. Eat less grains when doing less exercise.

For Meals

- Roasting vegetables caramelizes the natural sugar. Roast sweet peppers with onions, mushrooms, and green vegetables. No need to peel the skins. The skins have healthful nutrients. Brush with vinegar or tomato sauce to marinade. Season with any number of healthy seasonings.

- Instead of pouring oil on salad, try balsamic vinegar, pureed cucumbers, seasonings, and hot sauce. Seasoned Japanese rice-wine vinegar tastes sweet and rich enough to seem like oil. Make a vinaigrette with healthy grapeseed oil.
- Instead of cream on a potato, try lemon-pepper seasoning (without MSG or additives), real brewed soy sauce, hot pepper, horseradish, or wasabi. Prepare it so you can eat the skin, too.
- When you cook vegetables, don't use sugar, butter, cream, or sauce. Throw in onion, scallions, chives, shallots, nuts (like sunflower seeds and almonds), and hot peppers, and season with ginger, tamari, garlic, or curry.
- Make brown rice with lentils, peanuts, barley, green beans, peas, onions, or leeks, and hot sauce. Cook rice in fresh peaches with ginger. Cook in unsweetened pineapple and curry. Try tamari sauce. It is different every time.
- Put soft, cooked sweet potato in many foods you want to make sweet—your morning hot cereal, the morning blender drink, afternoon sandwiches, pies, baked goods, rice, or lentils. Make it sweeter with apples or spicy with onions. Don't overdo. Sweet potato still has calories. Don't add sugar glaze or butter. Good for days of high activity.
- You may be surprised how good onions can taste cooked with a sweet vegetable.
- You can do a lot with mangoes. They can sweeten vegetables, both cooked and raw. Mix chili peppers and mashed mango pulp into a sweet and tangy sauce. It is easy and fast.
- Substitute lentil and vegetable dinners for meat. With all the fruit, vegetables, legumes, beans, and grains available, you can eat a different, healthful, good-tasting meal every day.

For Baking

Common baking recipes use large amounts of fat and sugar. Your baking can be sweet and moist without the cholesterol-raising kinds of fat, sugar, or eggs.

- Mash apples, bananas, or soaked prunes and substitute them for most or all oil and sugar. Substitute approximately 1:1 by volume, or experiment on your own.
- Use walnuts milled in your blender or pounded to powder in a bowl, instead of oil and eggs.
- Add a sweet potato instead of oil or sugar for creamy, moist, good taste.
- For icing, spread fresh mashed apples (homemade applesauce) easily made in a bowl using a pounder, or putting fresh apple slices in a blender. Use edible flowers or even (non-edible) real or plastic flowers as decoration instead of icing.

- Instead of taking a cake-decorating class, take a decorative-vegetable-carving class, or get a book and try your own.

For Desserts

- For sweet desserts, try fruit and frozen, whole-juice popsicles instead of pie and ice cream. Make your own whole juice in a blender instead of drinking sugar water in commercial juices. For a simple dessert, chew fresh green mint leaves.
- Quickly make your own applesauce without added sugar or syrup. Cut apples into manageable cubes and mash them in a bowl to get exercise, or put whole apples into a grinder. Add cinnamon or nutmeg. Use over oatmeal instead of sugar, and over fruit for dessert and snacks.
- Make baked apple with cinnamon instead of sugar or honey. It will be sweet.
- Instead of ice cream, it is quick and easy to make your own frozen dessert. Add a scoop of unsweetened, undutched baking cocoa to a frozen mashed banana and crushed walnuts for a healthy sweet wonderful treat that tastes better than you would expect. For exotic flavor and more health benefit, add fresh grated ginger root. Real unsweetened cocoa (not processed, sweetened, chocolate candy) is a healthful food. It contains theobromine, an antioxidant, weak diuretic, stimulant, and mood booster. Compounds in cocoa open breathing airways and relieve coughing. Dark chocolate has more theobromine than lighter chocolate, with flavonoids and phenolics, plant substances that are good for the heart. People who get a kind of vascular headache called migraine do better not to eat chocolate.
- Substitute talking with your friends, or stretching, or appreciating the dinner centerpiece instead of eating dessert.
- Dessert does not have to be simple sugar and fat. Something can be good for you and still be a treat.

More ideas for healthy substitutes can be found in Chapter 18.

Don't Go Hungry

It is not true that dieting makes you fat because you get hungry and eat more. If you eat more, that is your decision. The idea is to be happy eating healthful things, not to be hungry and unhappy. Eating junk food and eating too frequently can keep insulin levels too high in the body, which is not healthy and can make you feel you want to eat. Relax and enjoy changing to healthier habits. Stand up straight over the counter with shoulders back to cut sweet peppers for snacks, instead of hunching over a bag of chips.

Don't just eat "low-fat" cakes, cookies, and sweets. They are full of simple sugar, which will make you hungry within a few hours—usually sooner. Get protein from nuts, seeds, grains, vegetables, and legumes like lentils.

Eat Less Simple Sugar

"Simple" or "refined" sugar is just about everywhere in prepared foods. The label may say "no sugar," "natural," or "organic," but don't be fooled. They can be full of refined "empty-calorie" sweeteners, like dextrose, high-fructose corn syrup, maltose, grape juice, rice syrup, galactose, and in refined flour products in crackers, biscuits, bread, and other processed foods that don't list added sugar.

Eat complex carbohydrates like fruit, red peppers, and brown rice for snacks instead of candy. Don't eat donuts and Danish or packaged cereal for breakfast. When you stop eating sugar, a magic thing happens—you crave less. Keep a list if you have to, to see what you eat every day. Find out where all the extra sugar you eat is coming from. You will save money and your health by not buying prepared snack foods. They are not good for you.

Don't buy candy or cakes or keep them in the house. They are refined sugar and hydrogenated fat. Don't give them to children. It is not parental love. It is the same as giving them cigarettes or addictive drugs. Change that. Parental love is giving them beautifully functioning, self-control brain centers.

Be Prepared

Food away from home at fast-food places, restaurants, the workplace, public events, and snack machines are high fat, high sugar, high calorie, and low nutrition. Go prepared. Pack fruit, sliced sweet peppers, and nuts to snack on, so you don't wind up with fries, shakes, and candy. Pack a brown rice and lentil lunch (cooked without oil or cream sauces) mixed with vegetables and seasonings, rather than oil.

Avoid most commercial sports nutrition bars and drinks. They are no more than candy with a sporty name. Sports bars and drinks are not magic energy potions; they are regular food, and often junk food, in a wrapper. Chapter 16 tells how to make your own sports bars and drinks. This chapter provides guidelines for more easy food to make on your own that is cheaper and healthier.

Improve Your Mindset

A better body and spirit come more from healthful movement in daily life than from an eating disorder. Stop eating junk soda and candy because you want to be healthier, and to practice having control, instead of acting on every impulse.

It is not being a good parent to give young children candy any more than it is being a good parent to give them cigarettes. To be a good parent, give them self control and good self-image though healthy lifetime habits.

Involve the People You Cook For

If you cook for people who don't eat healthful meals or understand about healthy eating, involve them. Learn together about good-tasting, healthy food and how to prepare it. Have them find things on their own that they want to try. Learn to cook together in fun cooperation. It is healthier than isolating yourself and feeling burdened by people who don't cooperate or understand. Young children need the life-skill-building practice of learning to choose good vegetables and to wash and prepare them in healthy ways.

Make It Easy

It seems easier to reach into the refrigerator or cupboard and pull out a cookie or cake than take the time to fix a healthy meal. Have healthy food ready and easy to get to. Keep a bowl of fruit handy. Keep a container of cut vegetables within easy reach. Get and make healthy snacks ahead of time for when you know you will eat impulsively, and put them on the top shelf of the refrigerator and in the front of your cupboards. Get rid of unhealthful food in the refrigerator and cupboards.

Make It Healthy

Instead of hunching shoulders and rushing to get the cooking done, straighten, breathe, and use each stroke of washing and cutting as a relaxation or meditation. While standing to prepare food at the counter, don't slouch over the counter. Put your shoulders back with chin loosely in and your back held in neutral spine (refer to Chapter 22). Even if you need to hurry to prepare and cook, remember to be happy that you are fortunate enough to have things to prepare and cook. Don't ruin it with paying to put unhealthful food in your body.

Think Long Term

Food items are not worked off in single death bouts. Don't become discouraged if your body is not remade by the end of a week or a month. Small, daily calorie expenditures multiply over time. An easy 150-calorie-a-day walk translates into about 15 pounds a year. It works both ways—one extra 150-calorie-a-day piece of candy can mean you weigh 15 pounds more in one year. Think of the benefits of the walk plus not having the junk food. Make walking work for you with slow, steady reduction that does not tax your system. Slow weight loss is more likely to stay off, is easier on your heart, and spares bone and muscle.

Check for Extra Calories You Don't Need

For people who think they don't eat much and don't feel their weight reflects calories eaten, or think they don't eat unhealthy food, one way to check is keeping a list over a week or so.

- Count small amounts. You can cut many calories by not tasting foods as often when you cook, not licking icing from spoons, or not "just" breaking off halves of cookies to snack throughout the day. It can add up to hundreds of calories each day.
- Alcoholic drinks can add several hundred calories, plus hundreds more from bar snacks.
- Remember soda when you tally calories. Drinking soda is not healthy, whether diet brand or not. You don't need to harm your body in that way.
- Gum, mints, and small candies can have 10 to 15 calories each. It doesn't sound like much until you remember you eat a few dozen a day. Give some thought on why you have to keep your mouth moving so much of the time. Create more peace in your body. For better breath and stopping dry mouth, chew fresh green mint leaves or fennel seeds.
- Eighteen calories for a teaspoon of sugar doesn't sound like much until you count up all the two-packs in several coffees and teas a day. Milk, honey, and creamers add hundreds more.
- A big bag of chips, caramel corn, snack crackers, or cheese curls has over 1,000 calories, as does a can of roasted nuts. This amount accounts for more than half the calories most people need in a day.
- Trail mix and granolas are deliberately made to be high-calorie to sustain extended efforts in difficult terrain. They are not a low-calorie food or a food for daily life or regular snacks in a sedentary day. Half a cup of granola usually has over 200 calories. A big bowlful can have three to four times that. Adding milk or milk substitutes can add up to a 1,000-calorie snack. Many granolas are not healthful snacks; they contain refined flour and sugar. It is usually better to have fruit and nuts.
- Salad bars often have vegetables with large quantities of dressing and mayonnaise. Add cheese, croutons, nuts, olives, bacon bits, meats, and the like, and you can easily eat 3,000 calories in a single meal.
- Sports bars average 200 to 300 calories. They don't make you healthy or able to do sports just by eating them. Eating several is more than you need for exercise.
- Don't eat unhealthy foods thinking they are healthful for containing a little fruit or vegetables. Packaged fruit cups are full of sugar and syrup. French fries are not good for you, even though they are made from potatoes.

- Stop snacking while watching television.
- Sometimes all it takes to lose the 10 or 20 pounds you want is to cut out one regular bedtime snack. Stopping just one 300- to 400-calorie-a-night snack will make a large difference.

Remember That "Diet Food" Is Food

Foods labeled as "diet food" are not magic potions that remove fat and calories from your body. They do not make you thinner by the action of eating them. They are food. Regular food. They have calories. Many have high sugar and fat content. They can make you fat if you eat too much of them.

What about meal replacement drinks? They also do not remove fat from your body just by drinking them. They are called "meal replacers" because you have one instead of anything else. You eat nothing else at all for that meal. Then you don't snack or sneak food before the next meal. It is better to learn healthy eating habits. Have real meals that have fiber and all the combined nutritional components that can't come in a can. Use a meal replacer when you are rushing somewhere and are really missing a meal. Don't have it in addition to your other meals as a snack. The extra calories will store as fat.

Increase Physical Activity

A major factor in becoming overweight is a sedentary lifestyle. If you reduce activity enough to gain only one pound per year, think how much heavier you will be in 20 years. Think about only two pounds per year. You will probably not notice these gains on a day-to-day basis. Small things add up. Responsible plans for long-term weight loss include exercise. Exercise, in almost all cases, is a healthier, more effective weight-loss method than starving yourself. A University of California study found that most of those people able to remain slimmed down were those who started exercising regularly.

If you think that not having time to exercise is the problem, you have good news. Thinking that your life and your health are two separate things is the problem. You don't have to stop your life to get exercise.

Some people prefer organized exercise classes. They will drive to a gym and take the elevator to an exercise class, but hate to go out for a walk. They may not be getting the functional movement that develops their body in the way it needs for real-life movement. You do not need a gym or special clothes or equipment to get aerobic or weight-lifting exercise. It is more "natural," now called "functional" exercise, to get healthy exercise outside of a gym.

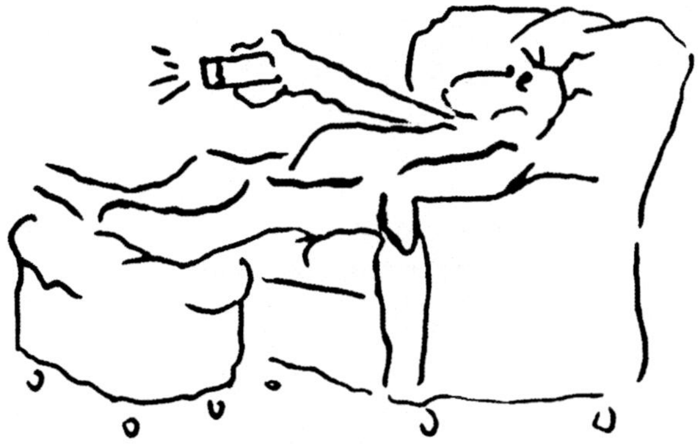

Figure 19-1. A major cause of becoming overweight is inactivity.

For both active and resistance exercise indoors and out, remember that daily healthful movement easily accumulates from your healthy bending, balancing while dressing, taking the stairs, and other daily, real-life movement. Find an activity you like anyway, such as going to a dance club, bicycling, or walking. Bend correctly for all the hundreds of times a day you need to bend. Make your life active. Try all kinds of things until you find something you love to do.

The modern inactive life goes against developmental human history and the design of the human body to be active. Going to a gym today is only a substitute for a natural active life.

- See if you would like to commute by bicycle, where feasible, to work, or various errands. Grocery shop by bike, and use a backpack or bike baskets to carry home groceries. If not as much fits on the bike as the car, then you will spend less money and eat less. Maybe you will make more frequent trips by bike for more exercise.
- Improve your legs on the stairs instead of only waiting for escalators and elevators You may beat the elevator.
- Go outdoors for a break every day that you can, for fresh air, sunshine, and fun movement. Instead of a smoking break, or donut-and-Danish break, take a walk-and-stretch break, and have an orange and some raw almonds. Bend properly all day. You probably bend hundreds of times daily for the files, the trash can, to jot a message while standing, to pick up mail, or any number of other things. Bending over at the waist is terrible on your back. Use your legs, keep your torso upright, and burn calories with every bend. Get free bending and spiritual exercise by cleaning your closets to donate clothing and household items to give warmth and help someone in need.

- Have fun—skate, bowl, cycle, walk, go dancing, work on your gardening, shoot hoops, take food to shut-ins and get them moving too, with improvised exercise of moving arms and legs, clapping, singing, and having fun.

The human body was designed for activity and was active through the eons. In much of the "developing world" today, people commute by bicycle, regularly lift and carry loads, and sit and rise from the floor often. Modern life became inactive, bringing diseases of inactivity with it. Going to the gym is just a substitute (and often a poor one) for having an activity level that seems to be programmed into the human body for health. With practice, you can find activities that are fun and do them often until they become a natural, healthy part of your life.

Being more active is important to weight control. Find ways to be more active as part of everyday life.

For attractive lips, speak words of kindness.
For lovely eyes, seek out the good in people.
For a slim figure, share your food with the hungry.

—Audrey Hepburn

Make It Fun

When you make a list of all the unhealthful food you eat, and how little you move as part of your real, daily lifestyle, weight gain is no longer a mystery to blame on metabolism or minor factors. Take a moment to breathe and think. Reflect on life as a brief gift, rather than something to harm through neglectful, undisciplined habits. Be excited about changing to good things. Don't just call it a diet to have to "stick to," but the way you want to live a quality life.

Eat healthfully and increase daily activity level by making common lifetime activities part of your exercise. Controlling weight without diets can become easy, safe, good feeling, and fun lifetime habits.

Resources for More Information

The Fitness Fixer
www.Healthline.com/blogs
Regular online health column for changing exercise and daily life to healthier ways

How to Control Your Weight

- *Reduce Fat and Refined Sugar.* You get too much fat and sugar in obvious ways, like fried food, rich desserts, and high-fat dairy products. You can also get too much fat and sugar in ways you don't always notice—in sauces, salads, packaged convenience food and snacks, and added to vegetables.
- *Make Your Own.* Homemade food is healthier and cheaper than "convenience" foods, and it can be quick and easy to make. It produces less litter, too.
- *Substitute.* Substitute good-tasting, healthy foods for unhealthy ones. Be creative, and find foods you like.
- *Eat Less Simple Sugar.* Stopping refined sugar and refined flour products is a factor in stopping food cravings.
- *Be Prepared.* Pack healthy food to take with you to places that have only unhealthy food.
- *Improve Your Mindset.* Check your ideas about what you think is healthful and why.
- *Make It Easy.* Have healthy food ready and easier to get to than junk food when you know you will eat impulsively.
- *Lose Real Fat Weight.* Rapid-loss fad diets concentrate on losing water and muscle. Steady weight loss with more movement and less bad food will reduce body fat weight, is easier on your heart and skin, and spares bone and muscle.
- *Check for Extra Calories You Don't Need.* Sometimes all it takes to lose the 10 or 20 pounds you want is to cut out idle snacking, foods that are terrible for you anyway, and late-night extra meals.
- *Remember That "Diet Food" Is Food.* It does not make you thinner by eating it. It makes you fat if you eat too much of it.
- *Increase Physical Activity.* A major factor in becoming overweight is a sedentary lifestyle.
- *Make It Fun.* Make your new, healthy lifestyle a fun one so you live it as a real life to enjoy, rather than making it something to do, and then stopping as soon as you can.
- *Eat More Slowly.* Put your fork or spoon down between bites. Breathe. Eat less.
- *Turn Off the Television.* Enjoy the quiet, or have a meaningful conversation with friends and loved ones over dinner.
- *Bend and Lift Properly.* Do you damage your back and knees all day, every day with bad, bent-over bending? Instead, you could burn hundreds of calories and exercise their legs by lifting with torso upright and knees bent. Examples include getting things out of the refrigerator, desks, low shelves, and closets; tying shoes; picking up mail, babies, papers, and laundry; vacuuming; making beds; leashing pets; and countless others.

Part III

HEALTH

When it comes to your health, I recommend frequent doses of that rare commodity among Americans, common sense.

—Vincent Askey

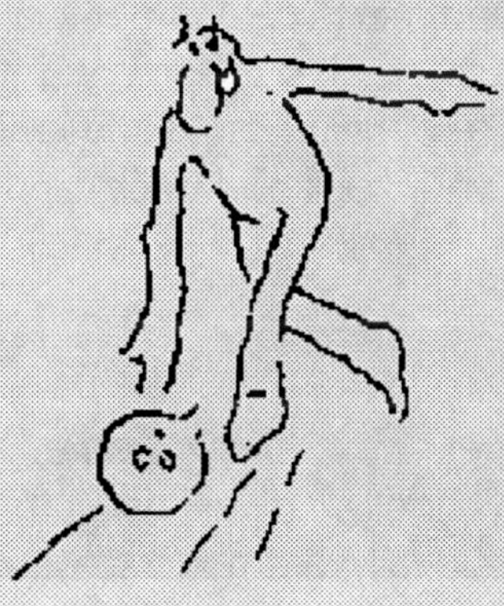

20

Back and Neck Pain—Why?

We sit at breakfast, we sit on the train on the way to work, we sit at lunch, we sit all afternoon...a hodgepodge of sagging livers, sinking gall bladders, drooping stomachs, compressed intestines, and squashed pelvic organs.

—John Button, Jr.

Although often thought to be a mysterious, permanent, unavoidable condition, back and neck pain are usually easily treated and easily prevented. Surgery is not necessary. This chapter will show you how to easily and quickly spot and stop the source of pain using sports-medicine techniques. Then, you no longer will get the pain, and your back and neck can heal.

An Injury, Not a Condition

"Upper crossed syndrome," "sacroiliac syndrome," disc disease, facet syndrome, swayback, a lower back that hurts with walking or running, or just "goes out" occasionally, are not diseases or conditions, nor are they caused by overuse. They are not genetic, or the way your skeleton is made, and they are not permanent. They do not require medicine, surgery, special devices, or treatments to fix.

The majority of neck and back pain is from bad movement mechanics that you do every day without knowing it. It is not true that once you have back pain you will be subject to lifetime bouts. Just as you heal after a sprained ankle or broken arm, you can heal from back pain and resume your normal life. Even if you have structural problems of arthritis, scoliosis, pain syndromes, things not being where they should, or other diseases, the same unhealthful daily movement habits that cause and worsen pain can be easily stopped.

> Someone who breaks their leg would not go around year after year saying they have a "leg condition." Back pain is an injury that can be treated, not a "condition" that cannot be changed.

Your Interesting Parts

Following are some quick vocabulary terms to help understand back pain.

Your Spine Bones. The bones of your spine are called vertebrae. The top seven vertebrae are your neck bones, called cervical vertebrae. Their names are C1 (from the top) down to C7. The biggest bump you can feel at the bottom of your neck is usually C7. Your next 12 vertebrae are thoracic vertebrae (T1 to T12). Your rib bones attach to these vertebrae, 12 on each side. Both men and women have 12 pairs of ribs, 24 total. The next five vertebrae do not have ribs attached. These vertebrae are your lower-back bones, the lumbar vertebrae (L1 to L5). Much back pain and disc injury occurs in these vertebrae because it is the place that is pushed outward the most the most when people sit and bend improperly. Below the lumbar vertebrae are your five sacral vertebrae (S1 to S5), fused into a single bone, the sacrum. The sacrum forms the bony back wall of your hip and lower back. When you stand with this area tipped forward instead of neutral position, the area can ache. No mystery. Attached to the bottom of your sacrum is the coccyx, your tailbone.

Your Discs. Discs are fibrocartilage cushions that sit like washers between bones in several areas of your body. The discs you hear about most often sit between each of your vertebrae. These intervertebral discs cushion shocks transmitted through your spine with every step, and prevent your vertebrae from rubbing directly against each other.

You also have discs in other areas of your body. Tiny discs cushion the joint between your head bone, called the temporal bone, and your lower jawbone, called the mandible. Sometimes, these little discs wear out from bad use, causing pain at the joint between them, the temporomandibular joint (TMJ). You have two larger discs, called menisci (singular is meniscus), in each knee. Injuring a meniscus is one cause of knee pain.

The discs most often involved in lower-back pain are your vertebral discs between L4 and L5, and between L5 and S1. The disc between lumbar vertebrae numbers four and five is called L4-L5. The disc between lumbar vertebra number five and sacral vertebra number one is called L5-S1. When you bend incorrectly and sit slouched, most of the leverage goes onto L4-L5 and L5-S1, instead of onto your leg muscles.

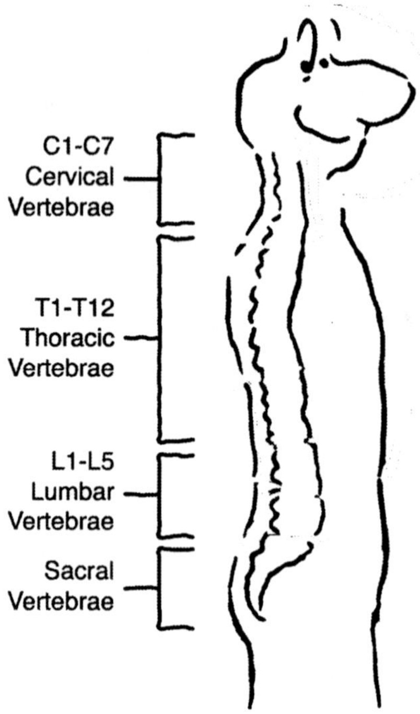

Figure 20-1. You normally have seven neck vertebrae (cervical); 12 upper-back vertebrae (thoracic); five lower-back vertebrae (lumbar); five sacral vertebrae fused into the bony back wall of your pelvis; and your small tailbone or coccyx, made of several fused rudimentary vertebrae.

Disc and Muscle Pain

If you do nothing more than stand and bend forward (bend incorrectly), you put hundreds of pounds of force on each vertebral disc, the most on L4-L5 and L5-S1. Twisting when you lean adds more damaging force. You have many opportunities to bend improperly while doing those things: picking up packages and children, lifting things out of cars and trunks, making beds, taking out the trash, doing laundry, doing crunches and Pilates exercise, stretching to touch toes in yoga class, retrieving bags at the airport baggage claim—many times during every day.

> The pressure of your own body weight on your muscles and discs over several years of poor posture is enough to injure your back as badly as a single accident.

Lifting weight, by itself, is not bad for you. Lifting properly is good for you. Even carrying loads, bags, backpacks, and shoulder bags is not the problem. Lifting and carrying with unhealthful mechanics is what injures. Your back is tough. Lifting and carrying improperly takes years to do enough damaged to begin pain "suddenly." Chronic bad positioning and slouching while standing, bending, and sitting can injure your back and neck over years as badly as a single accident. Good bending and not rounding when sitting is beneficial lifestyle exercise (refer to Chapter 8).

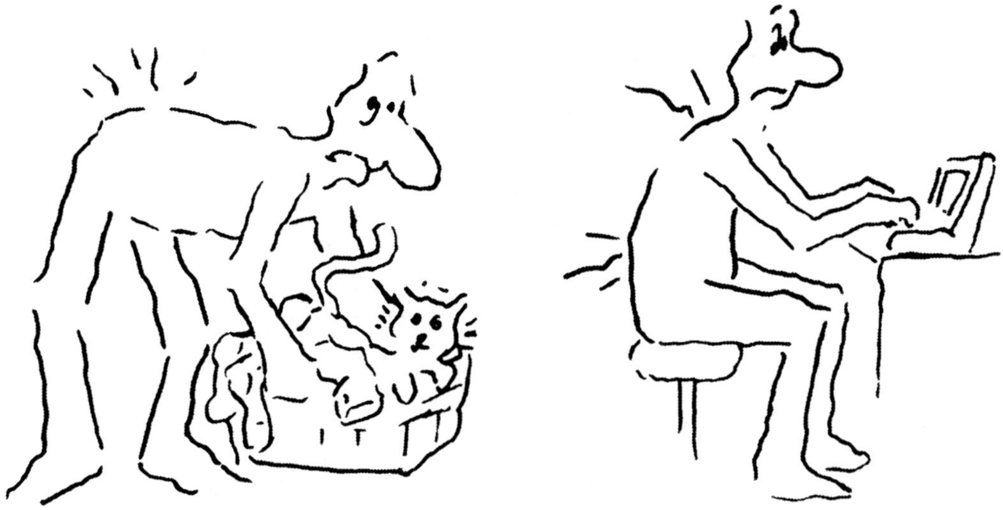

Figure 20-2. Improper forward bending.

The lower back is supposed to have a small inward curve. Bending forward reverses it so that you curve forward instead, like the letter "C." This bad posture is called lumbar flexion. Flexion is the action of bending a joint. Bending your elbow is elbow flexion. Putting your chin toward your chest is neck flexion. You do hip flexion when you bend forward at the hip or raise your leg. Genuflection (*genu* is the Latin word for "knee") is the term for bending a knee in church. Knee flexion is knee bending any other time. Sitting, standing, and lifting with a rounded back instead of maintaining the normal inward curve of your lower back is lumbar flexion.

Too much lumbar flexion squeezes and pushes your discs outward toward the back. The disc may eventually fray and give out like a worn tire. Discs are not like jelly donuts, as often said. They are tough. It takes years to break down (degenerate) a disc from bad habits. Bad rounded sitting, and continuous bad bending over for the hundreds of times you bend in a day around the house, job, and gym squeezes the discs outward toward the back each time, like squeezing toothpaste. Moreover, chronically holding back muscles, or any muscles, in a stretched position weakens them.

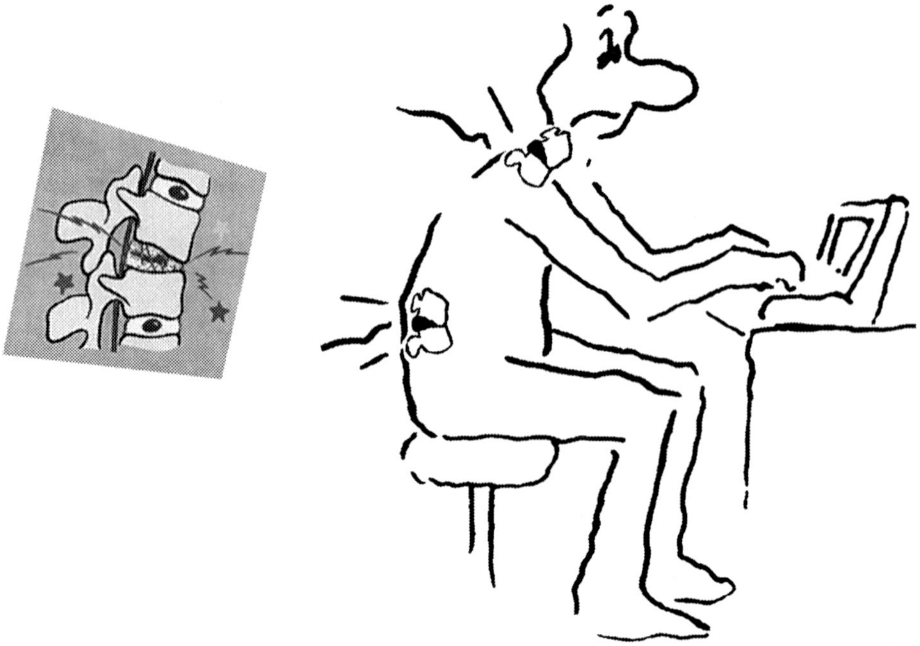

Figure 20-3. Too much spinal flexion, over years, physically breaks down discs (degenerates them), and moves discs outward, an injury process called slipping, bulging, or herniating.

Discs don't usually protrude straight back. Their path is blocked by a long, tough, vertically-running ligament called the posterior longitudinal ligament. It is good that their path is blocked because your spinal cord lies behind the discs. It also means that discs are likely to push out sideways. The long nerves serving your legs also exit your lumbar vertebrae to the side. When a disc bulges against these nerves, pain extends down your leg. One common nerve to be pushed on by bulging discs is the sciatic nerve. The sciatic nerve has both sensory and motor functions, meaning that if compressed, it will hurt down the back of the leg and can reduce the function of your leg. Compression of other nerves can make tingling and numbness in the front of the thigh. This injury can heal when you stop the bad movements that cause it. Occasionally, a disc can protrude backward against the spine, reducing or disrupting ability to move from that level down. In the most serious cases, control of bowel and bladder is affected. Continuous back flexion overstretches the long ligament down the back of your spine, weakening the back and allowing discs more room to protrude. Even these problems can be stopped with stopping the cause of poor positioning and doing some of the techniques in Chapter 21, giving it a chance to heal.

Neck Pain, Upper-Back Pain, and Upper Crossed Syndrome

Letting your upper body slouch so that your head tilts forward of your body is called a forward head. A forward head contributes to upper-back pain, pain between the shoulders, around the shoulder blade, and may also radiate down the arm and cause hand numbness. It is easily reversible. Although often given fancy and frightening names like "upper crossed syndrome," it is just mechanical pressure from slouching the head and neck forward, pressing on the structures within. The forward head can also make the middle and lower back hurt.

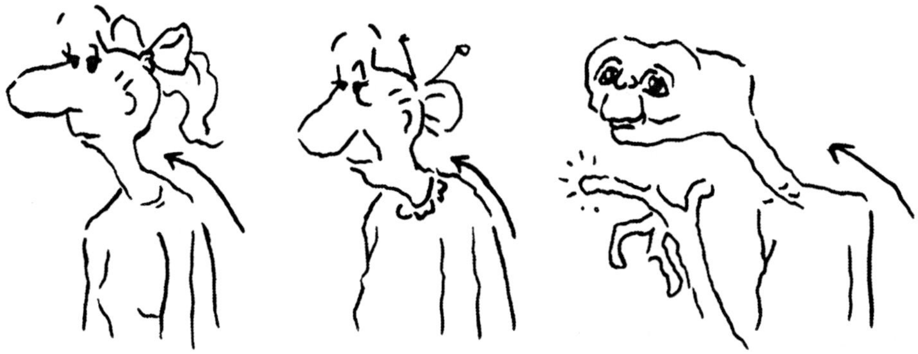

Figure 20-4. A bad position called the "forward head" is the major course of upper-back and shoulder pain and pain radiating down the arm. It is a poor posture that can be easily stopped, which quickly stops the pain.

The forward head can contribute to shoulder trouble. The forward-head posture brings the top of the shoulder bone over the top of the arm bone, limiting overhead reaching, and, over time, contributing to shoulder impingement problems. Pain and numbness can radiate down the arm to the hand. Each time you raise your arm with your head forward, you can compress your rotator cuff, contributing to injury over time.

A forward head can make you look older. A forward head is so common that it looks normal, and is just about taken for granted in older people. However, it is a posture that can be avoided.

Preventing this slouching posture prevents the cause of the pain. Taking medicine, getting shots, and using heating pads and special pillows do not treat the cause. Being too tight to stand straight is common, covered in Chapter 6 on stretching. Chapter 21 gives simple things to do to make straight upright neck and head positioning comfortable and normal.

Sacroiliac Pain, Overarching, Hyperlordosis, Swayback, and Pain With Long Standing, Walking, and Running

The main cause of lower-back pain after long standing, walking, running, reaching overhead, and carrying loads is allowing your lower back to exaggerate the normal inward curve. Too much arching, called hyperlordosis or swayback, is not an anatomical condition. It is just a bad way of standing. Both men and women can stand with too much arch in the lower back.

One way to overarch is to stand with the hip bent forward at the crease where the legs meet the body (Figure 21-6, middle and right). Tipping the hip forward in front and out in back is not standing straight. Another way to overarch the lower spine is leaning back to try to offset or balance a carried or lifted load (Figure 20-5). Both kinds of overarching are bad body mechanics, not an unavoidable structural adaptation. Many people lean the upper body backward instead of pulling their shoulders back when trying to straighten their upper body. Overarching does not cancel out problems from excess flexion, but creates much back pain of its own. Often, people who sit and bend with too much back flexion also stand excessively arched. The next chapter shows how to stand without overarching when lifting, walking, and carrying, which stops the pain of overarching. Too much arching irritates the soft tissue and joints called vertebral facets, where each vertebra attaches to the one above and below it.

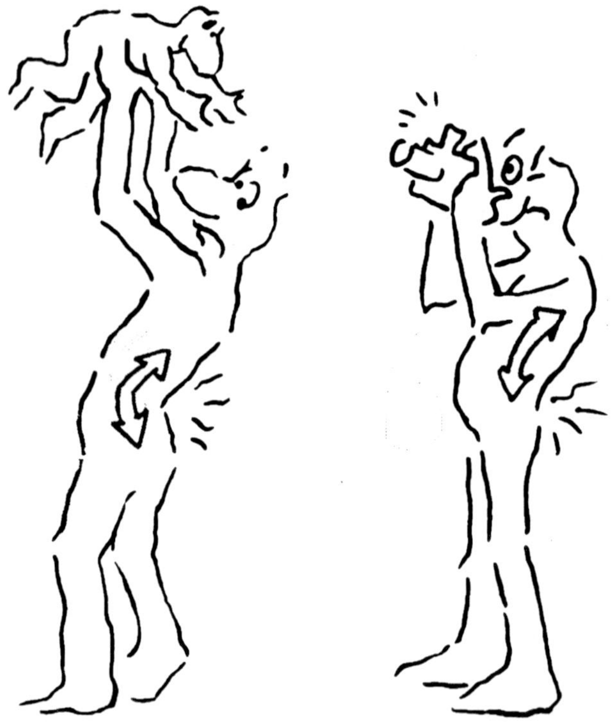

Figure 20-5. Tipping the hip out in back (left) and leaning the upper body backward (right) both increase the inward curve of the lower back. Overarching (hyperlordosis) is a poor posture that is a major cause of mystery lower-back pain during long standing, walking, and running, and sports done with much overhead arm motion. It is not a structural problem, just a slouching posture that can be easily stopped.

An Average Day of Making Your Back and Neck Hurt

You wake up and sit at the edge of the bed, curled in back and neck flexion. You then slouch over to the sink and bend over the sink. You lean your upper body backward while brushing and washing your hair, creating lower-back hyperlordosis. You bend over, twist, and lift to make the bed. You get dressed bending over while sitting. You sit curled forward in lumbar and neck flexion in a chair for breakfast, and again in the car or public transit to work, or curled over handlebars if commuting by bicycle, jutting your chin forward. You sit in flexion at work and during lunch. From your chair, you lean over, twist, and yank open file cabinets. You crane your neck forward at your desk to view the computer monitor. If your computer monitor is in the usual low position on your desk, you hold your head both forward and down, with your chin jutting forward. You stand, walk, and carry packages with excess lower-back arching (and forward head). You reach overhead for shelves by leaning backward, increasing the arch in your lower back. You pick up boxes by bending over incorrectly, and then lift them overhead by arching your lower back. You commute home, sitting in flexion. You sit in flexion at dinner, in front of the sink, and in a rounded chair or couch in front of the TV with your head craned forward. You bend improperly to pick up and carry the kids. You hold them with an overarched lower back while standing. You use flexion to tuck them in. You add chronic bad lifting mechanics during house and yard work.

> Just as smoking one cigarette at a time eventually can cause much trouble, you can gradually accumulate back pain from bad daily habits without knowing it.

If you had gone to the gym, you might have added the large number of conventional gym and fitness exercises that add to the problem of overflexion and overarching under load: abdominal crunches, weight lifting while leaning over; straight-leg dead lifting, touching toes from a stand, many Pilates exercises, rowing with a rounded back, swinging elbows down to opposite knees, repetitive back arching, like "donkey kicks" and "bird-dogs" that swing the leg overhead from a hands-and-knees position, lifting weights overhead while overarching your lower back, and curling over stationary bicycle handlebars with your head forward and back rounded.

It does not mean you should never get vigorous exercise. With good body mechanics, you can do more than before, without injury. Healthy ways are demonstrated in Chapter 6 on stretching, Chapter 7 on abdominal muscles, Chapter 8 on lifestyle exercise, and Chapter 9 on changing bad exercises into good ones.

What About Backpacks and Shoulder Bags?

Wearing backpacks and shoulder bags is not the problem in back pain. Most of the pain comes from how you lift them and how you stand when you carry them. A paper on "Asymmetrical Loads and Lateral Bending of the Human Spine" in the July 1993 issue of *Medical & Biological Engineering & Computing* reported that bags worn over one shoulder curl your spine slightly. The researchers concluded that such unequal forces contribute to the high percentage of school children turning up with scoliosis. They suggested switching to knapsacks to distribute the load. However, you do not have to curl your shoulder to carry a bag. Stand straight and you will not get the problems of curling, plus you will get the abdominal and core muscle work of holding straight against the load of the bag.

For anyone, child or adult, pain is not because of the bag; it is because of letting your posture sag. Stand upright instead of hunching forward or arching and leaning backward. Don't curl or lean to the side or hike your shoulder up. Stand right against the load. You could burn calories, and get an abdominal and back workout by simply holding good positioning against the pull of the bag, no matter where you wear it.

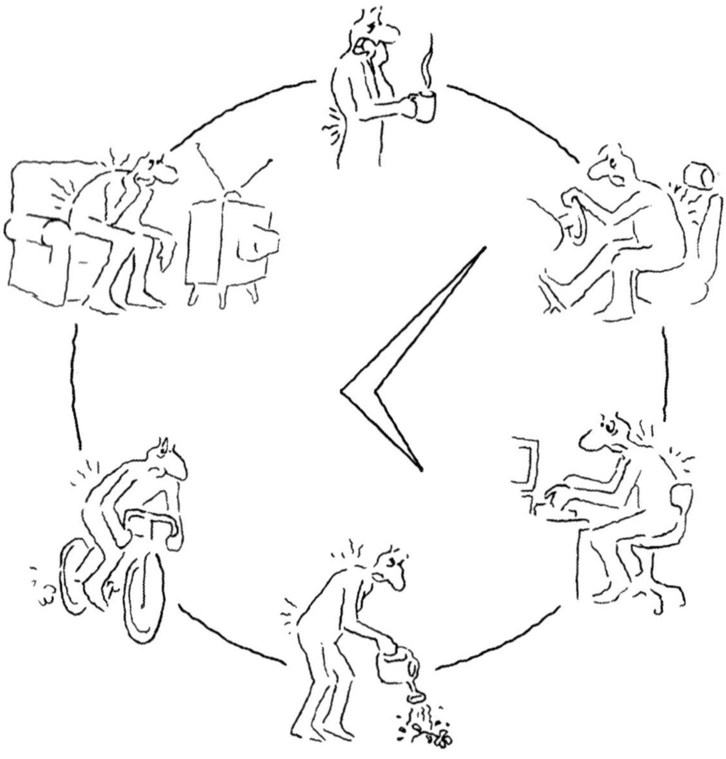

Figure 20-6. An average day of ruining your back with poor positioning and movement mechanics starts in the morning and goes on all day, every day for many people.

Do Not Reduce Activity

Unfortunately, once the back and neck begin to hurt, people are more likely to reduce activity or give up active movement that keeps them healthy, while they continue sitting, and bending with a rounded back, and standing with too much arch—major back-injury-producing actions. A particularly sad sight is back pain patients in doctor and physical-therapy waiting rooms, sitting in lumbar flexion and bad neck posture and worsening their condition while they sit, then increasing the flexion injury by doing abdominal crunches, and increasing the hyperlordosis injury by overarching the back to do leg lifts and other exercise.

Check the Medicines You Take

Not all pain is from unhealthful positioning and bad exercise. Common medications cause a large amount of serious pain. It used to be thought that muscle and joint pain was a small and minor side effect of common medications, only occurring with toxic doses. It is now known that major pain syndromes are common.

Main medicines that can result in body aches, muscle pain, chest pain, and joint pain include classes of the following: statin drugs for cholesterol, medicines for blood pressure, allergy, stomach acid, anxiety, depression, sleep disorders, erectile dysfunction, constipation, and irritable bowel, certain heart drugs, the antibiotics erythromycin and clarithromycin, some HIV medications, cancer medicines, and several others. Even medicines for pain, if taken often, can result in rebound pain.

Doing a few stretches or repositioning will not take away the pain these drugs cause. It is not necessary to suffer pain and injury as a result of health care. Look at the cause of the problem and fix it so that you do not rely on unhealthful drugs. It is often more straightforward and attainable than it seems.

The Major Causes of Pain Are Not Mysterious and Are Easy to Fix

This overview shows that most back pain is not mysterious, but simple mechanics that you can easily change. Although you may have specific back conditions (like arthritis, stenosis, or scoliosis), the bad habits described here increase anyone's risk of pain and injury.

> The pull of bad posture habits all day, every day on your back and neck will eventually reshape them, just like braces on your teeth. Only the result is not pretty or healthy.

Like braces on your teeth, the continuous pull of bad posture habits on your back and neck will eventually reshape your body—in unhealthy ways. Common gym exercises train bad bending and movement habits. They contribute to tightness in front of the body and overstretch back muscles until healthful standing and bending is not normal, or even comfortable. It is not just lifting wrong one day. The effects are cumulative, like smoking. Then, one day you bend wrong one more time to pick up a sock, and your back has had enough. It is no mystery. It does not require surgery or months of exercises and therapy to fix. As soon as you change bad bending, standing, and sitting, you should feel the difference. Chapter 21 tells what to try.

Resources for More Information

Fix Your Own Pain Without Drugs or Surgery
Jolie Bookspan
www.healthylearning.com

The Fitness Fixer
www.healthline.com/blogs
Health expert column on Healthline.com.
New fun techniques three to four times a week.

21

Back and Neck Pain—Prevention and Treatment

We don't consider a patient cured when his sprain has healed or he's restored to a minimal level of functioning. The patient is cured when he can again do the things he loves to do.

—Stanley A. Herring, M.D.

Almost all back pain is preventable and easily stopped. Chapter 20 described simple sources of most back and neck pain. This chapter shows how to stop the cause of the pain and injury. Then, it can heal, and the pain will stop. It is simple and quick. Even with problems you can't prevent, such as certain inherited back disorders or serious accidents, you can reduce or eliminate pain. Tendency toward arthritis, for example, increases with habits that contribute to wear and tear, and with lack of proper exercise. Scoliosis is aggravated by moving and carrying without postural control and using muscles to hold yourself straight. You can change many factors. This chapter shows what to try.

> Most back pain is easily stopped.

Stop Disc and Muscular Back Pain

Do you sit, exercise, and bend with your lower back rounded outward? Disc protrusion, called herniation, usually results from chronic outward pressure on discs. In your neck and lower back, this pressure occurs from the bad posture of slouching your torso forward into the shape of the letter "C" when sitting, bending, and lifting, rather than keeping the normal inward curves of the neck and lower back. Continually putting grinding, unequal pressures on your discs can cause them to break down (degenerate) over time. The curled posture also pushes discs further out over time. The edges begin to fray like a wearing tire. Eventually, one day, after even a small provocation, the disc finally protrudes far enough for a sudden onset of disc pain. You then attribute the injury of the "slipped disc" to the one event that brought on the pain, never realizing it was brewing all along from the way you sat, stood, and lifted, day after day, year after year.

> Years of poor sitting and standing posture can wear out your discs. One day, a disc finally "goes," while you are doing nothing more than sneezing or reaching for something. The "slipped" disc wasn't caused by the one event; it was brewing all along.

Although "slipped" or herniated discs used to be thought of as a life sentence, it is rarely the case. Most disc protrusions heal in days to weeks, if you let them, and you can go back to your life, as after any other injury

> Most disc herniations will heal with stopping the bad habits that made them herniate in the first place.

When You Wake Up. Disc pain is often worse upon waking in the morning because your discs swell a bit overnight, plumping up with water as part of healing. The thing you don't want to do when you wake is to sit at the edge of the bed with your back rounded in flexion. No one should sit in that way, particularly not anyone with disc trouble. It puts outward pressure on discs when they are the most vulnerable. Instead, turn face down and lie propped slightly on your elbows, in extension, for a few moments or so. Lying prone reduces pain and pressure, and unloads the discs. Don't stick your chin forward. Lift from the upper back, not the neck.

> When you first wake up, turn face down and lie propped slightly on your elbows for a few moments, instead of sitting. In most cases, it's better for your discs.

When making beds in the morning, don't lean over and lift. Bend properly. Keep your torso upright. Bend your knees, keeping your knees over your feet, not forward.

During the Day When It Hurts. Turn face down on the floor or bed, and lie propped slightly on your elbows for a few moments. The pain should diminish or stop right away. If it doesn't, check if you are straining or propping too high. Use the hip tuck to neutral if you feel pinching in your lower back, as described in Chapter 7 on abdominal muscles and in the hyperlordosis section of this chapter. Do this exercise several times a day.

Bending. The most important thing you can do to stop the cause of disc and muscular back pain and let it heal is to stop bad bending and do good bending. Do you pick things up by bending at the waist with your legs straight or nearly so? Don't do it that way. Keep your torso upright (not bent over), and bend your knees. A common complaint is that using the legs is difficult. Using your legs is free exercise and burns calories, and it will fix your back and knee pain, so be glad.

What is "lifting correctly"? One way to get healthy, built-in leg exercise and stop back pain by bending well every time you bend is the half-squat:

- Stand with your feet side-by-side, comfortably apart.
- Bend both knees. Keep both heels down, touching the floor.
- Keep your upper body upright, as if you don't want something to fall out of your shirt pocket.
- As you bend lower, peek down. If you can't see your toes, that means you are letting your knees slide forward, which shifts your weight to your knee joints.
- Keep your weigh back toward your heels, not toes, to keep weight on your muscles, not on the knee joint.
- Keep your knees back over your ankles to keep your weight on your leg muscles.
- Many people won't bend with their knees because it hurts their knees. This good bending stops knee pain, too.

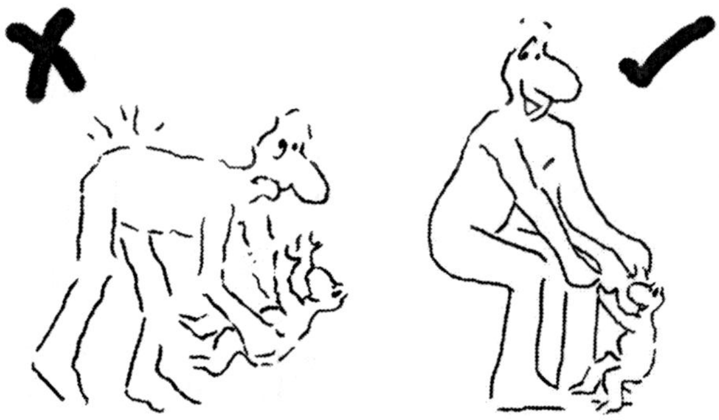

Figure 21-1. Good bending with the half-squat (right). Keep your torso upright and bend your knees, keeping your weight back over your heels and your knees over your ankles. Bend this way any time you lift anything—laundry, packages, or weights in the gym.

A second way to bend correctly is the lunge:

- Stand with one foot far in front of the other.
- Bend both knees.
- Keep your upper body as upright as you can, as if you don't want something to fall out of your shirt pocket.
- Keep the front knee in place over the foot, not sliding forward.

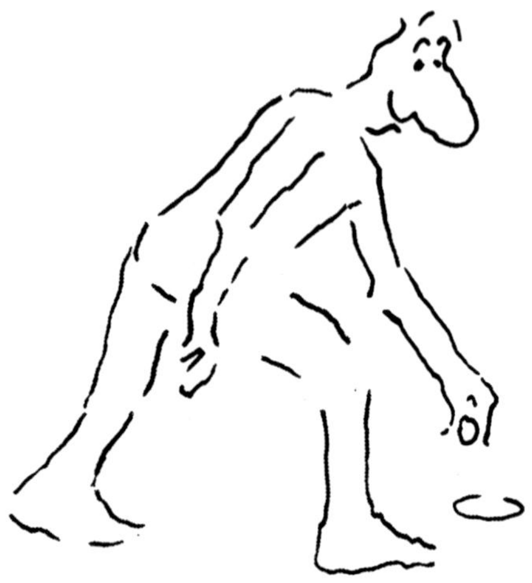

Figure 21-2. Good bending with the lunge.

The average person bends hundreds of times every day for daily activities like laundry, kitchen, pets, gardening, children, household chores, and everything else. Check to see if you are bending badly each time, hurting your discs and lower back. Check at the gym if you add more forward bending for toe-touches, weight lifting, and exercise class. Bad bending puts herniating forces on your discs hundreds of times every day. No wonder your back hurts.

> Any time you bend over, whether for a drink of water, to jot a note, wash your face, tie your shoe, start the lawn mower, or lift anything, bend your knees and keep your torso as upright as possible. It uses more muscles than bad bending, giving much built-in exercise, and prevents damage to discs.

If you lift dumbbells or other free weights, don't bend over to pick them up or put them down. You already know not to pick up a child or suitcase in that manner. Don't go to a gym and magically forget this. Don't lift weights while standing in a bent over or in a bent-forward position. Use the squat and lunge to pick things up and put them down.

Good Bending Should Not Hurt Knees. Don't use the excuse of bad knees to bend and lift straight-legged, or with bad knee positioning. If your knees hurt, check your bending habits. Many knee complaints result over time just like back and neck pain—from poor walking and standing habits that wear, tear, and unevenly load the knee joint, and from uneven muscle strength and flexibility. Proper bending should not hurt your knees. Proper movement and exercise is supposed to help the knee, not make it hurt more. Proper movement gives you the exercise you need for health, for feeling good, and weight control. When you bend properly, you will feel right away if it is helping. If it hurts, it is not right.

Different "camps" have different philosophies about knee pain management. Some camps believe any lunge or squat-like bending is bad. They prefer to restrict all bending and exercise the knee by having you sit with a small leg weight at the ankle and lift that with a straight knee. After doing that exercise, how are you supposed to stand up and walk away and have normal life function? Good bending, done with the brain and the aim of restoring function, retrains the motion to be healthful. Chapter 9 has details on good squat and lunge exercising without hurting the knees.

Good Bending Has Another Benefit. Muscles that are tight from inflexibility, and muscles that are tightly in spasm from bad posture habits, can compress nerves, mimicking the kind of pain produced by herniated discs pressing on nerves. One of several muscles that seems to like to compress nerves is the piriformis (or pyriformis) muscle. The pyriformis lies deep in your pelvis under your posterior hip muscles. In a small percentage of the population, the sciatic nerve goes through or close by the pyriformis. If the pyriformis is tight, it can compress your sciatic nerve, causing pain and sometimes weakness in the buttock and down your leg. Good bending is a functional, daily, built-in stretch for this area. Another good bending exercise is standing to put on shoes and hosiery with one ankle crossed over the other knee, without rounding the back.

Stop Upper-Back and Neck Pain, and Pain Down the Arm

Do you stand and sit with your neck sloped forward? That position juts your head forward of the center line of your body. A forward head is a common source of upper-back, neck, and head pain, pain between and across the shoulders, and pain down the arm. This bad posture is called a forward head. Many people have a forward head without knowing it. Think of a bowling ball. Imagine continuously holding that heavy bowling ball out in front of your body. Soon, your back and neck muscles that hold it will fatigue, and then hurt. That bowling ball is your head. The rounded position of the shoulder also can press on the nerve going down the arm, causing pain and numbness.

A forward head is so common that it looks normal, but it is a serious problem. Keep your ears and the corner of your jaw over your shoulders, not in front of them. Look at

Figure 21-3 and see if your head is forward (left). A common mistake is just lifting the chin up, which just compounds the pinching, rather than pulling it back and in. The ear may be over the shoulder, but the chin juts far forward. Keep the chin loosely back and in. Check by standing with your back and against a wall often. The back of your head should touch easily. If not, it is probably a forward head.

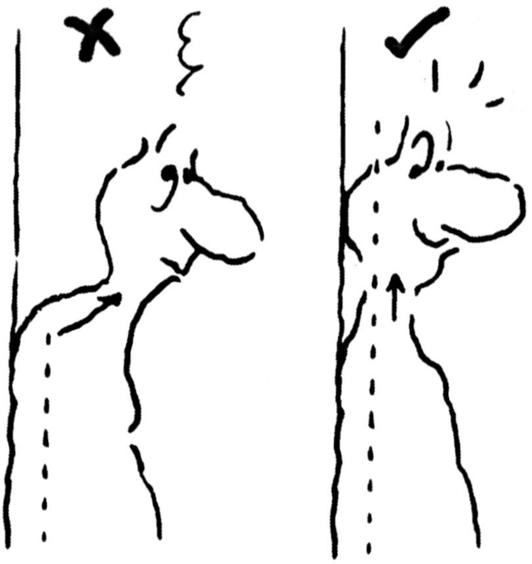

Figure 21-3. Correct a forward head (left) by lifting back and in, bringing your ears over the center of your shoulders without looking up or down (right). Lift up and back without strain or tension. Check yourself against a wall.

A forward head can eventually damage neck and upper-back structures when they begin to bend and rub at angles they were not built for. Your discs can degenerate or begin to protrude. Protruding (herniated) discs can press on nerves that go down your arms. Chronically holding your neck muscles, or any muscles, in an overstretched position weakens them. You wind up with shortened, contracted muscles down the front of your neck, and a stretched, weakened upper back. You may have seen this forward-head posture on older people and wondered how they got that way. The answer is: practice.

> Relieving back and neck pain does not mean giving up activities you love, or sitting and standing stiffly like a soldier. You can be more active than before using good body ergonomics (positioning).

An average day is filled with bad habit of the forward head:

- Sitting with your head craning forward in front of the computer screen
- Hunching over your desk

- Commuting in car, bus, or train seats
- Bending over the kids
- Walking
- Doing household chores
- Watching television
- Craning your head forward while exercising

In short: you do these bad habits all day, every day, at work and play, even at rest in a chair, and then all night if you sleep on your back with your head pushed forward with pillows. No wonder your neck and back hurt. The average person does so many things every day to damage their back and neck that it is amazing they don't hurt more. You can stop the pain as soon as you stop hanging the weigh of your head forward on your neck.

Put your computer monitor up on blocks, rather than sitting it on the desk, so that you can look at it straight on without looking down. Place your TV screen at head level. Reading and writing at a desk is no excuse to hunch over. Keep your body upright and your head pulled back while you look down rather than tipping your head down and forward.

Two Stretches to Make Stopping Neck Pain and Numb Hand Possible. To restore resting length to the neck, do the following two stretches first thing in the morning and throughout the day. Then, use the new proper resting length to hold healthful positioning so that the neck and upper-body pain will stop.

You should notice the pain and stiffness reduce as soon as you do these stretches. If not, check how you are doing them, and repeat correctly. Also, use these two stretches if you have lower-back pain to restore ability to stand comfortably straight. The stretches are not the cure for the tightness; how you use them is. If you do the stretches but then walk around with a forward head, what are the stretches for? The two stretches make it comfortable and possible to stand right.

- First, check yourself by standing with your back against a wall (Figure 21-3). See if your head is forward of the wall, and how comfortable it is to touch the back of your head against the wall without tipping your head back or straining.

- Do the pectoral stretch. Then, try standing against the wall again. It should immediately feel more normal to stand straight against the wall.

- Do the trapezius stretch, keeping the back of your head against the wall. Then, check yourself with the wall stand again. It should immediately feel more normal to stand straight. If not, check exactly how you are doing things.

Stretch 1: Pectoral Stretch. Stand facing very close to a wall—you can almost touch your face to the wall. Bend one arm to the side, with your elbow even with your ear and fingers pointing upward. Touch the inside of your bent elbow to the wall. Keep your shoulder down. Turn your whole body away from your arm so that your arm is stretched behind you by the wall (Figure 21-4). You will know it is right when you get a good-feeling stretch in your front chest muscles and no pain in the shoulder. If you do not feel the stretch in your chest, you are not doing this stretch as needed to restore muscle length.

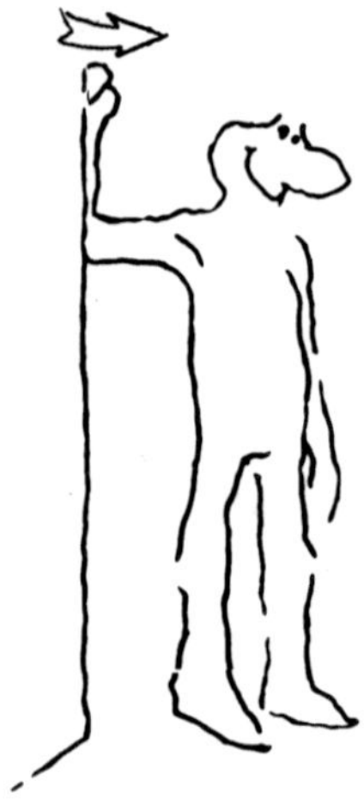

Figure 21-4. Pectoral stretch. Use a wall to brace your bent arm behind you. When done properly, the stretch will only be felt in the front chest muscles where it is needed.

Stretch 2: Trapezius Stretch. Put one hand behind you over your opposite back-pants pocket (or imaginary pocket). Gently tilt your head and body toward that hand, sliding the other hand down your leg (Figure 21-5). Look forward, not downward. To see if you are doing the trapezius stretch in the way it is intended, keep your back and the back of your head against the wall for the entire stretch. Then, you will not be doing it with a forward head, which would be missing the point.

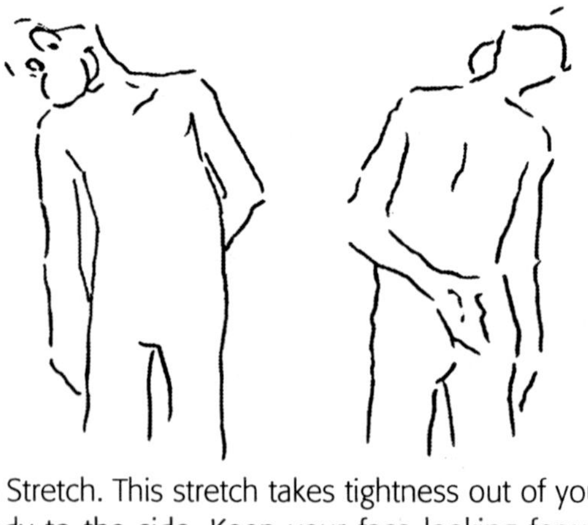

Figure 21-5. Trapezius Stretch. This stretch takes tightness out of your neck and shoulders. Tip your ear and upper body to the side. Keep your face looking forward, not down. Don't lean forward. It takes only a moment. Try it throughout the day.

The purpose of the pectoral and trapezius stretches is to restore resting length so that it feels normal to stand straight. Then, you use the new comfort to maintain your neck and upper body in relaxed healthy position, not bent forward. If you do the two stretches correctly, you will be able to begin standing right the same day. It may take a few tries. Do not continue keeping a forward head, or the pain will continue. Standing with straight upper-body position does not mean never to look up or down. Use full range of motion with chin in, instead tilting the neck forward.

Misunderstood Neck Exercise. A commonly prescribed exercise for neck pain and the forward head is called the "double-chin" exercise or "dorsal glide." It is often misunderstood. The way it is usually taught is to pull your head back in an exaggerated way, so that your chin becomes a "double chin." and hold for 10 counts, or to pull back 10 times a few times a day. The idea is not to "do" this stretch as an exercise, but to pull your head back to normal position one time and hold it all the time. Pulling back 10 times doesn't fix the source of the problem. The problem is not neck strength; it is position. Don't "do" dorsal glides and then go back to the forward-head position. Pull back loosely and comfortably one time, and hold upright positioning with the corner of your jaw comfortably over your shoulder.

Bad Neck Exercise. Forced neck stretches (such as shoulder stands) push discs outward to the back, increasing risk of herniation over time. Forced head turning and rotation by practitioners has been documented to sometimes result in stroke, even death from tearing neck blood vessels. The bones of your neck are not made to roll around each other, a motion called circumduction. Excessive rolling is just wear and tear, and can be uncomfortable for people with neck complaints. For a healthy range of neck motion, don't roll your head. Do the trapezius stretch (Figure 21-5). (Refer to Chapter 9.)

Stop Neck Pain When Looking Upward. A common bad neck habit is jutting the chin forward to look upward, or to look forward when on a bicycle or swimming. It presses one neck joint back forcefully, instead of getting the extension throughout the upper spine.

To look directly upward for all you need in healthful position:

- Keep your chin in, loosely and relaxed.
- Shoulders back.
- The back of your head lifts loosely upward without strain.
- Straighten the rounded-forward curve of the upper spine; get more upward gaze range from your upper back.
- Don't yank or force the head and chin back, or the corners of your neck will ache.
- Don't lean back by arching your lower back.

To look forward when on a bicycle or when swimming or scuba diving:

- Keep your chin in, loose and relaxed.
- Straighten the rounded-forward curve of the upper spine; get more upward gaze range from your upper back.
- Don't look forward by bending back one point in your neck. The neck is not a hinge joint.

Stop Lower-Back Pain During Standing, Walking, and Running—Overarching and Hyperlordosis

Standing with too much inward curve in the lower back (also called overarching, swayback, or hyperlordosis) is the largest source of mystery lower-back pain (Figure 21-6, middle and right). If your lower back hurts with standing, walking, running, or carrying loads, too much inward curve is the usual cause. If you feel you must sit to reduce the pain, bend over forward, or stand with your knees bent or one foot propped up, it is likely that your pain is from overarching the lower back. Aching lower-back pain is often labeled sacroiliac pain (SI syndrome), but the usual cause is the overarching of hyperlordosis.

Two Main Ways to Overarch, and How To Fix It. Standing with a large inward lumbar curve or leaning the upper body backward while moving or carrying any load, is not cute or the normal curve. It is a painful, injurious bad posture. Standing bent at the front of your hip where your leg meets your body is not standing straight (Figure 21-6, middle and right). Your hip should not tip forward in front and out in back. That position is not neutral spine, but an overarched spinal posture that often causes lower-back pain. Following is one easy way to learn to feel it:

- Stand with your back against a wall. Touch your heels, backside, shoulders, and head.
- Does it hurt the lower back to stand straight? Do you have a large space between your lower back and the wall?

A second way to overarch is to lean the upper body backward (Figure 20-5, right). If you stand with your back near a wall and back up, the upper back may be the first to touch the wall. Some people both tip the hip forward and lean the upper body backward (Figure 20-5, left, and Figure 21-6, right).

To change hyperlordosis to neutral spine:

- Standing with your back against a wall, press your lower back toward the wall to reduce the arch to neutral.
- One way to feel this is to put your hand in the space between your lower back

and the wall and press toward your hand. Do not flatten your back; just reduce the curve until you feel the lower-back pain stop.

- Use the new neutral position for all daily walking and activities. Then, you will no longer make the cause of the pain and can be active and do more.
- If you have to bend your knees to do reduce the overarching, you are probably tight in the front of your hip. It means you are probably keeping a large arch when you stand and walk. No wonder it hurts. Use the front hip stretches in Chapter 6. Stop the cause of the pain instead of having surgery and taking pills. It uses muscles, and it is healthy.

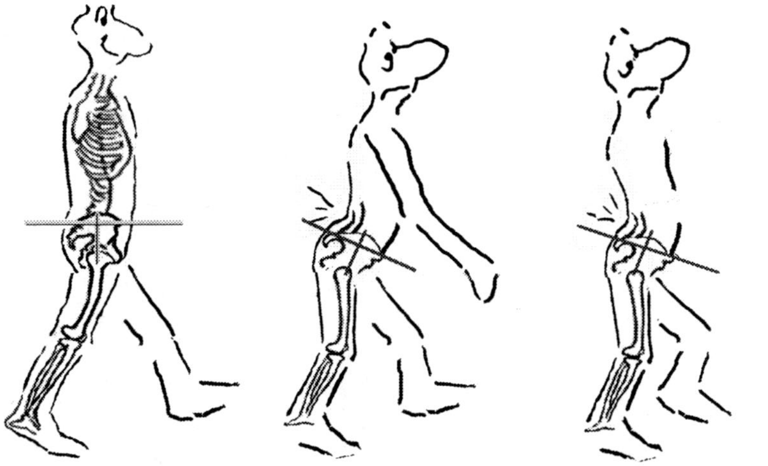

Figure 21-6. Neutral spine is shown on the left. Hyperlordosis is overarching the lower back. You have too much curve (middle and right), which pinches and presses the lower back when standing. Trying to lift up the upper body without changing the tilted hip (right) is not standing straight; it is still painful hyperlordosis.

Hyperlordosis is not a structural condition. Damage does not show on X-ray until the later stages when it shows as facet injury. It is easy to be fooled by unrelated X-ray findings that are not causing the pain, such as a bulging disc that is asymptomatic, and spend time and money treating the wrong cause. Injections are often prescribed for facet injury, but that treatment does not stop the cause. Hyperlordosis pain is easily stopped and prevented from ever returning by not standing that way, and simply using neutral spine.

Stop Lower-Back Pain

Stop Lower Back Pain When Reaching Overhead—Overarching and Hyperlordosis. Don't lean back to raise your arms and reach or lift overhead. Don't increase the arch in the lower back. To check yourself:

- Stand with your back against a wall. Touch your heels, backside, shoulders, and head.
- Reach arms overhead to touch the fingers to the wall behind you (or toward it).
- Does it hurt the lower back to reach up? Do you have a large space between your lower back and the wall? Did your ribs raise, increasing the inward curve of your lower back?

To fix the overarching and restore neutral spine:

- Press your lower back toward the wall, as previously described.
- Another way to feel the movement of how your hip should change position is to put your hands on your hips. Thumbs in back. Fingers in front.
- Roll your hip so that thumbs roll down in back. Feel the lower back press toward the wall, and your hip roll under you.
- Raise your arms to touch the wall overhead again, this time keeping the small neutral curve, not the large painful one.
- If you have to bend your knees to do reduce the overarching, you are probably tight in the front of your hip. Use the front-hip stretches in Chapter 6.

Stop Lower Back Pain in Golf, Tennis, Baseball, and Swimming. Use the hip tuck to achieve neutral spine previously described, instead of increasing the lower-back arch when reaching overhead for a golf swing, tennis serve, baseball swing, high brace in kayaking, and other sports. Get more reach from the upper body rather than the lower spine or shoulder joint. When swimming, use neutral spine when face down in the water for the front crawl. It will also give better streamline and speed.

What Is Neutral Spine? Think of a line through the crest of your hipbone from back to front. The line from the top bump in back (medical abbreviation is PSIS) to the top bump in front (ASIS) should be approximately horizontal (Figure 21-6, left).

If you let your spine slouch so that the front of the hip (ASIS) drops downward and the back of the hip tilts outward in back, the small, normal, inward curve of the lower back increases (Figure 21-6, middle and right). The lumbar spine is no longer neutral. It is overarched.

Another way to assess neutral spine is to look at the line from the ASIS to where the pelvic bones meet in front, called the symphysis pubis (PS). When you hold your spine in neutral, the line from ASIS to PS will be vertical. When looking at people, it is usually easier to see the line at the side, from the top of the leg bone up through the hip and waist. It is like the side seam in clothing. The line in the left drawing is vertical, showing the hip is straight and level (Figure 21-6, left). With hyperlordosis (overarching), the line from the leg bone to the center hip tilts forward. The hip sticks out in back (Figure 21-6 middle and right). The spine is no longer neutral. It is arched—hyperlordotic.

Another way to overarch the lower spine is to lean the upper body backward. Notice if you lean your upper body backward when you reach up, take photos, carry things in front (like a package, child, or chair), or during walking or running (Figure 21-7, left). Tilt your hip back to neutral and bring the upper body forward until straight. Compressive lower-back pain from hyperlordosis should stop then and there (Figure 21-7, right).

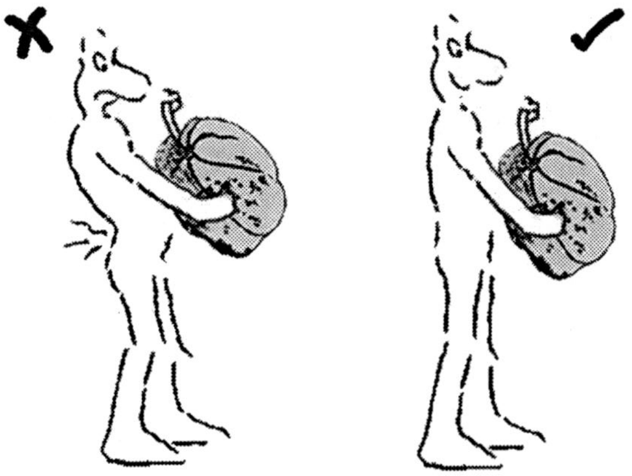

Figure 21-7. *Left:* Leaning the upper body back and/or tilting the hip forward in front and out in back increases the inward arch (hyperlordosis), creating compression and pain in the lower back. *Right:* This pain can be immediately stopped by tilting the hip to neutral.

Is Overarching Structural? It is not true that a "beer belly" or pregnancy by themselves cause the overarching (hyperlordosis) or the pain. The pain is from slouching—allowing the upper back to lean backward and/or the hip to tip forward to offset the load, instead of maintaining neutral spine. It is not true that the lumbar spine is shaped to overarch. It is shaped to have a small inward arch, not a large one. Leaning the upper body backward to offset a pregnancy (or any load carried) puts compressive loading on the lower spine, causing damage and pain. For more on how and why your abdominal muscles control posture and can be used for pain, refer to Chapter 7 on abs.

> Don't let bad postural mechanics grind your back structure down to where it will be harder to fix later. Good muscle support around the joint comes from proper use and educating the muscles how to support the area, not by stopping your activities and "resting it."

Stop Hyperlordosis Pain Coming From Tight Front-Hip Muscles

Muscles called hip flexors bend you forward at the hip. Hip-flexor muscles go down from your lumbar vertebrae (lower-back bones) and the crest of your hip bone to a knob on your upper leg bone, called the greater trochanter of your femur (Figure 21-8, left). When these muscles are tight, common in people who sit a lot and do much forward bending and leg-lifting exercise, it makes overarching feel normal and trying to tuck the hip to neutral feel difficult (Figure 21-7). The resulting overarch (hyperlordosis) is a large source of mystery lower-back pain when standing and lying down flat (Figure 21-8, middle and right). See the lunge hip stretch that follows in this chapter, and refer to Chapter 9 for more good stretches for the hip.

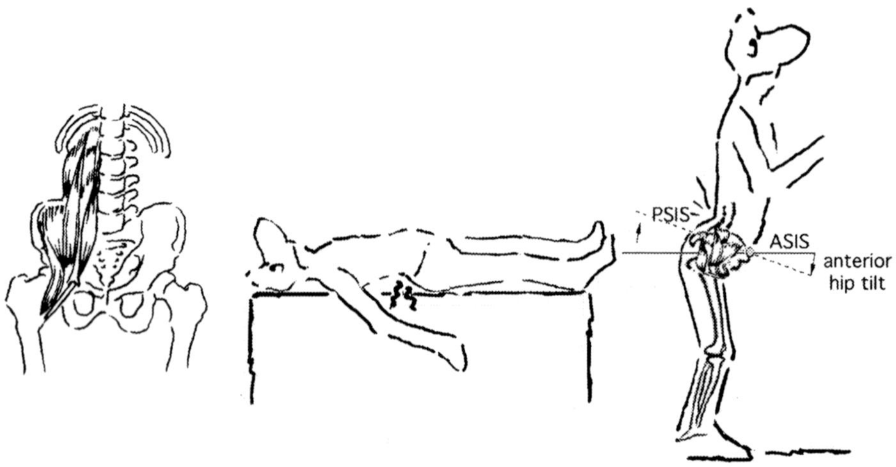

Figure 21-8. Hip-flexor muscles cross your hip in the front and attach to the top of your leg (left). When tight, they prevent normal lengthening at the hip, creating arched positioning and pain when standing (right) and lying flat (middle).

Wall Posture Test

The wall-posture check is a simple check using a wall (Figure 21-9). Do this check first thing in the morning and throughout the day. It is important to identify how your body segments line up in general.

- Stand very near a wall, facing away from the wall, but not touching it.
- Assume a posture that you feel is normal.
- Slowly back up and contact the wall.

- See what part of your body touched the wall first.
- Then, back up and touch your heels, hips, shoulders, and the back of your head to the wall. Do not try to flatten your lower back against the wall.

Look at Figure 21-9 of the wall-posture test:

#1. Did your behind touch first? You may tilt or lean forward.

#2. Did your shoulders touch first? You might be leaning the upper body backward, indicating hyperlordosis.

#3. Did the back of your head never touch? You probably have a forward head.

#4. Do you have to overarch your lower back or crane your neck to stand straight? That position is hyperlordosis, tight chest and neck, and probably tight front-hip muscles.

#5. Did your head, shoulders, back, behind, calves, and heels all touch at once? That position is standing straight.

Do this quick check first thing in the morning and throughout the day to make sure that you know how you are standing and why. Check yourself as you walk through doorways. Check yourself while waiting for things. Watch other people to see their positioning. Look sideways in a mirror to see if you lean backward or tilt your neck or hip forward. Fix everything using the methods presented in this chapter so that standing upright and straight feels normal and comfortable for all your daily movement.

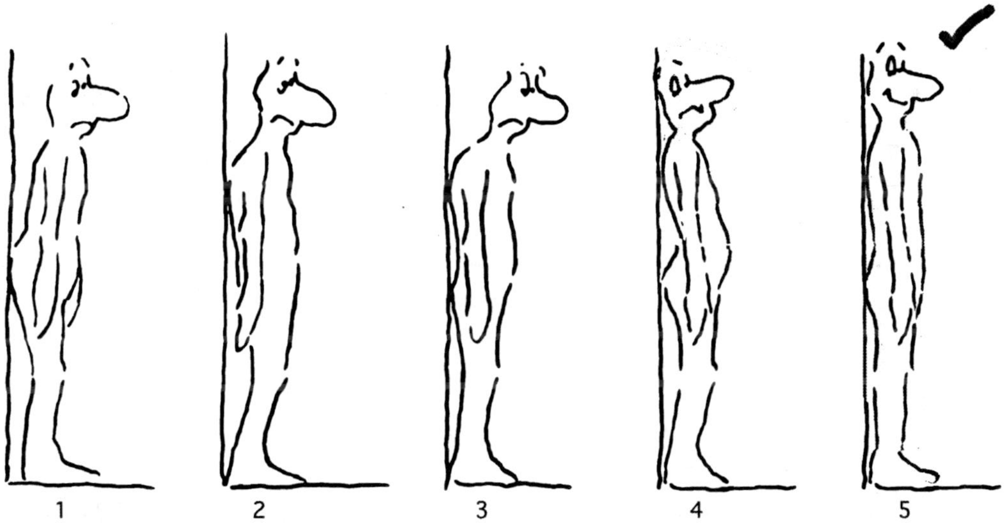

Figure 21-9. Check yourself first thing in the morning (and many times during the day) with the wall-posture test. Straight position is at right. This quick check can identify the source of pain.

Stop Pain From Sitting

The hollowed (concave) back of most chairs makes you sit with a rounded back and a forward head. Watch for bad chair engineering in office, bus, train, and plane seats. Other problem chairs are bench seats in restaurants and church pews. Plane and bus seats seem to be exceptionally bad. People worsen the problem by putting a pillow behind their head

> Sitting rounded makes muscles hurt and presses discs outward, putting herniating forces on them. It takes years, but eventually they may begin to move or "slip"

News reports of a study of spine pressure when sitting implied incorrectly that sitting up straight is not good for the back. What was meant was that it is less pressure to lean back than to sit vertically upright. It is still not good to round your spine forward. You don't need to sit at the edge of a chair, stiffly and uncomfortably:

- Sit with your hip against the back of the chair, not forward of it.
- Lift your upper back against the chair instead of pressing your lower back into a rounded position.
- Leaning back is helpful, if done with a straight, not curled torso.
- Keep your head up, not tilted forward.

Lumbar cushion. When you sit in a chair that is concave, use a small cushion or article of clothing in the space at your lower back keep a small inward curve in your lower back.

- To get the idea of what a lumbar roll does and what size is good, sit in your chair with your entire back against the back of the chair. Put your forearm behind you, between your lower back and the chair. Nestle your arm in the natural space. Lift your upper back against the chair. Your forearm is usually the right size to fill the space of your lower back. It should feel comfortable.
- Try a small rolled towel, a soft, small article of clothing, or a commercial lumbar roll between your lower back and the chair. Small inflatable pillows are inexpensive, and pack flat and light.
- Lift your upper back against the chair instead of pressing against the roll.
- Don't make too large an inward curve in the lower back, or too large an outward curve in the upper back.
- For airline seats and some office chairs with a large hollow in the upper-back area, you may need two pillows or small soft rolls made from soft handy

clothing or other items. Put one roll in the natural inward curve of your lower back, and a second roll behind your upper back—or use one longer pad placed vertically. Doing so will help you lean back in the chair, instead of forward. With sensible placement of the pads, you will sit upright to rest the back of your head against the headrest, instead of rounding forward.

What about "ergonomic" chairs, "ball" chairs, or kneeling chairs? You can sit poorly in any chair if you slouch and hold your neck tilted forward, no matter how expensive or engineered the chair. They do not "make" you sit up properly or burn more calories.

Avoid Bad Exercise

Several exercises common at gyms and exercise studios can do your back more harm than good. A few bad exercises now and then usually do little damage, but give it a chance. Like smoking, the repeated damage of the exposure can harm at a rate faster than your body can repair.

- *Straight-legged dead lifting and other continuous, weighted, forward bending.* It may strengthen the muscles and feel good, but it injuries the discs over time.
- *Standing and sitting bent over for toe touches.* You already know that sitting bent over your desk, steering wheel, and computer is unhealthy for your back. It is not magically different or healthy because it is called a stretch. Sitting and leaning forward to touch toes, even with your back straight, is a common hidden contributor to lower-back pain. It may stretch your back and legs, but sitting (especially sitting bent forward, even if it is for a yoga or Pilates class) puts high forces on the discs of your lower back. Sitting and bending forward is not even the most effective way to stretch your hamstrings, even though it is a common stretch, and has been done for many years. Many things that are common and traditional are also not healthy, like smoking and hostility. Use healthy ways instead. (Refer to Chapter 9.)

Modern lifestyle predominantly favors being bent forward, overstretching your back and tightening the front of your body until it becomes natural to slouch forward and uncomfortable to stand straight. Lower-back discs become increasingly squashed and pressed outward from all the forward bending. It starts feeling "normal" to stand and move with your back rounded in unhealthy position. Adding to it with forward bending exercise classes in counterproductive. (Refer to Chapter 9.)

Abdominal and Core Muscles Do Not Automatically Support the Back

It is a myth that strengthening the abdominal muscles will automatically stop back pain. Most pain is not caused by core weakness, but by spine positioning. Strong muscles do not automatically make you stand or bend right. Many muscular people have back pain. Crunches are the exercise usually thought of for ab exercise and back-pain control; however, they create a hunched-over posture, encourage a forward head, and are not how you need your abs in daily life. They do not automatically make your abdominal muscle work properly while standing, so they are not a form of good, functional exercise. Abdominal muscles can hold you upright and prevent hyperlordosis (overarching) of the lower spine, if you use them to do so (Figures 21-6 and 21-7). However, strengthening exercises do not hold you in this manner, and you will still stand overarched if you do not know how to reposition your hip and lower spine. Chapter 7 on abs explains this process in detail and what to do instead.

> Crunches are a common ab exercise; however, they do not train your core muscles to hold neutral spine, and they encourage the same hunched-over posture that creates more back and neck pain.

Posture (Biomechanics) Matters More Than You Think

Good posture doesn't happen automatically just from doing exercises. Healthful positioning can make a difference between a pain-free back and neck, and chronic misery. People don't take posture seriously as the main contributor to back and neck pain. Think of it as mechanics. If your car had crooked parts, you'd know right away that would cause grinding and early wear.

Good posture doesn't mean standing stiffly for a moment, then stopping because it doesn't feel natural. It means getting the flexibility and strength so that you are able to move into the right position and hold it. Most people don't have the flexibility even to stand straight. They crane their necks. Their tight chests and shoulders feel more "natural" slumped. That feeling is a signal that you have to stretch and strengthen, not slouch.

> Strengthening muscles through general exercises doesn't automatically "give" you good posture. Plenty of muscular people have terrible posture. Posture is a conscious muscular activity, so it burns calories and is good exercise by itself.

Notice Posture. Watch other people from the side as they stand, walk, and sit so that you can identify a forward head. At home, spend time to learn about your own posture. Stand sideways in front of a mirror. Use a second, handheld mirror to look at your profile, or use a three-way mirror. See where your ears are relative to the middle of your shoulder. See where your shoulder is relative to your back and hips, and so on.

Notice how often poor posture is represented in popular magazines, not only by models who do it as an art form, but by people shown in athletic activities. Begin to see how the poor postures put strain on their joints during their activity.

> Do you feel unnatural standing with good posture? When the postural muscles of your back and abdomen are so weak and tight that they cannot comfortably support you, that means you need to work them to be comfortable, not slouch to be comfortable.

Is it natural to slouch? As natural as wetting your pants. At first you make mistakes, but then you learn to "hold" it, even when you don't feel like it.

Healthy Exercises

Exercise alone will not fix back pain. Strengthening can put a stronger lock on a paper door. It does not solve the source of the problem if you go back to unhealthful, painful bad bending and sitting. Doing your back exercises a few times a week, but keeping the old, bad postures and habits that hurt your back in the first place is like eating cake and ice cream morning, noon, and night, and doing five minutes of exercise a few times a week, then saying you don't know why exercise isn't working. Use these exercises to improve strength and endurance, but more important, to get your back "unrounded" and retrain how to straighten.

Upper-Back Extension

- This extension is also good for your neck. Lie face down with your hands at your sides and off the floor. Slowly lift your upper body a few inches. This action is called back extension. Then, lower your back to the floor. Don't force. Don't tilt your head back. Keep your head in line with your body. If you feel any pinching, don't do this exercise, and see your doctor. If you feel muscles working, it is correct. Start with one or two lifts. See how you feel the next day. If you feel no pain, increase to 10 times, trying to do a few times a day.
- To progress, move your arms from your sides to overhead.

Lower-Back Extension

- Lie face down with your chin on your hands. Lift one leg off the floor, and keep your knee straight. Hold and lower several times before switching legs. Breathe. This exercise unloads the discs. It does not compress as sometimes feared. Do not lift so hard that it hurts. If it pinches the lower back, you may be overarching. Tuck your lift and get the lift more from the back and upper-leg muscles.
- To progress, lift both legs together.

> The point and benefit of "doing" back exercises is lost when you just do back exercises without thought to using the exercise to retrain your muscles and brain how to hold good posture all the time.

Hip Stretch Using the Lunge

Hip flexors, the muscles that bend your hip and raise your leg, as in walking, were covered Chapter 6 on stretching. Tight, short hip flexors are common. Hip-flexor stretches are important to back health, but unfortunately neglected. If you have a hip replacement, do not do any exercises without clearing them with your hip team. You can dislocate the prosthetic (the artificial hip).

A good, functional way to stretch your hip flexors is the lunge. The lunge is often done improperly so that little or no stretch is accomplished on the hip flexors. To do the stretch properly:

- Stand with your feet comfortably apart, then slide one foot in back of you as far as you can do comfortably.
- Don't lean forward or backward.
- Tuck your hip under you (pelvic tilt to be straight).
- You will feel the stretch in your forward leg where it normally creases in front.
- Lower gently straight downward by bending your knees and keeping your body upright. This step turns the stretch into a combined dynamic stretch and leg strengthener.
- This stretch is also a healthy way to pick up things. Many people bend improperly all day to get things—bending at the waist. Use the lunge instead and get free exercise all day.

Tests, Treatments, and Surgery

Your body works to make continual small (and large) repairs all the time, while you may be continuing bad bending and exercises that make pain return. This tug-of-war makes back and neck pain seem to come and go on its own. Much confusion results about what relieved it.

You may do a bad forward-bending stretch because your back hurts from too much overarch backward. You may feel temporarily better; however, the bad forward bending adds to conditions that set you up for pain later.

Address the Cause. Many people take back-pain remedies, and then go back to the standing, sitting, and lifting problems that gave them the trouble in the first place. Pain eventually returns. The person doesn't understand it. They call it stress. They try chiropractors, acupuncture, prescription and over-the-counter medications, herbal remedies, psychotherapy, and prayer. They do everything except to change the positioning and movement habits that created the problem. Some wind up in surgery, yet their pain persists. They are told they have to learn to "live with pain." Luckily, it does not have to be that way.

> People take back-pain remedies, then go right back to the bad habits that gave them back pain in the first place. They don't understand when their pain returns, because they thought they were "fixed." They didn't fix the cause.

Beware the Structural Diagnosis. The Greek word gnosis means "knowing" or "recognizing." Dia is a word element that, in this context, means "completely." It is crucial to know completely. Getting rid of pain and the disability that goes with it means treating the cause.

Someone with back pain may go to a doctor and get an X-ray or other imaging. The pain is from all the poor body mechanics all day, not any organic problem. The scans show nothing. What they need is muscle and posture retraining, but they are told they are imagining it, or that it is stress, or age, or that they need to exercise or stretch their hamstrings. They continue all their poor habits, stretch by forward bending, and their pain continues or worsens.

The scans may show arthritis, a bulging disc, or degenerating or slipping structures. Just like car tires that are mid-life but perfectly good, an exam may show some wear that is completely unrelated to performance or pain. The pain is falsely ascribed to the structure, even though the pain is from all the poor mechanics over the years. They may be told to give up activities or have surgery, and be put on medicines that cause a variety of other pain and problems, when what they need is exercise and muscle and posture retraining.

Sometimes, the scans show a major structural problem. Poor mechanics may be contributing to the pain, or even causing the problem. The person goes for surgery. The pain persists or returns because of uncorrected poor mechanics. A person may have had a herniated disc removed, and then herniate a disc in another area, due to the same uncorrected poor mechanics.

Pills and Adjustments. Most back and neck pain is not inflammatory in nature. For this reason, anti-inflammatory medications often do little to help the pain over the long run. Serious narcotic medicines are often prescribed. They do not remove the cause of the pain, and can continue a dangerous progression of movement that injures the area. The drugs themselves are unhealthful. For muscles that are tight with pain or spasm, specific stretches can lengthen the muscle back to normal resting length. Muscle-relaxant medications are meant to be used only for the first day or so. Muscle relaxants are not appropriate or healthful for long-term use. The purpose is to knock out the spasm right away, then let your body heal. If you have back muscles in spasm, the pain can be crippling, but it can be a simple matter to get out the spasm. A trained massage therapist, physical therapist, or osteopath can identify spasm and stretch it out with special release techniques. The relief is quick and seems to be miraculous, but it is often a simple matter. Muscles are not supposed to be left in spasm or produce a long-term condition. For more on muscle spasm, refer to Chapter 30 on leg cramps.

Identify the things you do that caused the problem. Don't just injure your back, allow it to go into spasm and pain, and go to someone to "fix" it. It is not a fix. Make easy modifications in your routine to avoid the whole problem in the future. Then, as pain subsides, begin a good back-exercise program to increase your resistance to future injury. Use ice after your workouts and at the end of every long day. The old thinking of long bed rest for back pain has been found to be counterproductive. It just further weakens and deconditions you. You need activity done with healthful joint mechanics, not just the usual 10 back exercises then get sit, stand, and move badly thereafter.

What About Shots? These shots are usually a special anti-inflammatory and or anesthetic, delivered right into the area. The idea is to reduce space-occupying swelling and pain, and stop the pain/spasm cycle. Two important cautions are that corticosteroid injections temporarily stop the healing process and make the area weak and susceptible to tearing. You need to stop exercise and regular strong movement for a few days after these shots to avoid harming the temporarily weakened area. The shots do not stop the cause of the pain and do nothing to change your movement habits. With the pain gone, you may go on to continue to damage the area far more by not changing to healthful mechanics. It is more effective and healthier to stop the source of pain with good movement habits.

Avoid Surgery. Surgery for disc herniation, sciatica, stenosis, facet-joint damage, and other problems is rarely necessary. Moreover, many problems can result from surgery—including the strain of the surgery itself and deconditioning from the recovery period. Your bones need your discs for cushioning and to keep from grinding bone directly on bone. After surgery to remove all or part of a disc, you are subject to early wear and tear, possibly predisposing you to early arthritis. A worse situation follows fusion surgery. It is a belief that stopping motion in a joint via fusion surgery will stop pain, but it also stops function. If you want an active life, it is setting you up for more problems. Even if you do not value being active, because fused back bones cannot move when you bend and sit and move, the vertebrae above and below the fused site must move more than usual, squeezing the discs and bones more than they are designed for. Fusion surgery is often a predisposing factor to more pain and loss of function, leading people to be pushed into future back surgeries.

An alarming number of people have pain that continues after surgery, or their pain stops initially while on pain medications and rehab following surgery, but then returns. The reason is, except for unusual situations such as bullet wounds (for example), surgery does not stop the root cause of back pain. Because the cause continues, you continue doing harm to your back until it hurts again.

Spinal fusion is surgery to fuse one vertebra to the next. It is the extreme, last resort. The area no longer moves at all. The immobile area does not function normally and transfers compensating strain to other areas. The vertebrae and discs above and below the fused sites must move more for you to have even close to the function you had before your surgery. The result is much more wear and tear on those sections than they were designed for. A problem with spinal fusion is that the adjacent area is subject to wear out from the trauma of working overtime next to a fused segment. The person is sometimes pushed to have the next segments fused too, which leads to more unnecessary pain and bodily trauma.

Facets are the joints at the back of each vertebra (spine bone). In one back surgery procedure for damage to the facets, the facet joint is cut off and replaced by "lumbar position preservation hardware," rigidly attached so that the area can no longer bend or arch backward. Surgical facet rigid fixation surgery is considered innovative because it replaces the drastic spine fusion. Why does the surgery want to prevent arching the lower spine? The facets are in the back of the vertebrae. Chronically letting your lower spine overarch (too much inward curve in the lower spine) squashes the facets in back. The overarching, called hyperlordosis (or slouching backward), is a chief factor in damage and pain to the facets and surrounding soft tissue. It means that you can stop this condition yourself, and quickly, without the surgery. By standing without overarching, you prevent the crushing force on the facets, and distribute the weight of your upper body through your core muscles instead. It is a simple positional adjustment that takes seconds (explained previously in the section on hyperlordosis and facet pain). Following rigid fixation surgery, you will no longer be able to stretch your lower spine as far backward, even when you want to stretch in healthful ways for range of motion and better disc health. You will still be able to slouch your body weight backward—onto the implants. They may eventually wear, along with adjacent bone, from the chronic crushing. Because the surgically fixed area can no longer overarch, increased forces occur on the joints above and below, which have to bend more. After years, those facets may be next to break down. It is no surprise "when the pain comes back." The cause of the pain was never removed.

Back-pain patients often go for several opinions and are told each time that surgery is the only answer. However, back pain—even chronic pain, sciatica and disc pain—are simple to stop with quick and non-surgical methods. Patients are often told that if they don't have the surgery, they might become paralyzed. A November 2006 *New York Times* article stated, "Many surgeons had long feared that waiting would cause severe harm, but those fears were proved unfounded." The *Times* article quoted Dr. Steven R. Garfin, chairman of the department of orthopedic surgery at the University of California, San Diego, "I think this will have an impact. It says you don't have to rush in for surgery."

More important to your health is what is not being reported. The *Times* article said, "No one who waited had serious consequences, and no one who had surgery had a disastrous result." It is important to know what is meant by "no one who had surgery had a disastrous result." It is not considered "a disastrous result" if you go through the pain and fear of surgery and still have back pain, or are worse after surgery. It is not considered "a disastrous result" if you lose your job because of the time lost to surgery and recovery, and your family won't talk to you because they think you're a complainer. It is not considered a "disastrous result" if the medicines given during and after surgery cause problems you didn't have before, or worsen existing problems, and then you are given more medicines to counteract the first ones, each with their small (or large) health drawbacks. It is not considered a "disastrous result" if you get far more out of shape and gain large amounts of weight because you could do less after your surgery, and your overall health declines from it.

No national database keeps track of people who have the same or worse pain after surgery. No clearinghouse is set up to help or count people who get new problems because of the surgery. Often, surgeons have no way to know that their patients still have pain years later. Patients may be referred to physical therapy, but as their pain, disability, and misery grow, they are "lost to follow-up."

Exercise programs for back pain frequently fail because they do not stop the cause of pain. Personal trainers and Pilates instructors frequently suffer herniated discs because they do unhealthy bending and stretches for their exercise. You can do far better exercises and stretches instead. You don' t need surgery to stop the pain. You can stop the pain without surgery, often better and faster.

Herniation, Stenosis, and Facet-Joint Injury Can Heal. Most disc herniations will heal, shrink, and go back into place—if you let them, and that big "if" is up to you. Most stenosis will stop, and even begin to reopen. Facet-joint injury is due almost entirely to overarching the lower back when standing. This kind of pain is usually immediately stopped with tilting the lower spine back to neutral away from overarched. Refer to the overarching section in this chapter, Chapter 7 on abdominal muscles, and Chapter 9 on changing bad exercises to good exercises. These chapters show you what to notice and how to change your positioning while sitting, bending, reaching, and standing.

> What's the most effective treatment for back or neck pain?
>
> Not drugs, not surgery. Just stopping the unhealthful body mechanics that causes the damage. The source of the pain stops right then, and the area can quickly heal. It takes only days to stop most disc pain.

Is Leg Length an Issue?

It is a myth that everyone has unequal leg length. For those people who do have unequal leg lengths, the difference is not always in bone length. Simply slouching more on one leg than the other or letting one ankle roll in more than the other results in dramatic leg length differences that are not in the bone. Muscle spasm can pull on your hip and lower body, making a "functional" leg-length difference, rather than a true structural one. These spasms can be easily dealt with by a good physical therapist, orthopedist, physical-medicine physician, osteopath, or massage therapist with appropriate training. Most often, leg length is not the root cause of the pain. Fixing the other conditions can relieve the tightness that creates all the problems together. Don't just slap in a shoe insert without stopping the cause.

Walk Softly

Walking "hard" shocks your spine (and hip and other joints) and adds to early wear and tear. Some people come down so heavily on each step that the skin on their face jiggles. Think of your car. Without good shock absorption, your frame will wear out early. You have several ways to add to your necessary, natural shock absorption:

- Your major bodily shock absorbers are your thigh and buttock muscles, the quadriceps and gluteal muscles. Exercise them for better back health.
- Strong back muscles are shock absorbers, much more so than weak back muscles, another good reason to do your back exercises.
- Wear a soft sole in your shoes.
- More important than "external" shock absorption, like soft shoe pads, is to maintain good posture by keeping the normal inward curve of your lower back. Your spine is like a spring, and it absorbs shock through its normal curves. Straightening out the curve by slouching removes the normal spring action.

Accentuating the normal curve through too much arching also reduces shock absorption.

- Walk softly all the time. Roll heel to toe, don't walk on tiptoe. Bend your knees when walking, descending stairs, and stepping off curbs.

> Your legs and feet have posture, too. How you stand and walk makes a big difference between getting healthy exercise, and putting extra pressures, shocks, andwear and tear on your joints.

Sit Down Softly

When you sit down, you should be using your leg muscles to decelerate so that you don't wham down onto your behind. The shock jolts you throughout your spinal column and wears out your discs. Watch people for this tendency, and check yourself. Do you need your arms to help you lower into a chair? Do your knees come together? If so, your leg muscles are critically weak. You need to strengthen them. Practice rising and lowering with good form. Don't lean forward since it puts weight on your knee joints. Push off your heels to use your leg muscles. Work up to several sets of 10 for a simple, free exercise that directly benefits your life.

> Do you let yourself flop down in your chair without using your leg muscles to decelerate? That behavior jolts your spine and loads your discs. It may be just a bad habit, or your leg muscles may be too weak. Lower yourself with strength and ease.
>
> People do things 23 hours a day to tighten, weaken, and cause back and neck pain. They spend an hour exercising and wonder why it doesn't "work."

Resources for More Information

Fix Your Own Pain Without Drugs or Surgery
Jolie Bookspan
www.healthylearning.com

The Fitness Fixer
www.healthline.com/blogs
Health expert column on Healthline.com.
New fun techniques three to four times a week.

Back and Neck-Pain Myths

All of the following statements are false.

- Back pain is usually from lifting something the wrong way one day.
- Once you have back pain, you'll always have back pain.
- Women get more back pain than men.
- When you get back pain, it is important to get bed rest—the more, the better. You should not get out of bed except for bathroom activities, if that.
- For back-pain rehab, forward-bending abdominal exercise is the best exercise.
- You can herniate a disc just from sneezing or getting out of bed in the morning, so it is practically unavoidable; therefore, it doesn't matter how you lift things.
- When you have back pain, it is important to take it easy, and sit down often to conserve energy.
- Back pain is a normal part of getting older.
- Pregnancy or beer guts automatically cause changes in the back. Leaning back to offset a load carried in front is good.
- Eventually you will need surgery.
- If you have back pain, you should sleep on a board or a hard mattress.
- You should be an adult and stop complaining about back pain. You must learn how to cope and live with it. You should go to a pain clinic to learn how to accept the pain.
- The back is a very different system anatomically than the rest of you, so it is very difficult to fix.
- No one knows what causes back pain.
- If back pain is caused by a bad disc, it is permanent.
- Disc degeneration is a disease.
- "I don't need to know about back pain because I do yoga (Pilates, tennis, karate, swimming)."
- "I don't need to know about back pain because I went to the doctor and got it fixed."
- "I don't need to know about back pain. The last time I had back pain, I took vitamin xyz (or meditated, or rubbed on a potion, or did deep breathing)"
- The X-ray shows nothing, which means you are a lying, complaining, wimpy, whining, attention-seeking hypochondriac.

None of these statements are true. Each claim is covered in this chapter and Chapter 20. Understanding the mechanics of back pain is key to changing the cause, instead of just doing "remedies." You can do a lot to easily prevent back and neck pain so that you don't need to treat it. Good mechanics is the key to keeping your back and neck healthy and pain free.

22

Calcium, Protein, Space Flight, Exercise, and Your Bones—A Detective Story

Current recommendations for the prevention of osteoporosis may actually be detrimental to health.

—J. Strain, researcher at the Biomedical Sciences Research Centre, University of Ulster (Med. Hypotheses. 1988 Dec; 27(4): pp 333-8)

Join me on an international detective story. The beginning is deceptively simple. Your bones need calcium; milk has calcium. Then, questions begin creeping in. Why do some vegetarians have a lower incidence of osteoporosis than the general population? Why do some groups of Japanese people, whose calcium intake is historically low, develop osteoporosis, while others don't? Why do African Bantu women, who eat relatively little calcium, have low rates of osteoporosis? Why doesn't the very high-calcium diet of Inuit and Yupik people prevent their suffering the highest rate of osteoporosis in the world? Why do astronauts lose bone in space, no matter what they eat?

The detective story opens with four separate studies. Researchers at the Mayo Clinic found no correlation between calcium intake and age-related bone loss after bone finishes forming in early adulthood. Then, at Tufts University, researchers concluded that calcium had no effect on preventing bone loss in the first five years or so after menopause. From Cornell came a study in 1989 reporting: "It was not clear that increased calcium intake has a significant impact on osteoporosis or other chronic diseases that have been linked to calcium nutriture." More work published in the Journal of the American Medical Woman's Association concluded that calcium intake alone will "neither guarantee optimal bone growth nor protect against bone loss if other critical factors are missing."

The search for these critical factors begins with a trip back in time and the realization that calcium not only can be excreted from your body before it has any chance of connecting with your bones, but it can be driven from existing bone.

Your Changing Bones

Your bones are alive. They continuously break down and rebuild. Throughout your life, you make new bone cells, and break down and assimilate old ones. That recycling process is your body doing its normal business of cell maintenance.

How you use your muscles causes them to pull differently on the bony attachments. Bones found years after death can still give clues about ways the person might have habitually moved. Your bones grow and shape themselves to facilitate your motion. Someone who habitually slouches can change the shape of their bones, eventually deforming them. This process can occur in the spine, knees, hips, ankles, shoulders, feet, and toes—everywhere you pressure your bones. Changing to healthier positioning habits can, in many cases, reshape the bones back to healthier shape. Think of braces on your teeth. It is human bonsai. In cases of extreme dystrophies of the muscles, someone who sits without function of their trunk muscles to hold the spine upright can eventually deform their spine until their ribs sit on their hip bones. How are you sitting while reading this book? You literally shape your own health. Use the information throughout this book to use healthful positioning for all movement and exercise so that your bones stay healthy.

You exchange about three to five percent of your bone cells every year this way. All is well as long as you replace at least as much in the same place as you lose, like money in your bank account. As you age, you may do less bone making and more bone losing, depending how much you exercise. That process isn't bad by itself. It depends how much bone you start out with and how much you lose. The amount you lose is something you can control to a good extent.

What Is Osteoporosis?

With osteoporosis, you lose too much bone, leaving spaces in your bones, making them porous and fragile. *"Osteo-"* is a Greek word element meaning "bone." *"Porosis"* means "porous." Osteoporosis is a serious degenerative bone disorder. Because bone loss is painless until you break a bone, you probably won't know that bone loss is happening in your body. Fractures then easily occur from little or no noticeable cause. Healing is long, sometimes never occurring.

The Toll of Osteoporosis

- Osteoporosis-induced hip and spinal fractures are a major cause of illness and death among older men and women.
- One woman in three over the age of 65 will suffer fractures of the spine.
- Following hip fracture, half of those patients surviving a hip or spine fracture never walk unaided again, become sedentary, even bedridden, leaving about a quarter of the elderly female population of the United States disabled by severe osteoporosis. These risks exceed a woman's risk of developing breast, uterine, and ovarian cancer combined.
- About 24 percent of hip fracture patients over age 50 die. The death rate in the year following a hip fracture is nearly twice as high for men as for women.
- One in eight men over age 50 will have an osteoporosis-related fracture. This risk is greater than his risk of prostate cancer.

The two top documented causes of death following osteoporotic fracture are the associated problems of not moving enough—pneumonia and cardiac events. These deaths include those that follow "successful" hip surgery. The risk of death rises when complications occur from the surgery and the months of recovery, directly leading to death or indirectly by reducing their ability to move, taking them back to the first two causes. Hospitals are a top source of antibiotic-resistant infections. Germs are concentrated in hospitals and health-care facilities, with staff invasively touching patient after patient, giving many antibiotics, thus furthering resistance.

Hip replacement is not a success if the person has pain reduction but can do little more than sit in a chair or shuffle to the bathroom, or becomes unable to stretch his legs in ways that allows straighter positioning for fear of displacing the prosthetic—all ways to become unhealthy from health care. Unhealthy reduction in activity is preventable with a mindset that movement is crucial to recovery, and a program to regain more function, not be made to be content with less.

Why Young People Need to Know About Bone Health

Osteoporosis is not something that just happens to old people; it begins in youth. Your bone density in later years depends on what you are doing right now. Risk factors and practices during youth can reduce the bone density of a teen, 20-, or 30-year-old to the equivalent of someone in his seventies.

Until your mid-thirties, your bones are in an active-growth phase that will determine your peak amount of bone. Building high peak bone mass in youth is like saving more money in the bank now for retirement later. It allows you to lose bone later in life through normal processes, without falling to dangerously low amounts as you make "withdrawals." After a variable plateau period up to around age 50, bone loss may begin, varying from your genetically determined potential, depending on your food and exercise habits.

Like heart disease, bone loss is a gradual process. The time to actively direct its course is now, to prevent it from becoming serious later. Once bone loss becomes serious, it is not easily reversible. By the time osteoporosis is usually diagnosed, 50 to 75 percent of bone may be gone from your skeleton.

Developing the most bone mass you can by the time your skeleton matures in adulthood is an important protection against bone loss and fractures later on. It may be that low peak bone mass, not average bone loss, causes osteoporosis.

Where Does Osteoporosis Affect You?

Three sites are most at risk for osteoporosis:

- Wrist
- Upper back
- Upper leg bone (femur) where it joins your hip

The femur bends and narrows at the femoral neck before widening into the ball that fits in the hip socket. The femoral neck is what usually breaks when you hear of someone "breaking a hip."

When bone thins too much in your upper-back bones, they slowly begin to crush. Because of many forces on these bones, the front of each vertebra crushes more than the back, giving a wedge shape to each bone, like triangles of cheese. Wedge fractures create the classic humped-back or "dowager's hump," with height losses up to five inches. The Hunchback of Notre Dame may have had osteoporosis.

Falls may fracture a wrist that would not have otherwise broken. A broken wrist may be a warning sign of osteoporosis impending in the hip or back. Tooth loss is another early warning sign. So much bone is lost from the jaw that teeth loosen, and then they are lost.

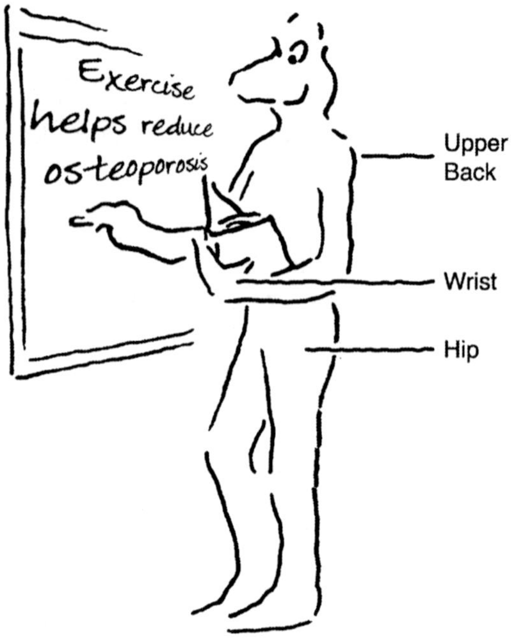

Figure 22-1. The main sites of bone loss with aging in both men and women are your upper back, wrist, and hip. The time to prevent problems later is now.

Why Are These Particular Sites at Risk?

About 1 percent of your skeletal calcium is readily available to supply your daily body processes. This bone pool is stored mostly in your spine bones, called vertebrae, and the ends of your long bones in a spongy, supportive mesh called trabecular bone (tra-BECK'-you-lar). When your body needs calcium, it takes it first from these stockpiles. The result of too much loss is fractures of the wrist and vertebrae.

In men and women over age 75, both trabecular and cortical bone are lost. The dense surface of your bones is called cortical bone. Long bones like those in your arms and legs are mostly cortical bone. Loss of too much cortical bone causes hip fractures. These fractures occur easily, even from normal stresses, because of the weakened bone structure. Men and women have the same trabecular thickness, so when values are adjusted for bone volume, men and women have similar peak bone mineral density (BMD).

Factors Affecting Risk

Many factors influence risk of osteoporosis, not all of which are completely understood. The following factors are major determinants of how much bone mass you can achieve in younger years, how much you later lose, and consequently, of fracture risk: heredity, nutrition, drugs and medicines, hormonal factors, and exercise.

Heredity

Different ethnic and racial groups differ in natural bone density. Everyone can lose bone with age, but the bones of Caucasian people are typically less dense than those of African-American, Hispanic, and Asian people at all age levels.

Bone density in healthy mother-daughter pairs seems to match well. Daughters of women with osteoporosis may have lower bone density in similar body sites as their mothers. Peak bone mass and density may be influenced by fathers, too. These tendencies can be countered with exercise and other practices to protect bone density, described in this section.

Nutrition

The role of high calcium intake in adulthood is not clear. You not only need to get enough calcium, you need to avoid things that cause you to lose calcium from your bones, and things that interfere with calcium absorption.

Protein. A succession of well-controlled studies published since 1920 showed increased urinary calcium loss with increased meat in the diet. In 1988, a published study by the Center for Mineral Metabolism and Clinical Research in Texas concluded that calcium loss due to the animal protein of milk raises the risk of osteoporosis. Studies find that animal protein in meat and dairy increases calcium loss, even with high calcium intake, and even when the animal versus vegetable diet is the same in sodium, potassium, calcium, phosphorus, magnesium, and total protein. The high sulfur content of animal protein raises acid production in your system. The acid increases bone calcium loss and reduces your ability to absorb it. Small losses build, like spending money here and there until you don't know where it all went. The less animal protein, the less loss of calcium is likely.

One study found that by age 80, 1,600 women on a lacto-ovo vegetarian diet for at least 20 years had lost only 18 percent bone mineral compared to closely paired meat-eating women, who lost 35 percent. The effect of animal protein to increase urinary calcium loss and decrease bone density is also thought to raise risk of another disease of bone loss—tooth loss from gum bone ridge resorption. The less animal protein, the less the loss of calcium is likely.

Wheat Gluten and Celiac. People with Celiac Sprue disorder, an autoimmune reaction to foods with the gluten protein, have higher rates of osteoporosis. Main gluten-containing grains are wheat, rye, and barley. It is not certain if a reaction to oats by some people with celiac is due to a something in oats or that they are processed in the same machines that process wheat, leading to cross-contamination. Symptoms can be painful and baffling until identified as coming from gluten. Check for wheat intolerance.

Copper. A 1988 study from the University of Ulster linked mild dietary copper deficiency with osteoporosis in both humans and animals. Medical literature states copper is abundant in normal diets but doesn't consider common barriers to copper utilization. The lactose in dairy products can interfere with copper metabolism. High sugar intake increases urinary excretion of both calcium and copper.

Vitamin D. Calcium does not absorb or work well without Vitamin D and other key minerals. Availability of Vitamin D, required for calcium absorption in the small intestine, diminishes with aging, as the kidney reduces Vitamin D synthesis, and the function or number of Vitamin-D-binding receptors in your intestine decline. Get a safe amount of sunshine every day. Don't overdo so much that you sunburn, obviously.

Sunshine. Sunshine is needed for many health aspects and disease prevention. Sunlight exposure is increasingly documented as crucial to bone density, healthy immune function, positive mood, sound sleep at night, physical development in children, relief of symptoms of rheumatoid arthritis, MS, tuberculosis, diabetes, eczema, and other health issues. It is more effective and healthful to get nutrients from sun and good food than supplements. Warnings on the dangers of overtanning are important for preventing skin cancer for people who work outdoors, people who overtan for cosmetic purposes, and a few other populations. Another group to consider is people who spend too little time outdoors. Darker-skinned people need longer sun exposures daily than lighter-skinned people, as darker skin filters exposure. Eating food with good antioxidant content regularly, such as vegetables, helps keep sun exposure safe for the skin.

Caffeine. Caffeine may make you excrete more calcium in your urine, but relation to risk is not certain.

Alcohol. Osteoporosis is more common in alcoholics than in non-alcoholics of the same age. Alcohol is directly toxic to bone cells. Alcoholism contributes to bone loss through poor nutrition, liver disease, poor calcium and Vitamin D absorption, and by interfering with parathyroid gland function. Your parathyroids are four little kidney-shaped glands near, or on, your thyroid gland. They secrete a hormone you need to metabolize calcium and phosphorus.

Smoking. Smoking, like alcohol, is directly toxic to bone cells. Cigarette smoking also interferes with calcium absorption and estrogen, and is associated with earlier menopause and bone loss more frequently than in non-smokers.

Anorexia Nervosa. Anorexia nervosa is a condition of abnormal loss of appetite and refusal to eat. It results in emaciation and malnutrition. Anorexia nervosa is a major risk factor for osteoporosis in both men and women for several reasons. The diet is severely calcium deficient, and the loss of muscle and total body weight decreases resistive forces on bones. Bones need a physical stimulus for maintaining thickness. Anorexia can lead to decreased reproductive hormones in both men and women. Estrogen and testosterone both help maintain bone density. The malnutrition of anorexia can lead to loss of regular menstrual function, which is another risk factor for osteoporosis.

Calcium. The issue of calcium requirement provokes much debate. Many factors affect calcium absorption and excretion, making it difficult to pin down just how much calcium you need. In the 1960s and 1970s, major textbooks of medicine did not consider calcium important in osteoporosis development or prevention, or only considered calcium malabsorption disorders. In the 1980s and 1990s, a calcium mania swept the public. Although much is still unknown, it is established that adequate calcium intake influences bone-mass formation until adulthood. In this way, calcium reduces subsequent osteoporosis risk since someone with high bone mass at age 30 may lose bone through normal aging, yet have sufficient bone remaining at age 75.

However, studies seem to show that calcium alone does not guarantee optimal bone growth in youth. Neither will it prevent bone loss with age in men, with estrogen withdrawal in women, with immobilization (such as a cast or bed rest), or with amenorrhea (ay-men-or-REE'-ah), which is absence of the menstrual cycle. It is also not even a sure bet that increased dietary calcium affects bone density once you reach adulthood. Therefore, instead of just eating calcium, you should use other techniques to have healthy bones.

> Just drinking milk or taking calcium pills will not stop osteoporosis. Bone density depends on many things. One big factor is how much exercise you get.

Other Nutritional Factors. Many nutritional components are involved in the health of any body system. Other vitamins and minerals (for example, Vitamin K and boron) are important to your continually changing bones.

Drugs and Medicines

Antacids. A class of drugs that reduce stomach acid, called proton pump inhibitors (PPIs), have been shown to greatly increase risk of hip fracture. Proton pump inhibitors include Nexium®, Prilosec®, Prevacid®, Zoton®, Inhibitol®, and others. The common practice of using proton pump inhibitors, as well as ordinary antacids, has long been identified in accepted studies to reduce calcium absorption. Chapters 20 and 21 on back pain show how to easily fix the cause of several pain syndromes so that you don't need pain medicines and the acid medicines often prescribed with them. For minor stomach complaints, use ginger root to sooth stomach pain, rather than medicines, and refer to Chapter 15 on healthy digestion.

Steroid Anti-Inflammatories. Long-term corticosteroid (non-anabolic steroid hormone) treatment may be prescribed for various conditions, including respiratory and endocrine disorders, skin conditions, autoimmune diseases such as lupus and multiple sclerosis, rheumatoid arthritis, cancer, and others. With continued use, steroid anti-inflammatories can cause cataracts and bone loss, weaken connective tissue, and increase risk of bone fracture for both men and women. It is counterproductive when people are put on these medicines for joint pain, while it is harming their joints. Long-term oral glucocorticoid therapy accounts for nearly one in six cases of male osteoporosis. Osteoporosis prevention is an important issue for anyone taking steroid anti-inflammatories for long periods of time. Use good body mechanics to stop the cause of body aches and joint pain instead of taking medicines that do not stop the cause and have unhealthful effects.

Non-Steroid Anti-Inflammatories (NSAIDS). Nonsteroidal anti-inflammatory drugs are commonly prescribed for arthritis or "aches and pains." Studies are mixed, but evidence suggests they reduce bone healing in bones already fractured or injured. In the case of patients receiving a bone-ingrowth type of hip or knee prosthesis, bone ingrowth can be inhibited, which may result in a loose prosthesis. The bone effects of NSAIDS are believed to be reversible if the medication is stopped. Avoid long-term use of non-steroidal anti-inflammatories like ibuprofen (Advil®, Motrin®, Nuprin®), naproxen (Aleve®, Naprosyn®), and COX-2 inhibitors (Bextra®, Celebrex®).

Depo-Provera®. The contraceptive Depo-Provera (medroxyprogesteroneacetate) reduces estrogen production. Women taking Depo-Provera can lose bone mass in the early years of use, and can have bone density values below normal. Bone loss in the later years of Depo-Provera use normally levels off until it approaches the normal rate of age-related fall.

Endometriosis Treatment. Treatment with nafarelin for endometriosis increases bone loss. Adding norethisterone (NET) to nafarelin treatment seems to have a bone-sparing effect. Ask your physician if this treatment pertains to you.

Other Drugs. Regular use of SSRI antidepressants, such as Prozac® and Paxil®, double the risk of bone fractures. Medicines for thyroid and anticonvulsant medications such as phenytoin (Dilantin®) and phenobarbital decrease calcium absorption. Numerous medications used to treat different cancers may produce osteopenia (bone shortage) and osteoporosis in long-term cancer survivors.

Hormonal Factors

Several hormones influence bone density and risk of osteoporosis in both women and men.

Menopause and Amenorrhea. One effect of the hormones estrogen and testosterone are to increase calcium retention in your bones. Estrogen (and to a smaller extent, testosterone) levels drop with amenorrhea (loss of periods before menopause) and with natural and surgical menopause. Surgical menopause removes the ovaries, called oophorectomy (oo-for-EK'-tuh-mee), causing abrupt losses regardless of calcium intake. During the first years of natural menopausal, withdrawal of the body's estrogen production is a gradual change. It takes time to adjust to the loss. Without exercise, much loss can occur.

Many things may cause menstrual irregularities, or loss of the menstrual cycle entirely (amenorrhea) in premenopausal women. It is popular to blame vigorous exercise, with some authorities going as far as stating that athletes who experience amenorrhea should be banned from further training. Exercise alone is not sufficient to cause amenorrhea. Greatly decreased body fat and poor nutrition are involved. It seems to be an obvious and natural safety feature that, in evolutionary times, if conditions were harsh with lack of food and constant, difficult travel, then conditions were unfavorable for reproductive survival. Physical resources were better reserved until easier times.

Physical exercise is important to preserving bone mass. Stopping an amenorrheic athlete from exercising is counterproductive. Investigation into other contributing factors can allow the athlete to continue vigorous training, with all its benefits of health and well-being.

Hormone levels affect bone density in men too.

Reduced Hormone Levels in Men. Testosterone has many functions, including regulating bone mass. The stress of extended periods of extreme exercise on the body seems to send a signal to the brain to decrease levels of two hormones that stimulate the testes to produce testosterone. Declining estradiol (an estrogenic hormone) in men is more strongly correlated with decreased bone density than is declining testosterone level. As hormone levels go down, risks of various reproductive and bone-density problems go up, just as in women. Much attention in the literature is paid to the role of hormones, exercise, and bone density in women, but unfortunately little about the phenomenon in men.

Exercise

Resistance exercise builds bone at any age, even elderly. Exercise is crucial in osteoporosis prevention. The job of your bones is to support your body against the pull of gravity. Your bones develop more when you have more need for them to resist gravity. The physical stress of muscle pulling on bone during exercise stimulates bone to thicken and strengthen. Throughout your entire life, when you exercise, you stimulate growth of new bone cells. The physical pull of muscles thickens your bones where the muscles attach. Using your arm muscles thickens arm bones. Using your legs strengthens leg bones, and so on. It is a main mechanism of how exercise prevents osteoporosis. Without exercise, you don't stimulate enough new cells to counter the normal loss as old ones break down. Your bones thin no matter how much calcium you eat.

Lack of mechanical stress from lack of exercise, prolonged immobility during bed rest, being in a cast, paralysis, a sedentary lifestyle, and weightlessness during space flight leads to bone loss, regardless of how much calcium you eat. Bone loss from extended immobilization may become greater than can be completely reversed after about six months of inactivity. Bed rest so effectively reduces bone density that it is used as a model in scientific studies for bone loss in the microgravity of space.

Animals that hibernate go without activity for long periods. Their bodies produce chemicals that prevent bone loss. Humans lose bone from inactivity and need resistive exercise to keep bones dense and strong. Like muscular atrophy from lack of exercise, the bone atrophy of osteoporosis is a "use it or lose it" disease. Sedentary lifestyle is a major factor.

Osteoporosis is "bone atrophy" from several causes, including lack of exercise. Sedentary lifestyle is a major risk factor for osteoporosis.

Physical activity can increase bone mass in all age groups. Movement alone is not enough; it must include active muscular resistance. Weight-bearing activity, for example, walking or jogging, increases bone density, primarily of the lower body. Weight-loading exercise, usually weight lifting, can increase bone density at all sites, including the upper body. Weight-resisting activity includes moving, pulling, and lifting your own body weight, such as fun activities as handstands, hanging from a bar, trying pull-ups, and safely loading wrist joints with good mechanics for push-ups and holding the plank position. You can load your upper leg at the hip, a major site of osteoporosis, by bending right using your legs for all the many times you need to bend every day. Weight lifting can include lifting groceries, children, and packages around the house. Like nutrition and unlike genetics, physical activity is an easily controllable risk factor.

What About Water Sports as Exercise?

Swimming is not a weight-bearing activity. It is a point of great interest to swimmers and scientists whether swimming can increase bone mass. Muscles still pull on bone to move you through the water, but is it less than during weight bearing? It depends how hard you work. Studies report that tough swimming workouts give plenty of bone-building resistance. If the only exercise you get is a casual swim, it is wise to augment that with weight lifting and weight-bearing activities.

Like swimming, scuba diving is not a weight-bearing sport, except when carrying gear. Regularly lifting scuba gear is weight-loading activity for healthy backs. If you are able, carry your own tanks to get weight-lifting exercise. If your back is already osteoporotic, it is a question of how close to fracture risk you are before you carry or wear your tank before you get into the water. The weight could further compress fragile vertebrae. In this case, don your tank in the water. Buoyancy underwater helps offset the weight of a tank. Check with your physician about diving safely if you have osteoporosis and what exercise will safely load the site enough to help heal it safely.

How Much Calcium Do You Need?

With so many interacting variables, calcium need varies. You need more calcium if you lose calcium from smoking, drinking alcohol, and eating high amounts of animal protein. High intake of animal protein may cause calcium levels to become inadequate in situations where a tendency to low dietary calcium already exists. You may do well with less calcium if you exercise and reduce factors involved in calcium loss.

Although much is unknown, it is established that calcium intake influences bone mass until adulthood. In this way, calcium reduces subsequent osteoporosis risk, since someone with high bone mass at age 30 may lose bone through normal aging, yet have sufficient bone remaining at age 75. After the skeletal maturation of adulthood, you still need calcium daily, although it is not known if calcium intake over a certain minimum amount of time influences bone density.

Dr. Neal Barnard, President of the Physicians' Committee for Responsible Medicine (PCRM), reminds us that, "Excessive calcium intake does not fool hormones into building much more bone, any more than delivering an extra load of bricks will make a construction crew build a larger building." PCRM filed a complaint with the Federal Trade Commission against ads showing celebrity milk mustaches, stating that some deceptively imply that just drinking milk will prevent bone loss. Whether or not extra calcium will help, it is important to get enough calcium.

For children, the American Academy of Pediatrics recommends the following daily minimum amounts of calcium:

- 500 mg/day (children 1 to 3 years)
- 800 mg/day (children 4 to 8 years)
- 1300 mg/day (ages 9 to 19)

For adults:

- 1000 mg/day
- 1200 to 1500 mg/day during pregnancy and lactation
- In 2000, NIH consensus was 1,000 to 1,500 mg per day for osteoporotic men
- In 2007, the North American Menopause Society updated recommendations for women to a target calcium intake of 1,200 mg/day.

Some authorities feel that most people do not get enough calcium. See your physician to determine your calcium needs.

Calcium Sources

What are good sources of calcium? Where do cows get theirs? You can't fully digest grass, but dark green vegetables like spinach, collard greens, bok choy, broccoli, Chinese cabbage, mustard greens, okra, and kale are good sources of calcium. It used to be often stated that certain components of these plants, called phytate and oxalic acid, would depress calcium absorption, making them far less effective than dairy sources. However, calcium absorption from both low- and high-phytate soybeans has been found to be close to that of milk, with absorption from low phytate soybeans slightly higher than that of milk. Another recent study found interference by oxalic acid to be less than previously thought. Use fermented rather than unfermented soy. Fermenting grains like tempeh reduces phytic-acid content, which increases absorption of calcium.

Broccoli has more calcium per calorie than any other food. Seaweed is another good, yet frequently overlooked, source. Fruit has calcium as do almonds and sunflower seeds. Better yet, fruits, vegetables, nuts, and legumes have the element boron, and leafy green have Vitamin K, both of which participate in preventing osteoporosis. Milk has little boron. Meat and eggs have none. Because calcium absorption goes down with increased intake, spread out your daily dose into spaced intervals to increase absorption.

Can You Get Enough Calcium Without Dairy?

Although dairy products are the prevailing calcium source in many Western countries, they are not the only source, or the best source:

- Dairy is one of the most potent causes of allergy.
- Dairy is a major source of fat and cholesterol, increasing risk of several chronic diseases of the heart and blood vessels.

- Capacity to break down the milk sugar galactose decreases with age, and some people just have low levels of the enzyme that breaks it down. Galactose is associated with cataracts and prostate and ovarian cancer.
- Increasingly, dairy cows are given hormones to increase milk production, as well as antibiotics and medicines which pass into the milk, contributing to a world problem of antibiotic resistance and other health effects still to be understood.
- The heat process to kill germs in dairy products also kills many nutrients.
- Dairy is a major contributor to reflux.
- Dairy products contain lactose. Most people lose the ability to digest lactose after childhood, causing gas, abdominal swelling from bloating, and pain. In most of human history, people did not consume milk after weaning.
- Lactose may interfere with copper metabolism. Mild deficiency of copper, common in Western diets, is related to the development of osteoporosis.
- Dairy protein can promote a specific auto-immune reaction in susceptible people that hurts insulin-producing cells in the pancreas, raising incidence of insulin-dependent diabetes.
- Cow's milk is not chemically like human milk. It has toxic effects on human babies, and possibly older children. Cow's milk must not be given to human infants.
- The animal protein in dairy directly increases urinary calcium loss.

It is not difficult to get adequate calcium without dairy products.

Many non-Western people get more calcium than the average American, from non-dairy sources. Peruvian Indians eat cereal mixed with powdered calcium carbonate rock. Contemporary hunter-gatherers have a high calcium intake, three times higher than the average middle-aged American woman, without eating any dairy. Getting enough healthy calcium and protein without dairy is easy with vegetables, seeds, legumes, and fermented vegetables. Fermenting increases protein and reduces phytates that reduce calcium absorption.

Calcium Supplements

Calcium supplements are major sales items, even though major health organizations recommend getting calcium from food, not supplements. The U.S. Food and Drug Administration recommends checking the labels of many kinds of bottled calcium pills, to avoid bone meal and dolomite sources because of their high content of lead and other toxic metals. Calcium carbonate and calcium citrate are alternatives.

High-Calcium Foods

Source	Milligrams of Calcium (mg)
1 cup tofu processed with calcium sulfate	868
1 cup dulse seaweed	600
1 cup navy beans and 2 corn tortillas	370
1 cup cooked collard greens	357
1 cup amaranth	280
1 cup tempeh	215
1 cup spinach	200
1 cup kale	200
1 tablespoon blackstrap molasses	200
1 cup broccoli	180
1 cup soybeans	175
1 cup fortified orange juice	120
1 cup dried apricots	100

Calcium absorption among the various supplement tablets is generally good, particularly between meals, except in people who underproduce stomach acid and people taking antacid drugs (refer to Chapter 15). For these people, an apple-cider-vinegar drink helps, adding lemon to food and water, and getting your calcium with a meal benefits absorption. Absorption fraction should be assessed by a trained dietitian or physician before beginning a supplement regimen. Not all supplements are easily absorbed. A common test is to put the calcium tablet in a glass of vinegar. It should dissolve within 30 minutes.

How to Reduce Your Risk of Osteoporosis

- One of the most important things you can do to reduce your risk of osteoporosis is to get regular exercise. One effective bone-building exercise is lifting weights, including packages and bags. Also important is resisting your own body weight during weight-bearing exercise like walking, dancing, running, skating, and skiing. Rest weight on your hands by doing push-ups, handstands, and arm balancing, because your wrist is one of the three main sites of bone loss. Carry groceries, bend correctly by bending knees with torso upright for all daily bending.

- Get adequate calcium from a variety of vegetable sources.
- Spread calcium intake throughout the day.
- Get healthful sunlight every day, over more of your body than just face and hands.
- Avoid meat and a high-dairy diet.
- Don't smoke.
- Drink less alcohol.
- If you drink a lot of alcohol, get screened periodically for Vitamin D, parathyroid hormone (and other deficiencies), and bone loss.
- Avoid chronic use of medications that cause bone loss, such as anti-inflammatory steroids (cortisone, prednisone, prednisolone), antacids, thyroid medication, some anticonvulsants, and Depo-progesterone.
- Limit consumption of sodas, since they contain phosphates.
- Plain raw flax seeds and walnuts have been found to be effective to help bone health as vegetarian sources of omega-3 (n-3) fatty acids. Don't overdo flax seeds, as they are estrogenic and can enhance estrogenic problems.
- Check to see if you have reaction to wheat products, an immune action called Celiac Sprue. Celiac is one of several predisposing factors for osteoporosis.
- Don't crash diet. Rapid weight loss is shown to lower hipbone density.
- Talk to your health-care providers about non-drug osteoporosis treatment and prevention programs.

Osteoporosis Drugs

Medicines exist to stop bone loss and build new bone in both men and women. About a third of hip fractures occurs in men.

Estrogen replacement was originally considered the only way to maintain bone mass in the first five years after menopause. However, bone density is more complicated than just estrogen or estrogen's several forms, and estrogen replacement may increase risk of uterine or breast cancer in some women, and stroke or heart disease in others. Testosterone replacement for elderly men may cause increased prostate size or increase the risk of prostate cancer.

New medications were developed to act like a combination of estrogen, progesterone (which balances estrogen's effects), and testosterone. These medications were hoped to prevent problems like hot flashes, skin atrophy, and mucus membrane drying, without the old problems of estrogen replacement, but questions and problems remained about which hormonal medications may increase risk of cardiovascular disease and other problems. The menopausal symptoms were found to be better relieved by exercise than medicine, and the medicines were found to have sometimes serious side effects.

Non-hormonal drugs were developed in hope of slowing bone deterioration without the problems of hormone replacement. Bisphosphonates and teriparatide (recombinant parathyhroid hormone) have been approved for use in men. Bisphosphonate therapy included alendronate sodium (Fosamax®) and risedronate (Actonel®). Some drugs were found to have serious effects on gums, causing tooth loss. Various calcitonin nasal sprays (like Miacalcin®) use a synthetic form of calcitonin, a hormone your body produces in several forms. "Designer estrogens" like raloxifene (Evista®) are selective estrogen receptor modulators (SERM). It means they select some parts of your body to help the same way estrogen does, but not other parts of your body that don't need it or could be harmed by it. In that way, they were hoped to have bone- and heart-saving benefits without the risks of breast and uterine cancers. Ideally, a selective medication would have all the good effects of hormones, and none of the bad. Nothing is available like that yet, not even in your own body.

Plant-based remedies are under investigation as commercial pharmaceuticals. Various "herbal" products sold over the counter in health-food stores claim to help avoid osteoporosis and menopausal symptoms. These products are not regulated the same way as pharmaceuticals, meaning any claim can be made for them. (Some people would argue the same is unfortunately true for pharmaceuticals.) Some products interfere with other medications you may be on, or cause you to bleed too much if you have surgery, even dental surgery.

Anyone with risk factors for osteoporosis and a history or risk of stroke, heart disease, or any cancer should weigh the risks of the various medications with their physician. Develop a complete program that includes doing regular, fun physical activity, regularly getting out in the sunlight, and changing bad nutrition and other habits that contribute to an avoidable spectrum of bone loss and related health problems.

Important Answers

The detective story, while not solved, reveals crucial clues. African Bantu women eat less than half the currently recommended calcium, and have low rates of osteoporosis. They eat predominantly plant protein. Their genetic relatives living in the United States eating the Western diet of high animal protein and getting less sunlight suffer rates of osteoporosis and fractures similar to those of other North Americans. Inuit and Yupik people have a high-calcium diet (nearly twice the recommended amount), are physically active, and have high Vitamin-D intake from animal sources, yet suffer the world's highest rate of osteoporosis, which scientists relate to their high-animal-protein diet. How much is related to low exposure to sunlight remains to be investigated.

Osteoporosis Risk Reduction

Reduce	Increase	Consider
Inactivity and sedentary lifestyle	Physical activity, weightlifting, weight-bearing activity	Osteoporosis prevention program
Animal protein	Vegetable sources of calcium	Bone-density evaluation
Alcohol, colas, smoking	Sunlight if deficient	Nutritional assessment, including check for celiac
Antacids, certain anti-inflammatories, and other medications that decrease calcium and bone density	Use walnuts for vegetarian sources of omega-3 (n-3) fatty acids, rather than animal based products	Reducing caffeine, salt

Populations in Japan whose low protein intake comes primarily from plant sources have normal bone growth and low rates of age-related osteoporosis, even with calcium intakes half that recommended in the United States. In their genetic relatives eating a modern diet, high salt and protein intake aggravates calcium deficiency in old age.

> Calcium is not the whole story in bone health. Getting enough calcium is crucial, but without other critical factors, it is not a cure-all.

Osteoporosis affects both men and women. Attaining high peak bone density when younger reduces the chance of lowering bone mass to unhealthy levels in later life.

Factors affecting your risk of osteoporosis:

- How much exercise you get
- Your total nutritional picture
- Heredity
- Hormonal status

Reducing calcium loss may be as important as getting enough calcium. Factors that increase your calcium and/or bone loss include:

- Lack of exercise
- Smoking
- High alcohol intake
- High-protein diet
- Antacids
- Celiac Sprue disorder
- High-meat diet
- Lack of Vitamin D
- Steroid medicines
- Cola drinks (The high phosphorus content in both regular and diet colas is not good for your bones.)

To build bone and reduce bone loss:

- Increase physical activity.
- Get healthful nutrition.
- Get a healthful amount of sunlight on a regular basis.

> The most important message is to not wait until later. Preventing osteoporosis later depends on what you are doing right now.

Resources for More Information

Physicians for Responsible Medicine
www.pcrm.org
P.O. Box 6322
Washington, DC 20015
202-686-2210
www.worldveganday.org

Includes a nice summary of sensible vegetarian food choices on their nutrition link.

23

Body Fat

Am I fat? I've fallen down and not even known it.

—Pat McCormick

Some people worry when they don't fit into their tightest suit. Others don't worry until they can't fit into the car, and sometimes, not even then. An informal look around reveals that being heavy seems to be common. Is that phenomenon bad?

When Does Fat Help You?

You could not live without a certain minimum of body fat. Fat is a necessary part of every cell in your body. Your nerves could not conduct signals rapidly enough for you to function without their fatty wrapping.

Body fat keeps you warm in the cold. Without a certain minimum of body fat, you lose your reproductive ability. Fat helps shield blows to your internal organs. High body weight, whether from fat or lean, provides the loading your bones need to stay dense and strong. Heavier people can have lower rates of osteoporosis.

Success in different sports depends on characteristic body sizes and compositions. Football linemen usually have more-than-average fat compared to other athletes. Fat weight is an advantage to linemen for the added mass and padding for blocking ability.

Increased muscle mass accompanies the extra fat weight to carry the whole package around.

Sumo wrestling is another sport where extra weight helps. Linemen and sumos don't have to run much. It's not as big of a sports disadvantage to carry extra weight. They have extra muscle, which helps their sport. Other sports where the players have more fat than average for athletes are baseball, discus throwing, and ice hockey, although trends are changing for track athletes.

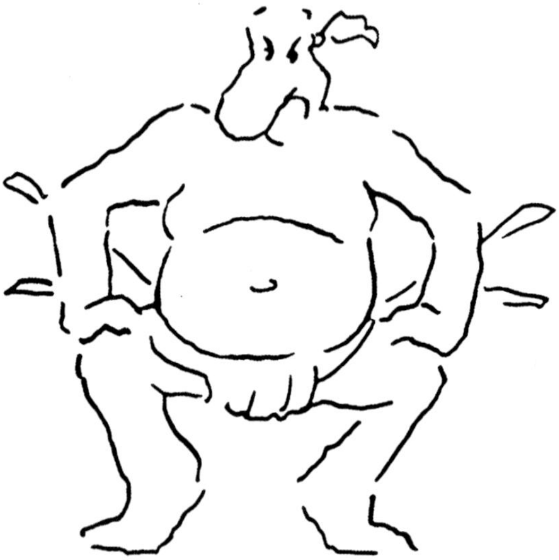

Figure 23-1. High body weight benefits some activities, like sumo wrestling.

Studies confirm a relation between body fat and keeping warm in the cold—helpful in sports like swimming, ice hockey, ice fishing, skiing, and other cold-weather activities. You don't have to be obese to experience thermal benefits. Any amount of fat adds insulation.

Because of the extra work of carrying extra fat, a heavy person generally develops extra muscle mass. Heavy people not only have more pounds of fat than lighter people, but more pounds of muscle. Extra muscle comes in handy in work like lifting things, and keeping warm in the cold. Consider the extra fat as a built-in daily weight-lifting regimen.

Fat increases buoyancy in the water, adding safety and comfort to swimming. A little fat on your legs lets you float more horizontally, which is a better body position for moving efficiently through the water for scuba diving and swimming. Skinny legs tend to sink, making streamline more difficult.

When Does Fat Hinder You?

Extra fat weight is a burden to carry across distance or against gravity. Extra fat weight is more work to carry around. The high-calorie cost of transporting extra weight makes low body fat advantageous to gymnastics, climbing, and any sport where you have to run around. World-class distance runners and boxers usually have low body fat. The same fat that keeps you warm in the cold makes you warm in hot weather, too. One predisposing factor to overheating is being large, round, and fat. A common question is: can you be fit and fat? Someone who has extra fat, but high cardiovascular conditioning can lower their risk of heart disease as low or lower than a lighter out-of-shape person, but other disease risks are high, and too much fat weight makes problems. Having enough fat for health, comfort, and optimal performance in your sport is important. Chapter 24 describes the problems of too much fat.

Body Fat of Athletes in Different Sports
(in no particular order)

Higher-Fat Athletes	Lower-Fat Athletes
Baseball players	Distance runners
Football linemen	Gymnasts
Sumo wrestlers	Acrobats
Ice-hockey players	Climbers
	Boxers
	Wrestlers

Why You Have Fat and Most Plants Have Little

With exceptions like avocados, coconuts, and nuts, plants don't store their energy in the form of fat. People do. Why?

Fat is lighter than an equal volume of protein and carbohydrate. The same volume of fat weighs less than muscle protein. One of fat's prominent traits is ability to float well. Fat has twice the calories as the same quantity of carbohydrate or protein by weight. In that way, fat stores more energy than carbohydrate or muscle. This lightweight, energy-dense storage form is the reason animals use fat as a storage vehicle. If you have to carry your energy around with you, it makes sense to make it a lighter package.

Plants don't go places often. Their storage medium does not require weight control. They store most of their energy as carbohydrate. The extra weight is not a metabolic burden. Avocados and coconuts, like other seeds and nuts, are the portion of plants that must move. They travel to new locations to germinate. They typically store fat to make their energy suitcases lighter.

Your muscles stock a small amount of carbohydrate called glycogen that you use to increase exercise levels. Muscle glycogen cannot release glucose for use by any other tissues. If you eat muscles (if you eat meat, you are eating muscles) you get some protein, a good deal of fat (even in lean cuts), but no carbohydrate that helps your exercise.

> Plants store their energy as carbohydrate, which is heavier than the same volume of fat. The extra weight is not a burden since most of these plants don't travel. Avocados and coconuts, like other seeds and nuts with healthful fat, are the portion of plants that move to new locations to germinate.
>
> Animals carry their energy around with them, so it makes sense to carry it in the lighter weight package of fat.

Why Extra Fat?

Humans have fat, but why so much in some cases? The difference between fatter and thinner people is mainly the amount of exercise they get and what kind of food they eat. It is easy to be sedentary, particularly in a lifestyle geared around the automobile and television. Modern daily life is hectic, but not active. Humans evolved to move as part of all activities needed for life, producing food, building shelter, and dancing and moving for fun. Modern habits take away the daily movement needed to stay healthy. Movement has become artificial and something you have to stop your life to go do. Many people become so unaccustomed to movement that they get too tight-jointed to tie their shoe without rounding the back, to bend properly to retrieve things from the floor, or to cut their own toenails. They don't use their muscles enough to stop their body from slouching during all sitting, walking, and even during exercise. Weekend exercisers rarely exercise enough for it to count as regular exercise. Exercise classes consisting of swishing the backside side-to-side are not enough real movement to burn many calories. It's easy to gain weight if you don't routinely move as part of your normal, daily activities. Weight gain is not a mystery.

> Being fat usually results from too little exercise and too much food. Active movement is an ongoing part of normal life, but has become artificially segregated into stopping your real life and "doing exercises."

24

Problems of Being Overweight

Those who think they have no time for bodily exercise will sooner or later have to find time for illness.

—Edward Stanley

Having a small amount of fat is necessary, as covered in Chapter 23. Too much fat creates many health problems. A person can be considered normal body weight, yet still carry a high percentage of it as fat. Debate continues over the difference in disease risk between being fat, but with good cardiovascular capacity, and having low cardiovascular capacity at any weight, which is a high risk factor of cardiovascular diseases. Fat cells are more than suitcases for energy stores. They are hormonally active and interact with various processes involved in many diseases. In general, it has been found that too much fat percentage has drawbacks, such as increased risk of orthopedic problems, stroke, diabetes, certain cancers, gastrointestinal problems, complicated pregnancy, even snoring.

More Work

It takes extra energy, work, and calories to carry extra fat around, depending on the workload. A heavy man may work harder and closer to his maximum than a lighter man or woman to do physical activity that moves his body against gravity—for example, walking, running, climbing a hill, ascending stairs, and dancing. This situation is often the case even if the lighter person has a lesser physical capacity.

On one hand, you could say that extra work is free exercise and you could be happy about burning more calories for the same work as a lighter person. For heavy people in good physical shape, the extra work falls within their comfort range. For those in so-so to poor shape, this work can be beyond the capacity of the out-of-shape heart to supply itself and the body with oxygen, beyond the capacity of fat-narrowed blood vessels to conduct enough blood, or past the ability of the joints to continually support the weight.

Illness and Injury

A 2007 study by the World Cancer Research Fund making news as "a landmark study" found that keeping slim is one of the best ways of preventing cancer. Heart disease, stroke, cancer, osteoarthritis, and gall-bladder trouble all become more common as weight increases.

A large percentage of adult-onset diabetes cases is triggered by obesity. Diabetes can cause deterioration of the blood vessels, sometimes ending in blindness and loss of your legs, and can cause serious health problems, doubling the risk of death compared to someone of similar age without diabetes.

Being overweight is one of several factors that promotes diverticulitis, a painful inflammation of the large intestinal wall. Extra weight raises the risk of the most common type of stroke in both men and women. Being overweight is a contributor to hernias. Hernia affects one out of eight men.

Snoring

High body fat is a key contributor to serious snoring and its more problematic consequence, sleep apnea. Sleep apnea is a disorder where the snorer stops breathing during sleep, sometimes hundreds of times per night. The large, heavy neck and throat of an overweight person can lead to intermittent upper-airway obstruction during sleep. Bouts of oxygen starvation occur during sleep, and the person may frequently wake up gasping and snorting. Over time, lack of oxygen to the blood vessels results in fatty deposits in the blood vessels of the heart and brain. This result is thought to be one of the mechanisms for the higher incidence of stroke and cardiac irregularities in people with this sleep disorder.

Repeated awakenings from the snoring and apnea result in chronic daytime sleepiness. This sleepiness greatly increases the risk of automobile accidents, up to seven times the normal risk, according to some estimates.

Sleep apnea is sometimes called the Pickwickian syndrome, after the "Fat Boy" in Dickens' The Pickwick Papers, who was obese and sluggish in the daytime. Various degrees of sleep apnea, from mild to serious, are sometimes called Ondine's Curse. In

Greek mythology, Ondine (alternately spelled Undine) was a water spirit who cursed a poorly behaving man to thereafter breathe only voluntarily, not automatically. When he fell asleep, he stopped breathing and suffocated. The ancient Greeks knew that you have two different controls for breathing. One is voluntary, meaning you can deliberately breathe more, less, or differently. Your involuntary center keeps you breathing when you don't think about it (for example, when you are asleep). In a small number of cases, genetic mutation prevents the involuntary breathing centers from working properly. For others, Ondine's curse is more a factor of "body habitus," which means body build, especially as it relates to risk of disease. Losing weight is often the first line of medically prescribed treatment.

Death

A man 20 percent overweight is twice as likely as a normal-weight man to die before age 50 from a weight-related disease—just 20 percent. As an example, a man who should weigh close to 170 pounds (77 kilograms) weighs over 200 pounds (91 kilograms).

Brain Function

"Cognitive decline" was linked to circulatory disorders resulting from obesity in a Cornell Medical College study published in the February 1992 issue of *Clinics in Geriatric Medicine*. Data reported in the September 1992 issue of *Hypertension* indicate that men with long-term high blood pressure lost more left-brain tissue than men with normal blood pressure. A high percentage of high-blood-pressure cases link to being overweight, even without high salt intake. The researchers suspect the specific areas of brain tissue loss affect memory, language, and "finding your way around."

What to Do

Several of the disease risks are related to low aerobic capacity. At whatever weight, regular aerobic exercise, done safely, helps reduce risks. Regular exercise of all the several aspects of fitness (Chapter 2 and 3) helps reduce body weight, making exercise important in a weight-control and disease-control program.

25

Body-Fat Tests

You know you're getting fat when you can pinch an inch on your forehead.

—John Mendoza

Many people carry more than a healthy amount of body fat. How do you know if you are one of them? Of the many tests, some you can do yourself at home or the gym with simple equipment. Some tests require only minimal training; other tests need sophisticated measurement machinery run by skilled operators and interpreters.

Reducing your fat weight helps to lessen your chance of the diseases and problems mentioned in Chapter 24, particularly if you are already at risk for them. In general, focus on the ideas, rather than the specific numbers. Still, finding out what the tests are and how they are done is an interesting story.

Apples and Pears

Where you carry your fat is as important as—or some say, more important than—how much you have. The apple versus pear test requires only a mirror. Carrying fat primarily in the upper body and abdomen gives an apple shape to your figure. Lower body fat distributed on the hips and thighs makes a body more pear-shaped. Apple-shaped people seem to have a greater risk of obesity-related disease like heart disease, colon cancer, diverticulitis, diabetes, and high blood pressure than pear-shaped people.

Waist-to-Hip Ratio

The waist-to-hip ratio test further defines the apple-versus-pear test. It looks to see if your waist is large compared to your hips. You find this ratio by measuring your waist and hips, and then dividing the waist by the hip measurement. Answers above 0.8 for women and 1.0 for men indicate a tendency toward the more problematic apple shape. For example, waist 37 inches, hip 36 inches (94 cm and 92 cm). The answer is 1.03, which is not good for anyone.

Insurance Tables

One way to predict health, according to insurance companies, is to check your weight against values in their insurance-company tables that tell the ideal weight for your height. According to the height-and-weight tables of the Metropolitan Life Insurance Company, if you are more than 20 percent above their supposed ideal weight, you are considered obese. Exercise scientists recommend against relying on insurance tables, as they had problems in the procedures for developing them, and like other tests limited to height and weight, the tests ignore that you could have any amount of body fat for your height and weight.

Body Mass Index

The body-mass index (BMI) compares how heavy you are relative to your height. To calculate BMI, divide your weight in kilograms by your height in meters squared. According to this test, if your BMI is over 25, you are fat. Above 30, you are considered obese. This test, like insurance tables, does not distinguish very muscular people from those overfat, and misses light, yet high-fat people. For example, at 5′10″ (1.78 meters), a weight above 174 pounds (79 kg) is fat; weight above 209 pounds (95 kg) tips your BMI over 30. At 5′4″ (1.63 m), your BMI passes 25 at weights above 146 pounds (66 kg), and 30 at weights above 175 pounds (80 kg).

Somatotyping

Height and weight tests do not account for your musculature and body dimensions. Somatotyping is a method of classifying your body according to three characteristics—thinness, fatness, and muscularity. Thinness is called ectomorphy. Fatness is called endomorphy. Muscularity is called mesomorphy. Each type has specific characteristics of limb and body dimensions, with varying proportions of fat, bone, and muscle.

No one is only one somatotype. Everyone is a mixture of the three types in differing amounts. Some people predominate in one type, giving them the long, linear, and

Feet and Meters, Pounds and Kilos?

The United States uses units of measurement historically based on royal anatomy and pottery: the foot, gallon, pound, and so forth. Much of the rest of the world uses the metric system, with comparable units of the meter, liter, and kilogram. How to convert one to the other?

- Kilos to Pounds: 1 kilogram is about 2.2 pounds. Multiply the number of kilos by 2.2 to get pounds.
- Pounds to Kilos: 1 pound is about 0.45 kilograms. Multiply the number of pounds by 0.45 to get kilograms.
- Meters to Feet: 1 meter is about 3.3 feet. Multiply the number of meters by 3.3 to get feet.
- Feet to Meters: 1 foot is about 0.3 meters. Multiply the number of feet by 0.3 to get meters.

delicate appearance of the ectomorph; the round, soft, and short-necked look of the endomorph; or the hard, square, and rugged muscled body of the mesomorph. In football, many players score high in both mesomorphy and endomorphy. Swimmers are usually endo-mesomorphs. Gymnasts are often ecto-mesomorphs. Sprint runners score higher in mesomorphy than distance runners. Coaches may use somatotyping to identify those who would excel in different sports.

Casual somatotyping is done by the eyeball technique. Complete somatotyping requires trained analysis, photographs, or close inspection of naked subjects in three planes, caliper skinfold measurements, reference tables, and equations.

Anthropometrics

As part of somatotyping, or as a separate assessment, the size of the body's frame is determined with calculations using measurements of bone lengths and widths. Knowing frame size helps determine optimum weight. One test, the Heath-Carter, measures elbow width, knee width, biceps circumference, and calf circumference. Another anthropometric test, the skeletal frame technique, measures widths of the shoulder and hip. The Tipton technique computes the minimum healthy weight for a given frame based on width and depth of the chest, and width of the ankle, wrist, and hip at two sites.

Index Tests

The Ponderal Index is your height divided by the cube root of your weight. Ponderal Index is used to determine degree of endomorphy. The Quetelet Index is another simple index of general body proportion. The circumference test is nothing more than the familiar tape measure around the waist, hip, chest, leg, arm, or whatever.

The Jiggle Test

It is just a common-sense general estimate. If your body is overfat and not strong with musculature, you will not be firm. The overly soft flesh will "jiggle" when moving. For example, a person may look slim, but have higher fat and less musculature to stop the upper arm from "flapping" during arm movement. More good arm exercise for the area plus more overall exercise is needed.

Measuring Percentage of Body Fat

The different assessments talked about so far give an indirect estimation of fat distribution. If you want to find out how much fat is actually attached to your body, you can use body composition tests. These tests estimate what percentage of your total weight is just fat weight.

Why Measure Percentage Body Fat? A slender-looking person of normal weight can have a high amount of body fat. Another person weighing above average for their height may have heavy musculature and little body fat. The second person is above average weight, yet has low body fat. The first is normal weight and overfat, even though they don't seem to be. The difference is in their amount of body fat relative to their total weight, or percent body fat.

What Is "Average" Body Fat? For comparison purposes, a healthy body fat is often given as 10 to 15 percent for men and 15 to 20 percent for women. Lower percentages are considered thin. Higher figures are considered to be getting fat. Figures very much above those are considered to be very fat. As an interesting note, recent studies reveal the average American, male or female, is closer to 26 percent fat.

Body Fat Percentage Tests—Body Composition Analysis

The most direct way to find out the specific amount of body fat you have would be to cut your body apart and try to scoop out all the fat stores. Even this direct method would miss fat deep inside and scattered around internal organs. All the other body fat

Are You Fat?

Apples and Pears. Is your body apple-shaped with fat primarily in the upper body and abdomen, or pear-shaped with fat mostly on the hips and thighs? People with the apple shape tend toward obesity-linked disease.

Waist-to-Hip Ratio. Take your waist and hip measurements. Divide your waist measurement by your hip measurement. Stay below 0.8 (women) and 1.0 (men).

Insurance Tables. Compare your weight against values in tables. More than 20 percent over this weight range indicates that you are considered obese. Test is less reliable than other methods.

Body Mass Index. The body mass index (BMI) measures how heavy you are compared to your height. Divide your weight in kilograms by your height in meters squared. If your BMI is above 25, you are considered fat. If over 30, you are considered obese.

Somatotyping. Somatotyping classifies your body according to three characteristics—thinness (ectomorphy), fatness (endomorphy), and muscularity (mesomorphy).

Anthropometrics. Measuring bone lengths and widths at specific joints tells the size of your body's frame—small, medium, or large, which helps determine optimum weight.

Index Tests. Several different index tests measure body proportion.

The Jiggle Test. With higher fat and lower muscle amounts, movement increases in the flesh when walking, running, and jumping.

tests are estimates, although newer techniques are getting better at estimating. Several methods estimate your percentage of body fat. Accuracy of some tests is poor, others moderate, some accurate to within a few percent.

Calipers. Calipers measure the thickness of your folds of fat. This procedure is also sometimes called the "pinch test." Calipers are a small, simple, and inexpensive instruments. Several caliper tests use different sites and different numbers of sites on your body. For example, different caliper tests include the 7-site and the 10-site tests, and the less accurate 5-site and 3-site tests. Simple equations translate the sums of different sites into percent fat. Caliper measurement is painless unless the tester too enthusiastically grabs and squeezes. A tester may grab the muscle under the fat, making an erroneously high measurement. They may pull up the skin over the fat, missing the true fat measurement entirely. They may pull up the actual fat layer correctly, but squeeze it between the calipers tightly enough to reduce the measurement.

The error of measurement of testing percent fat with calipers can be large, up to about 3 to 7 percent, varying greatly with the experience of the tester, and the quality of the caliper used, making it not a true measure but a gross estimation. Caliper testing is often misused, particularly in health clubs. If a first reading shows 25 percent fat, then weeks later after an exercise program the second reading is 22 percent, it does not necessarily mean the person lost 3 percent fat. The large error of measurement makes it impossible to tell. It is like a bathroom scale that weighs you at 160 one time, at 170 the next, and at 150 the third time. Calipers have error with each testing.

Hydrostatic Weighing. Hydrostatic weighing, also called underwater weighing, is currently the gold standard of body-composition-analysis techniques. It has a low percentage error among body-composition tests. Two main methods of underwater weighing can be used with several different equations. One underwater weighing method uses Archimedes' principle. Density is mass divided by volume. You know your mass, and can find your volume with water displacement.

Another method obtains body volume by subtracting your weight in water from weight in air. You sit on a scale in a tank of water and exhale as fully as you can with your head under water. The air that is left in your lungs after you exhale maximally is called residual volume. Residual volume can either be directly determined before the underwater weighing, or estimated with population charts. Your body density is determined from equations of your weight under water minus your residual volume. The final reading can be off if you are unwilling to exhale completely underwater and hold the exhale for as long as it takes for the tester to get a good measurement. Being gassy can also affect your results.

Near Infrared Interactance (NIR). NIR is a technique based on the absorption of light in your fat versus your lean mass. A beam of infrared light is shined through the skin, usually over the biceps muscle. Light is absorbed by the fat and reflected from the muscle. DXA measurements claim low error and good correlation. Generally, manufacturers haven't burdened themselves with input from scientists in developing it, and some professionals feel that the technology has a long way to go. Some units claiming to use infrared interactance don't use it, rendering the unit even less accurate.

Bioelectric Impedance. Various home and commercial impedance units are available—both in handheld form, and models that are stood upon like scales, with varying error of measurement. A painless electrical signal passes either from hand to hand or foot to foot. The faster the signal travels, the more muscle you are thought to have because muscles have far more water than fat. The method can have a margin of error of about 4 percent. Results are affected by your skin temperature and how well hydrated you are.

DXA (or DEXA). DXA stands for dual-energy X-ray absorptiometry. DXA is used to measure bone density to assess fracture risk in osteoporosis. It also measures body-fat percentage and distribution. You lie in a whole-body scanner for 10 to 20 minutes. Two different x-rays read bone mass and soft-tissue mass. It has a 2 to 3 percent margin of error, which is considered low.

Other Tests. Other body composition analysis includes potassium ion determination, ultrasound, CAT scans, creatine absorption, proton absorptiometry, and nuclear magnetic resonance imagery. These tests require expensive equipment and need further validation to know how helpful they are.

26

Diabetes

Clearly, if a disease is manmade, it can also be man prevented. It should be the function of medicine to help people die young as late in life as possible.

—Ernst Wudner

More than 20 million people in the United States have diabetes (colloquially called "the sugar disease"), with 2 million new cases diagnosed every year. Simple dietary changes can make large improvements in control of blood sugar. In addition, exercise has been found to be a top factor in preventing, treating, and lessening the effects of diabetes.

Kinds of Diabetes

Three main types of diabetes are type 1, type 2, and gestational:

- In type-1 diabetes, the body does not make enough insulin in the body organ called the pancreas. Type 1 is treated with injected or inhaled insulin, although nutrition and exercise changes are a fundamental part of management.
- An estimated 90 to 95 percent of cases of diabetes in North American are type 2. Type-2 diabetes is also called non-insulin-dependent diabetes and obesity-related diabetes.

- Type 2 was rare until modern sedentary habits combined with mass sales of unhealthful food.
- Gestational diabetes is generally a form of type 2 during pregnancy.
- In the recent past, type-2 diabetes developed only in adults as they gained weight, reduced activity, and increased packaged, commercial, unhealthful foods. An escalating phenomenon of type-2 diabetes in children is now occurring.

Problems of Diabetes

- Diabetes causes such serious health problems that the risk of death is twice as high for someone with diabetes compared to someone of similar age without.
- Diabetes greatly increases incidence of heart disease, stroke, kidney failure, blindness, and limb loss.
- Diabetes is a major risk factor in impaired wound healing, making foot wounds one of the major problems of diabetes. Fifty percent of lower-limb amputations in the U.S. are due to diabetes
- It is estimated that every 30 seconds, someone in the world has his foot amputated because of a diabetic foot ulcer.
- Reduced blood supply to the feet and lower legs in people with diabetes delays wound healing and increases infection and chance of gangrene.
- Foot infection worsens the situation of inadequate blood supply by increasing the area's need for oxygen but decreasing blood supply.
- Poor blood supply further decreases ability to fight infection.
- Diabetic ulcers treated with antibiotics can become colonized with drug-resistant bugs.

How Does Exercise Help?

Approximately 85 percent of adults and children diagnosed with type 2 are overweight and less active than they could be. Type 2 is increasingly being found to be best treated with more fun movement and less bad food, a win-win situation.

Benefits of regular exercise for people with diabetes include:

- Helps your body burn more sugar.
- Increases the number of insulin receptors on your cells and increases the sensitivity of your body to insulin.

- Helps your body grow new blood vessels and improve circulation.
- Reduces high blood-fat levels (cholesterol and triglycerides), which lead to early aging of blood vessels.
- Increases blood flow to the feet, which helps prevent diabetic foot problems.
- Improves oxygen levels to areas to help them heal.

If you attach a machine called an oximeter to the skin, it will assess oxygen levels through the skin. If you attach an oximeter to the skin on the limb of someone with compromised circulation in that limb due to diabetes, and have them exercise their limb, you can see that movement makes rapid, effective increases in oxygen levels.

In the past, people with diabetes were cautioned not to exercise because it was felt that they would injure themselves. It is now known that exercise is an important part of preventing injuries from diabetes, and preventing or curbing diabetes itself.

- Increasingly, studies confirm that exercise is a top factor to prevent and reverse diabetic problems. According to Dr. William Kraus of Duke University Medical Center, "Failing to prescribe exercise to patients with diabetes is simply unacceptable practice."
- Several studies have found that exercise can reduce need for oral and injected medications.
- Other studies show that exercise and healthier diet are more effective than medicine for people with type-2 diabetes.
- A randomized, controlled Canadian study published in 2007 in the Annals of Internal Medicine found that people with type-2 diabetes who began exercising developed better blood-sugar control, both from aerobic exercise and resistance training. Not exercising yielded no improvements in sugar control. People who combined aerobic exercise, and also lifted weights had the biggest improvement. It is not known in this study if results occurred because of the type of exercise mattered, or because the duration of exercise was greater in the combined exercise training group.
- According to an editorial co-published with the study, "Doctors should prescribe exercise to all type-2 diabetes patients who are healthy enough to work out."

Hyperbaric Oxygen for Problem Wounds From Diabetes

Supplying oxygen to compromised areas, such as problem diabetic wounds, is important to restoring health. Hyperbaric oxygen treatment is one accepted treatment for that purpose. Hyperbaric treatments are done by putting the entire person in a special chamber and increasing the pressure inside so that the person breathes oxygen at higher pressure. Patients with severe diabetic foot ulcers treated with hyperbaric oxygen have higher chance of healing and reduced chance of amputation. Hyperbaric oxygen therapy is also shown to enhance stem-cell mobilization in people with diabetes.

What Changes in Diet Help?

Studies of changing diet to eating plant-based food showed weight loss and improved glycemic control in type-2 diabetes, and reduced cholesterol and need for medicines. It was not known at first if the results were from the change in diet, or from the weight loss it characteristically produced, or exercise done with the diet. All three factors of diet, weight loss, and exercise reduce several dangerous aspects of diabetes. Studies specifically looking at the effects of a vegetarian and vegan diet showed positive results. Vegan is a vegetarian diet without any animal-derived products, such as eggs or dairy. Several aspects of a vegetarian and vegan diet reduce and reverse the contributing causes of diabetes:

- Changing eating habits to vegetarian food and soluble fiber instead of unhealthful food reduces cholesterol and improves glycemic control
- Eating less total fat and saturated fat increases insulin sensitivity
- A vegan diet provides iron in its non-heme form, also examined for its role in improving insulin sensitivity.

According to a 2006 study published by the American Diabetes Association, participants on a vegan diet lowered blood sugar and cholesterol to a greater extent, improved kidney function, and lost more weight than people on a standard American Diabetes Association diet. Participants said the vegan diet was easier to follow than the ADA and other diets because they did not measure portions or count calories.

Have fun making a new healthier life. Keep moving, and enjoy trying food that will help you avoid disease, as well as the secondary effects from disease. You will change your health for the better.

- You do not need a gym or special clothes or equipment to get aerobic or weight-lifting exercise.
- Go outdoors for a break every day that you can, for fresh air, sunshine, and fun movement.
- For both active and resistance exercise indoors and out, remember that daily healthful movement easily accumulates from your healthy bending, balancing while dressing, taking the stairs, and other daily real life movement.
- Have fun. Skate, bowl, cycle, walk, go dancing, work on gardening, shoot hoops, take food to shut-ins and get them moving too, with improvised exercise of moving arms and legs, clapping, singing, and having fun.
- For fun exercise-as-lifestyle ideas, refer to Chapter 8.
- Stop eating junk food and processed sugar foods, and substitute vegetable meals.
- For advice on developing a healthy, nutritional mindset, recipes, and ways to start, refer to Chapters 18 and 19.

27

Cardiovascular Disease

The trouble with heart disease is that the first symptom is often hard to deal with: sudden death.

—Michael Phelps, M.D.

What condition kills more people than any other in the Western world? Cardiovascular disease. It is the number-one non-injury cause of death, beginning at age 30 for men and 40 for women. Nearly half of all deaths in the United States each year are from cardiovascular disease, which includes heart attack and stroke. It kills twice as many men and women as cancer. Most men dying a sudden death during physical activity have been found to have underlying heart disease. Cardiovascular disease develops largely through unhealthy habits, making it largely preventable.

How Does Cardiovascular Disease Affect You?

Cardiovascular disease keeps you from enjoying your life in several ways:

- It can end your life at a young age.
- It reduces your physical capacity to deal with exertion.
- It limits your ability to go out and enjoy life.
- Environmental stresses on your body from weather extremes of heat and cold are hard enough on your cardiovascular system. Cardiovascular disease greatly

limits your ability to cope with these extremes safely. Even men with no underlying heart disease usually show greater blood pressure and other cardiovascular responses (such as irregular heartbeats) than women during activities in the cold.

- For men with cardiovascular problems, the combination of poor health, work, and cold in activities like shoveling snow or just having fun in the snow can be lethal.

Cardiovascular Disease Affects More Than Just Your Heart

Your blood vessels can become narrowed and blocked all over your body, not just in your heart. One common place is your brain. Reduced blood flow to your brain can hurt your mental processes. "Hardening of the arteries" may explain an older person's senile behavior. An often-missed warning of heart attack and stroke is confusion and change in reasoning powers.

Blood vessels clogged with cholesterol plaques in your lower leg cause pain and problems when walking. Oxygen can't reach the muscles, and they cry in pain. Sometimes, they just stop working, causing a limp, a condition called claudication, which comes from a Latin word meaning "to limp."

Another place is your Achilles tendon, the large "string" that attaches your calf muscle to your heel. High cholesterol levels can stiffen the area and predispose it to injury, increasingly common in middle-aged men.

Another body site also concerns men. An often-ignored warning signal of dangerously narrowed arteries is decrease in erectile function. High blood pressure, high cholesterol, and smoking are major risk factors. Men with this warning sign should check the possibility of cardiovascular disease with their physicians. According to the guidelines released by the American Urological Association at the World Meeting on Impotence in San Francisco, "One of the major risk factors for erectile dysfunction is smoking."

All these injuries are more common in industrialized nations because of the link to vascular problems from Western diet and sedentary lifestyle. Seventeenth-century English physician Thomas Sydenham summarized it: "A man is as old as his arteries."

How Your Blood Vessels Are Involved

Your blood vessels aren't just inert pipes. They are living and responsive. The lining of your blood vessels is a layer of flat cells called endothelium. Your endothelium regulates how your blood vessels dilate and constrict. Normally, the endothelium makes a chemical called nitric oxide, which relaxes vessels and prevents spasms. When fat, diabetes, smoking, and other stresses upset your endothelium, it stops making nitric oxide. Constricted vessels make your blood less able to flow smoothly and more likely to cause heart attacks or blood clots.

Your endothelium knows when cholesterol enters your bloodstream. Cholesterol slows your lining's ability to regulate cell growth, which builds up plaque. Lowering your cholesterol lets the endothelium function well enough again that heart-disease symptoms subside—even with the plaque.

Surgically removing the plaque that blocks arteries is a common medical treatment. However, in many patients the blockage comes back when they don't change their diet and they still don't exercise. In addition, other factors are involved. Plaques also build outside the blood vessels (not just inside), and constrict from the outside. Procedures to remove plaque seem to make the body react as if an injury has occurred to the endothelial wall. White blood cells come to the rescue at the site of the removed plaque as if it were a wound. It is like relatives barging into help you when you don't want them. Inflammatory proteins build up tissue that blocks the artery again. Healthy diet and exercise can reduce plaques without this injury process so that your blood vessels stay clean and open.

Heart Disease Begins in Childhood

Markers of cardiovascular disease are showing in increasingly young populations. Cardiovascular problems can be stopped and even reversed with good nutrition and regular exercise.

> *Children who grow up getting nutrition from plant foods rather than meats have a tremendous health advantage. They are less likely to develop weight problems, diabetes, high blood pressure and some forms of cancer.*
>
> —Benjamin Spock, M.D.

Dr. Spock was a pioneer American pediatrician. His 1946 book, *The Common Sense Book of Baby and Child Care*, outsold all other nonfiction books. His nutritional guidance is not trendy overstatement or groundbreaking news. It is long-known important information that urges simple, common sense health.

Risk Factors for Cardiovascular Disease

Major and minor indicators can help determine your chance of developing cardiovascular disease. Although some factors are more serious than others, all are cumulative, meaning the more you have, the greater your risk.

Four Top Risk Factors. These four factors are the most predictive factors of your risk:

- Cigarette smoking
- High blood pressure
- High blood cholesterol
- Lack of exercise

Other Common Risk Factors. Your risk usually increases with:

- Age
- Family history of cardiovascular problems
- Diabetes
- High body fat
- High-sugar and high-fat (particularly animal fat) diet
- Lack of fruits and vegetables in your diet
- Being male (Men develop cardiovascular disease, on average, about 10 years younger than women.)
- Cocaine use (Even with no other risk factors present, you may have a sudden heart attack if you use cocaine.)

Too Much Iron. An intriguing risk factor is high blood-iron level. Iron in the body is usually found in a form tightly bound with a protein, as in hemoglobin. Iron is an oxidant, and when it becomes available in unbound form, it turns on several harmful reactions with oxygen that damage your cells. People with high iron levels have been found to develop high rates of heart disease. Conversely, premenopausal women who lose small monthly amounts of iron, and vegetarians and athletes who often run a bit low, have lower incidence of heart disease than the rest of the population. High iron levels may also be linked to unusual fatigue, and possibly cancer. It is another good reason to cut back on red meat, which has a high iron content.

A genetic disorder called hemochromatosis prevents a small portion of the population from processing iron. High iron levels that result sometimes cause heart failure. Even slightly high iron levels may raise risk even in those without the faulty gene, particularly men who don't have the benefit of monthly blood loss. It seems to be more common than previously thought. Dr. James Cook, an iron specialist at the University of Kansas Medical Center, states, "No one, unless he or she has been diagnosed with an iron deficiency, or belongs to a high risk group, should routinely take iron supplements." How common is hemochromatosis? Dr. Victor Herbert, chief of Mount Sinai's hematology and nutrition lab in the Bronx, states, "Only 6 percent of Americans have iron deficiency anemia. Twelve percent have a hemochromatosis-related iron overload."

Not Enough Fruit and Vegetables. A number of studies have linked the "Mediterranean" style of eating, which is high in fruits, vegetables, and nuts, and low in dairy foods and red meat, to reduced risk of death from cardiovascular disease. According to a 2007 study of over 300,000 people, smokers who were not overweight nearly halved their risk of death. The researchers stated that the smokers may have had the most to gain from the antioxidant and blood fat-lowering effects of following the Mediterranean eating pattern.

Aside from the association between cardiovascular health and healthy eating in general, many vegetables have folic acid. Folic acid, a B-vitamin, has several functions in your body. One function is to lower your levels of a substance called homocysteine. Homocysteine occurs naturally in your body and has many roles. In high amounts, it is associated with heart attack and stroke. The average meat-centered Western diet can result in deficiencies of common vitamins, including folic acid.

Folic-acid deficiencies might be responsible for 15 to 40 percent of heart attacks and strokes, depending on the study cited. Eating more folic acid won't make up for a sedentary lifestyle and unhealthy eating habits, but getting enough folic acid (about 400 micrograms per day) seems to be important to cardiovascular health. Supplements do not give the benefit of having the whole food. Nutrients need to work together with the other nutrients they occur with. Find folic acid in green leafy vegetables like spinach, Brussels sprouts, lettuce, and many fruits, including oranges and apples.

Vegetarians have the best diet. They have the lowest rates of coronary disease of any group in the country. ... They have a fraction of our heart attack rate and they have only 40 percent of our cancer rate.

—William Castelli, M.D., Director, Framingham Heart Study, the longest-running epidemiological study in medical history

Good Diet Helps You and the Earth

You can help your heart and the earth at the same time. A NewScientist.com headline reported in the December 17, 2005 issue, "It's Better to Green Your Diet Than Your Car." You could exchange your "regular" car for a hybrid Toyota Prius, and by doing so, it would prevent about a ton of carbon dioxide from entering the atmosphere each year, but according to the University of Chicago, being vegan is more effective in the fight against global warming. A vegan prevents approximately 1.5 fewer tons of carbon dioxide from entering the atmosphere each year than a meat-eater does. The math is simple: you could spend more than $20,000 on a Prius and still emit 50 percent more carbon dioxide than you would if you just gave up eating meat and other animal products.

Sleep Apnea. Sleep apnea was detailed in Chapter 24 on the problems of being overweight. "Apnea" means to stop breathing temporarily. In sleep apnea, the sleeper stops breathing, sometimes hundreds of times per night. They may make loud, labored snores and efforts to breathe. The episodes of apnea starve their bodies of oxygen. Low oxygen seems to make fatty plaques deposit in their blood vessels. Sleep apnea is a risk factor for stroke and heart attack. The many nighttime awakenings also cause chronic daytime sleepiness. This sleepiness greatly raises the risk of serious automobile accidents. Sleep apnea is a serious sleep disorder. One effective treatment for sleep apnea is losing weight.

What Is Your Risk?

Several pen-and-paper assessment tools can help you determine your own risk. The following page shows one from the Michigan Heart Association. It is one of the older assessments, but a good and easy one to start with. Circle the number in each category that best describes you. Then total your score.

If you scored:

6 to 11: Your risk is well below average.

12 to 17: Your risk is below average.

18 to 24: Your risk is generally average.

25 to 31: Your risk is moderate.

32 to 40: Your risk is at a dangerous level.

41 to 62: Your danger is urgent. See your physician now.

Reducing Your Risk of Heart Disease

Of the four major risk factors, you can directly control how much you exercise and smoke, and indirectly control high blood pressure and cholesterol with exercise and healthy nutrition. Most cardiovascular disease has a large nutrition and fitness component. You can reduce your risk through healthy eating and exercise habits.

Adopt Healthy Habits. Exercise more, quit smoking, and eat less sugar and unhealthful fat. It gets easier the more you do it. Many fatty foods are an acquired taste. After switching to healthier food, you'll be surprised to find how greasy fatty foods taste when you try them again. When you eat fewer sweets, you crave them less. You will also notice your weight and blood pressure drop, if they were previously high, further reducing your risk. If you have diabetes, you can usually reduce its effects with better nutrition and more exercise.

Cardiac-Risk Index

1. Age	10 to 20 1	21 to 30 2	31 to 40 3	41 to 50 4	51 to 60 6	61 to 70 8
2. Heredity	No known history 1	One relative over 60 with cardiovascular disease 2	Two relatives over 60 with cardiovascular disease 3	One relative under 60 with cardiovascular disease 4	Two relatives under 60 with cardiovascular disease 6	Three relatives under 60 with cardiovascular disease 8
3. Weight	More than 5 lbs below standard weight 0	-5 to +5 lbs standard weight 1	6 to 20 lbs overweight 2	21 to 35 lbs overweight 3	36 to 50 lbs overweight 5	51 to 65 lbs overweight 7
4. Tobacco Smoking	Nonuser 0	Cigar and/or pipe 1	10 cigarettes or less a day 2	20 cigarettes a day 4	30 cigarettes a day 6	40 cigarettes or more a day 10
5. Exercise	Intensive occupational and recreational exertion 1	Moderate occupational and recreational exertion 2	Sedentary work and intense recreational exertion 3	Sedentary work and moderate recreational exertion 5	Sedentary work and light recreational exertion 6	Complete lack of all exercise 8
6. Cholesterol or, if not known, % fat in the diet	below 180 mg No animal or solid fat in diet 1	181 to 205 mg 10% animal or solid fat in diet 2	206 to 230 mg 20% animal or solid fat in diet 3	231 to 255 mg 30% animal or solid fat in diet 4	256 to 280 mg 40% animal or solid fat in diet 5	281 to 330 mg 50% animal or solid fat in diet 7
7. Blood Pressure (Upper Reading)	100 1	120 2	140 3	160 4	180 6	200 or ove 8
8. Gender	Female under 40 1	Female 40 to 50 2	Female over 50 3	Male 5	Stocky male 6	Bald stocky male 7

RISKO® used with permission and courtesy of Michigan Heart Association. © Michigan Heart Association. Total score ________

Start Healthy Habits Young. It is not just older people who suffer heart disease. Autopsies on American soldiers killed in Vietnam and Korea showed that the majority already had moderately advanced atherosclerosis. Autopsies of children who die of causes other than cardiovascular disease reveal that artery clogging can begin as early as childhood, the product of a sedentary lifestyle and the modern diet of chips, fries, burgers, and ice cream. Habits developed early, both good and bad, are more likely to be kept throughout your life.

> Clogged arteries begin in youth. Heart disease is not just something that happens suddenly to older people.

Eat More Fruit and Vegetables. Make vegetables the main part of your meals, instead side dishes. Fruit can make easy and good-tasting snacks and desserts, and part of healthful breakfast and lunch.

Lower Your Blood Cholesterol. Two thirds of heart attacks happen to people with cholesterol readings over 200. Cholesterol slowly deposits on blood-vessel walls and makes blood vessels more likely to suddenly squeeze shut, contributing to mini-strokes that warn of serious illness to come.

Blood cholesterol can rise when you eat high amounts of saturated and trans fats, don't eat enough vegetables for good nutrients and soluble fiber, and don't exercise enough. The type of fat seems more important than total fat, although both influence health. Blood fats also rise with eating junk sugar. Changing unhealthful diet and getting more aerobic exercise are top factors to reduce high cholesterol. (Refer to Chapter 28 on good and bad cholesterol.)

Consider Different Options After Menopause. Hormone-replacement drugs—as well as the drugs replacing them, prescribed after surgical or natural menopause—have been found to have serious health risks. Speak with your physician about the benefits and risks of the different options that apply to your current state of health.

Donate Blood. Some experts recommend regular blood donations to avoid high blood-iron levels that may relate to disease risk. This option is usually only for certain people with abnormally high iron levels. The *British Medical Journal* reports on a study from Finland of 2,600 men. Nearly 10 percent of the men who had not donated blood in the two previous years suffered a heart attack. Only one of the 153 who had donated blood had a heart attack in the same period of time. Although it is possible that the men who had donated blood were more health conscious in general, the connection in the study seemed to be strong. Call your local Red Cross for information on donating blood—to help someone who needs blood, and possibly yourself.

Get in Better Physical Shape. Being out of shape is a vicious cycle. You are not able to do enough exercise to improve your health. Consequently, you become more out of shape and more unhealthy. Your risk of a problem brought on by exertion rises. Being in better shape lowers your risk of cardiovascular disease while exercising, and improves your ability to do the amount of exercise you need to become healthier.

Have a Social Support Network. Behavioral researchers report that having a social structure of friends is heart-healthy. Speculated reasons include that friends share health information, and that the support of friendship reduces physical and emotional stress. Many people socially isolate themselves. How can they develop a better network of friends? Writer and philosopher Ralph Waldo Emerson observed, "If you would have a friend, you must first be one." Make time for friends, accept people as they are, and respect their secrets. That advice will go a long way to developing and keeping friendships.

Get Your Blood Sugar Checked. Diabetes and heart disease often go together.

Know the Symptoms of a Heart Attack. If you get chest pain, chest tightness, shortness of breath, or pain down one arm, go immediately to a hospital emergency department. Don't dismiss these warnings as indigestion. Don't ignore these symptoms in a woman. Cardiovascular disease is the number-one disease of both women and men.

Get the Right Medical Care Right Away. Even if the pain goes away, it doesn't necessarily mean you didn't have something serious happen. How well the hospital can care for you if you are having a heart attack partially depends on how quickly you get there. Delay reduces the effectiveness of the many treatment options available. Quick treatment (within six hours) prevents more extensive, irreversible damage to your heart.

Have someone you can call in mind ahead of time, so you know who will help, instead of trying to get to an emergency room yourself, risking a serious automobile accident if driving. Call ahead to ask your doctor to meet you at the hospital. Before you need to ever call on emergency measures for a heart attack, check which doctors and hospitals offer the real care needed, in the manner that is healthy for you.

Be Proactive, Not Reactive

The reactive approach is to sit around, get clogged blood vessels, wait for the physician to prescribe drugs, worry, have surgery, have a stroke, and have a heart attack. Your heredity is not your destiny. If your father had heart disease, you are not doomed. On the other hand, another common approach is, "My father (or mother) didn't have heart disease, so I have nothing to worry about." Neither is completely true. Be proactive with preventive care.

Check Your Beliefs and Mindset

Don't dismiss exercise and good nutrition as, "It's easy to say, but hard to do." The same people who wait hours in the snow at 4 a.m. to shop for expensive holiday electronics sales that they have to put on credit say that eating vegetables is too hard, or requires too much discipline, or is expensive, or isn't convenient. Check your attitudes toward health. Discover if it is something you believe and want, and what you believe will help. When it is something you relate to what you want to have, you will suddenly find how much you can do it and how easy it is.

How to Reduce Your Risk of Heart Disease

- Adopt healthy habits. Exercise more, quit smoking, and eat less sugar and fat.
- Start healthy habits young. Habits developed early, both good and bad, are more likely to be kept throughout your life.
- Eat more fruit, raw nuts, and vegetables.
- Lower your blood cholesterol by exercising more and eating less unhealthful fat and sugar.
- Heart-attack risk rises after menopause. Menopausal medications may not reduce risk as hoped. Some medications may increase risk (refer to Chapter 22). Check with your doctor for healthier options.
- Donate blood. It's not certain, but possible, that regular blood donations help to avoid the high blood iron levels that may increase risk.
- Get in better physical shape. Being in better shape lowers your risk of cardiovascular disease while exercising and improves your ability to do the amount of exercise you need to become healthier.
- Have a support network of real friends.
- Know the symptoms of a heart attack.
- Get medical care right away. If you get chest pain, chest tightness, shortness of breath, or pain down one arm, go immediately to a hospital emergency department equipped to both help and care.

Resources for More Information

American Heart Association
www.americanheart.org
National Center
7272 Greenville Ave
Dallas, TX 75231-4596
1-800-AHA-USA-1 (1-800-242-8721)

American Red Cross
www.redcross.org
1-800-REDCROSS (1-800-733-2767)

Iron Overload Diseases Association
www.ironoverload.org
433 Westwind Drive
North Palm Beach, FL 33408-5123
1-888-678-4766
iod@ironoverload.org

28

Cholesterol

Avoid fried meats, which angry up the blood.

—Rule 1 of the six "Rules for Staying Young" by Satchel Paige

What Is Cholesterol?

Cholesterol is a necessary ingredient in your body in small amounts. It is a precursor of your steroid hormones, including all your sex hormones, and a precursor of your bile acids, which handle fat digestion. Your body uses it to make Vitamin D. Cholesterol is part of every cell membrane in animals, giving the outer cell area part of the structure it needs. Plants don't need cholesterol around their cells because they have rigid cell walls. It is why only animal products have cholesterol.

Too little blood cholesterol is not healthy. There is debate around the role of high cholesterol, both in the diet and in the blood. Cholesterol is found in atherosclerotic plaques in the cells lining your arteries and outside of your arteries, however, cholesterol is not the only contributor. There is also debate on what is a healthy cholesterol level.

Cholesterol and Lipoproteins

You may have heard of the different kinds of lipoproteins as "good cholesterol" and "bad cholesterol." Lipoproteins aren't just cholesterol. Lipoproteins are large molecules that your body makes out of cholesterol, fat (lipid), and protein. Lipids won't dissolve in your blood or travel through your blood on their own, so they have to be carried around by helpful proteins. Cholesterol is one of three lipids (kinds of fat) carried through your blood by lipoproteins.

Lipoproteins are divided into five types. High-density lipoprotein, abbreviated HDL, is often called good cholesterol. Low-density lipoprotein, or LDL, is also called bad cholesterol. The other lipoprotiens are VLDL, or very low-density lipoproteins, IDL, intermediate-density lipoproteins, and chylomicrons.

"Bad" Lipoproteins and Cardiovascular Disease

Low-density lipoprotein is sometimes called "bad cholesterol." Fatty plaques that narrow blood vessels are made of LDL and VLDL (very low-density lipoproteins). LDL picks up 60 to 75 percent of the cholesterol from the fats you eat and from your liver, which makes cholesterol, and takes it to the cells of your blood vessels and muscles. Because LDL carries most of the cholesterol, a high amount of LDL in your blood translates to higher risk of heart attack and angina pectoris (angina means "pain," and pectoris means "chest").

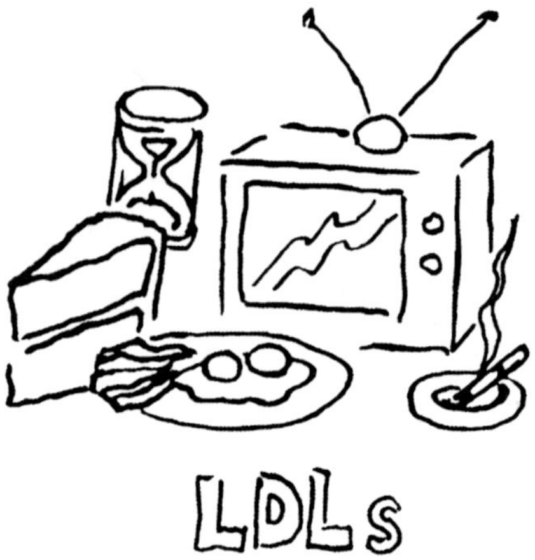

Figure 28-1. You don't eat low-density lipoproteins (LDLs); your body makes them. You can make too much LDL when you eat too much animal fat or saturated vegetable fat, smoke, take drugs such as anabolic steroids, and/or don't exercise

What "Good" Lipoproteins Do

High-density lipoprotein (HDL), popularly called "good cholesterol," removes cholesterol from your bloodstream and does not collect or stick to the inner linings of your arteries. HDL contains an enzyme that helps break down deposits and takes "used" cholesterol away from the cells back to your liver for recycling and excretion. The higher your HDL level, the lower your risk of cardiovascular disease.

According to a study reported in the November 27, 2007 issue of the journal *Neurology*, low blood levels of high-density lipoprotein ("good") cholesterol increase the risk of memory problems and greater disability after a stroke.

Dr. David Hsu of Stanford University Hospital describes the four main functions of HDL:

- It is an airport baggage handler that tags and de-tags chylomicrons, VLDLs, and IDLs (the very low and intermediate density guys) with protein tags that identify them and allow them to be picked up out of your blood (the conveyor belt) by the correct recipient at the correct destination. The tags are called apoproteins.
- It is a maintenance person, picking up garbage (free cholesterol) from peripheral tissue (e.g., from cell membranes of dead or live cells) and storing it, using an enzyme that makes the cholesterol even more willing to stay inside the HDL maintenance person.
- It is a porter that carries cholesterol back to the liver, where the HDL is broken down and the cholesterol released into liver cells to be used as needed.
- It is a trader, and trades cholesterol stores with VLDLs and LDLs for fats.

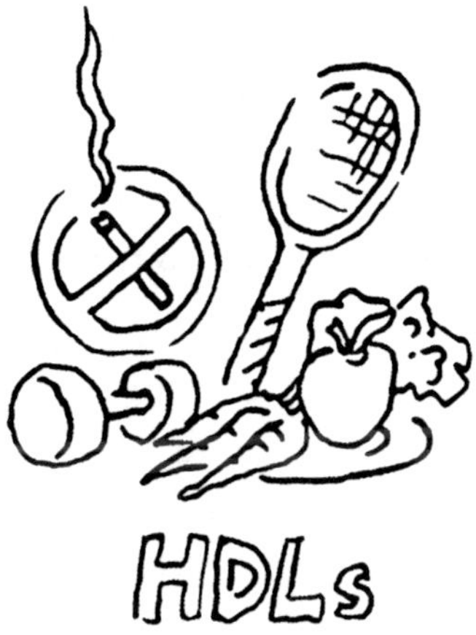

Figure 28-2. Increase good cholesterol, or high-density-lipoprotein (HDL) level, by avoiding smoking, avoiding drugs such as anabolic steroids, eating less animal fat and more vegetables, and exercising more.

What Distinguishes High From Low Density?

The names "high density" and "low density" come from two characteristics of lipoproteins. The first is lipid content. LDL has more lipid than HDL. Normally, when you call something "low," you think of a smaller amount. The higher lipid content of LDL decreases the density because fat is less dense than other body constituents. Think of cream floating on milk. Heavy cream has more fat than light cream, making it less dense. Although it weighs less than light cream, it's called heavy for its higher fat content. In the same way, LDL has more fat but lower density.

The names "high" and "low" also come from the way they're packaged. Loosely packed LDL cholesterol floats through the bloodstream to your cells. Cholesterol released from the cells tightly crams into HDL for the voyage back to your liver.

One way to remember which is which:

- HDL = Healthy
- LDL = Lousy

What Is Non-HDL?

Your non-HDL cholesterol count is the total of your various lower density cholesterols. They are the sum of LDL, VLDL, and IDL.

How to Get Less LDL and More HDL

Improving your ratio of good to bad cholesterol is not difficult. Lipoproteins ferry LDL and HDL to and from each cell in amounts determined by your food choices and activity level. Although blood vessel diseases like heart attack and stroke are the number-one killers in the United States and Great Britain, they are practically strangers in half the world. In those areas, intake of animal products and fat is lower, and activity level is higher. Cholesterol-reducing drugs are often not as needed as advertising may suggest.

Improve Nutrition

- A small relation can be found between eating cholesterol and blood levels of cholesterol. Cholesterol is found only in animal products, such as eggs, dairy, and meat. The average person makes about 75 percent of blood cholesterol in the liver and absorbs 25 percent from food. Your liver makes all the cholesterol you need—even if you eat no cholesterol at all. There is no need to eat any cholesterol.
- Eating foods with saturated fat raises total blood cholesterol more than eating foods that contain cholesterol. Eating saturated fat is found to raise good cholesterol, but also raises bad cholesterol in the body. Saturated fats are mostly found in meat, poultry, dairy, and certain hydrogenated vegetable oils.
- Trans fats raise the various bad cholesterols, lower good cholesterol, and are inflammatory—a process increasingly recognized as being involved in cardiovascular and other disease processes. Trans fats are made by heating liquid vegetable oils in

the presence of hydrogen, a process called hydrogenation. Trans-fats are found in most margarines, solid vegetable shortening, partially-hydrogenated vegetable oil, French fries, fried potato chips, packaged snack food, many fast foods (although bans in some areas are changing that likelihood), and many commercial baked goods.

- Trying to lower cholesterol with unhealthful, low-fat diets of primarily simple sugars does not meet with much success. Eating much refined sugar can also raise blood fat. Use common sense so that you do not eat junk sugar just because it is low fat. For example a breakfast of toast and jam with sugar and non-fat creamer in your coffee is low in fat, but high in sugar.

Cholesterol-Reducing Food. Lack of dietary fiber prevents normal removal of cholesterol, resulting in build-up. Accepted studies find that soluble fiber prevents cholesterol from being absorbed in the intestine, and moderates blood sugar after eating, which is helpful for people with diabetes (refer to Chapter 26). High sources of soluble fiber include: oatmeal, oat bran, apples, mangoes, plums, kiwi, pears, blackberries, strawberries, raspberries, peaches, citrus fruits, dried apricots, prunes, figs, dried peas, beans, and lentils. Other fruits and vegetables also contain soluble fiber in varying amounts. Other cholesterol-reducing foods include almonds, red yeast rice, and cinnamon. Results may also occur from the policosanol in citrus peels. Grate the insides and outsides of rinds into blender drinks, salads, baked goods, and cooked vegetables. Healthful amounts of essential fatty acids may reduce cholesterol (refer to Chapter 18). Good nutrition to reduce cholesterol is not a matter of eating junk food, then adding a supplement or snack food with added fiber or essential fatty acids, but involves reducing or stopping the consumption of cholesterol-raising foods and eating regular meals of vegetables, fruit, seeds, and legumes.

Quit Smoking

Among many reasons for you to quit smoking, smoking lowers HDL.

Avoid Anabolic and Non-Anabolic Steroids

The male hormone testosterone depresses HDL levels, which is one reason men's risk of heart disease is higher than women's risk. Taking male hormones, such as those found in anabolic steroids, greatly drops HDL levels. Corticosteroid medicines, such as prednisone, raise LDL bad cholesterol, total cholesterol, and triglyceride levels. Beta-blockers are among other medicines that raise cholesterol.

Exercise

Exercise more effectively changes HDL-LDL ratio than dietary change and weight loss alone. Endurance exercise increases HDL and its important enzyme, and decreases total blood cholesterol and LDL in both men and women. Altered blood-lipid profile may be one of the principal mechanisms of reduced risk of heart disease through exercise.

What About Cholesterol-Reduction Drugs?

Several common drugs for cholesterol, called statin drugs, can cause joint pain, leg cramps, limb twitching, loss of memory and libido, headache, and sore, weak muscles. Statin medicines for cholesterol are also a common cause of gas, heartburn, and painful upset stomach. Some of the stomach medicines given for these effects add unhealthful effects, explained in Chapter 15 on digestion and Chapter 22 on osteoporosis. A 2007 study from the University of California, San Diego, School of Medicine confirms, "Concerns about statins adversely affecting sleep in case reports and case series dating back to at least 1990, just after the release of statins." These side effects are not mild or rare, as originally stated by manufacturers.

Some cholesterol-lowering drugs have been found ineffective in older adults unless heart disease is already present. In several studies showing benefits, study authors were found to have direct financial ties to the statin drug manufacturers. In many cases, the drugs are not necessary to lower cholesterol. Although advertisements may imply that exercise and diet are often not enough, with changes in food habits, weight reduction, and regular exercise, blood fats often normalize. If not, check what you are really doing compared to what you think you are doing. If you are constantly eating unhealthful food and not moving in healthful ways throughout daily life, then adding a bowl of oats or a fiber supplement and going out for an exercise class a few times a week, you are not practicing healthy eating or using significant healthful movement.

Several studies published in accepted medical journals report that more exercise and less dietary fat may not only stop coronary artery disease from progressing, but reverse it.

Healthy Blood Fats

- Eat less total fat and trans fat. Although there is debate on specifically how much saturated fat and cholesterol affect blood cholesterol, eating high amounts is not necessary or healthy for many reasons.
- Eat less refined sugar.
- Eat fruit and vegetables.
- Quit smoking.
- Avoid anabolic steroids.
- Engage in regular, fun exercise.

Your Cholesterol Ratio

Your total cholesterol reading is determined by your LDL and HDL levels. You raise your risk of heart disease if you have too much total cholesterol and if you have too little good cholesterol (HDL). High levels of circulating HDL in relation to LDL are usually more important than your total amount of blood cholesterol.

Your total, and the ratio of good to total, is a number determined by blood testing. In general, the lower your cholesterol ratio, the lower your risk of heart disease. The optimal ratio is 3.5 or lower.

Cholesterol Ratio Before an Exercise and Better Diet Program:

$$\frac{\text{Total cholesterol 200}}{\text{Good (HDL) cholesterol 50}} = 4.0 \quad \text{This ratio is high.}$$

Cholesterol Ratio After a Program to Raise Good Cholesterol:

$$\frac{\text{Total cholesterol 180}}{\text{Good (HDL) cholesterol 60}} = 3.0 \quad \text{This ratio is good.}$$

Occasionally, people who eat very low fat diets, particularly vegetarian diets, lower total cholesterol—including their LDL level—so much that their cholesterol ratio becomes high. This result should not be mistaken for an unfavorable ratio. These people have a lower-than-average risk of heart disease. The big picture of blood fats is what is important.

A Priority

Much attention is paid to the few yearly deaths by sensational events such as plane crashes. At the same time, hundreds of thousands of people die every year by the frying pan. Heart disease is the number-one killer of both men and women in the "developed" world. To whatever extent cholesterol plays a role in that fact, what will change that outcome, more than any drug or fad health food, are simple, healthy food choices and practices and regular exercise.

29

Headaches

One man's food is another man's poison.

—Socrates

Foods or actions that cause no pain to some people can trigger a terrible headache in others. Two thousand years ago, physicians required their patients to fast as part of their medical exams. Often, the patients' symptoms would stop.

Many headaches are caused by things you can change, meaning that many headaches are preventable. This section is not intended for use as a medical diagnosis, and is not intended as a complete source, but is a look at possible mechanisms and things to try for relief.

Types of Headaches

A continuum seems to exist between the various kinds of headaches (for example, tension-type and migraine). These types of headaches may represent ends of a single continuum rather than being distinct from one another. Modern headache centers take an integrated approach to understanding the types of headaches, leading to better diagnosis and treatment. The types of headaches are described separately in this chapter to introduce them in an organized fashion.

Tension-Type Headache. Previously called muscle-contraction headaches, or tension headaches, these types of headaches can occur when you tense the muscles of your face, brow, scalp, and neck for lengthy periods: frowning and brow furrowing over paperwork; tensing over a desk, computer, or workbench; tightly shouldering a phone to your ear; or clenching your teeth. The pain is steady, felt on one or both sides of the head, or can feel like a tight band around the head. Since tension headaches can be triggered by stressing the head and neck muscles for long periods of time, tension headaches more often start late in the day and resolve with sleep. Tension headaches usually disappear after the stress is over, but if you habitually tense your muscles day after day, you can have pain from it day after day.

Migraines. Migraine headache is sometimes called a vascular headache because of its relation to inflammation of the blood vessels surrounding the brain. Nausea, vomiting, and sensitivity to light and sound may occur. The pain can be so terrible that even a word meaning "depression or unhappiness" (*megrems*) comes from a Middle English variant of migraine.

Migraine can occur with or without an "aura"—neurological symptoms appearing 10 to 30 minutes before a classic migraine. An aura may include flashing or zigzag lights, lines, and dots, dimmed vision, tingling in the face or hands, weakness of an arm or leg, speech difficulties, or confusion. Migraine usually starts on one side of the head and may spread to the other side. Left untreated, attacks can last up to three intensely painful days.

Migraine without aura used to be called common migraine, because it is more common than migraine with aura. When warnings occur, they might include fatigue, mental fuzziness, mood changes, or unusual fluid retention. These symptoms, as well as those of the aura, indicate that the generator of migraine is in the brain, not the blood vessels. Untreated, common migraine pain can last up to three days. If it lasts longer, it is called migraine status.

People can experience several other kinds of migraine. Hemiplegic migraine produces temporary paralysis on one side of the body (hemiplegia). Basilar-artery migraine is named for a problem in a major brain artery called the basilar artery. In ophthalmoplegic migraine, the pain is around the eye and causes droopy eyelids and double vision. Dr. William B. Young of the Jefferson Headache Center in Philadelphia explains migraine origins:

> Ten to 15 years ago, it was state of the art to say that migraine began with changes in brain blood vessels. Today, we have evidence that migraine sufferers have a lowered threshold of the 'migraine generator' within the brain. One theory is that this generator is in the brainstem, involving serotonin cells. Another theory is that an aura, or an aura-like phenomenon in the cortex of the brain, starts a cascade of events that

leads to migraine pain including inflammation of the blood vessels surrounding the brain.

Cluster Headaches. These headaches are rare. They are highly painful and have a characteristic pattern. They occur mostly in men. Cluster-headache sufferers experience severe bouts of pain on one side of the head for about an hour, one to three times per day. Often, cluster headaches occur at the same time every day, "clustered" into a period of weeks or months, then disappear for months to years, only to recur. Eye tearing, lid drooping, and nasal stuffiness are characteristic. Sufferers may pace, bang their heads, rock, and become irritable during the attack. The pain can be so intense that it has been called the "suicide headache."

> *Neurologist Jim Burke at Albert Einstein Medical Center in Philadelphia explains cluster headaches: "These headaches are different than migraine headaches. People who are experiencing a cluster headache will be pacing the floor holding their head, while a person experiencing a migraine will look for a dark, quiet room."*

Other Headaches. These headaches come from a variety of other problems, from stroke to sinus congestion. Traction headaches can result from pulling, stretching, or pushing the head, for example, with tight hats, collars, hair barrettes, earphones, and earbuds for electronic and wireless devices. Inflammatory headaches may come from elsewhere in the body, signaling problems like meningitis or tooth infection. Neural pain may come from trigeminal neuralgia, and pressure pain from glaucoma or the sinuses. Modern office work may involve long periods sitting in climate-controlled spaces without access to fresh air or unfiltered sunlight.

Common Headache Triggers

Common things in everyday life can trigger headaches.

Head and Neck Posture. A common and overlooked cause of tension headache is poor back and neck posture. Holding your head forward of the midline of your body is called a "forward head." The weight of your head held in front of your neck rather than over it fatigues and strains neck muscles, overstretches the ligament down the back of your neck, and gradually pushes cervical discs outward until they can bulge and herniate (Figure 29-1). Pain from a forward head is usually felt down the back of the head and neck, along the top of the shoulders, between the shoulders, and under and along the shoulder blade.

Do you have a forward head without knowing it? A forward head is if you crane your neck forward while driving, using computers, or watching TV. Many exercises common in gyms practice a forward-head habit: pulling your neck forward for abdominal work, craning and tensing your neck while lifting weights, and tipping your neck forward while lifting or pulling a bar in back of your neck. Healthier substitutes for these exercises can be found in Chapter 9. A forward head is easily prevented with proper posture. Bring your head into healthy alignment by holding your ears above your shoulders, rather than letting your head crane forward of the midline of your body. Stand with your back, buttocks, and heels against a wall and see if the back of your head touches the wall. It should touch without lifting your chin or arching your back. Similarly, you should be able to lie face up flat on the floor comfortably without a pillow. If these positions don't feel natural, you are too tight to hold your head and neck in healthy posture. You need to stretch your shoulders and chest more to the back so that they don't make a forward position feel natural. Chapters 20 and 21 show how to correct a forward head.

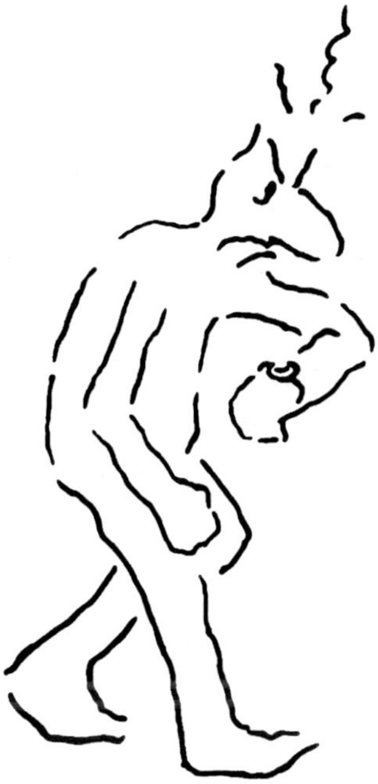

Figure 29-1. Unhealthful upper-body mechanics and positioning contributes to many upper-body pain syndromes, including upper crossed syndrome, disc pain, painful knotted muscle spots, and headache

Food. For migraines, food is often part of the cause. Classic food triggers are estrogenic food, nitrates, MSG, and foods high in tyramines. The plant-based estrogen in soy is becoming more recognized as a cause of migraines. Other estrogenic foods are listed in Chapter 17.

Tyramine foods include chocolate, red wine, beer, walnuts, peanuts, liver pâté, yogurt, lima beans, onions, salted and cured meats (ham, corned beef, sausage, bacon, lunch meats), dried meats, pickled herring, chicken livers, and aged cheeses (like bleu cheese).

Headaches come from processed meats, like hot dogs and lunchmeats. Processed meats contain nitrite compounds, which can dilate blood vessels in susceptible people, causing pounding head pain.

MSG (monosodium glutamate) is a widely used flavor enhancer. Annual worldwide demand is about 1.1 million tons. Some sources claim that no studies show causation of headache and other pain following eating foods flavored with MSG. At the same time, many people report chest pain, body pain, and headache after eating foods with MSG. Food labels may not list MSG and instead use other names such as hydrolyzed vegetable protein. Varieties of packaged foods contain it, as do various seasonings, packaged broths, bullion cubes, and other foods. MSG is sold as a stand-alone seasoning and flavor enhancer in the U.S. as Accent®, and under several trade names around the world.

Specific foods can set off an allergic reaction, resulting in headache. If avoiding certain foods does not reduce the number of headaches you get, it may be combinations. The difficulty in finding out which foods are problems is that migraines often take a day or two to "bloom" after eating trigger foods. By then, the connection is long forgotten. Write down foods and headaches for a while.

Alcohol. Non-migraine headache is common after too much wine, whisky, brandy, or rum because these drinks (unlike vodka) are high in headache-causing substances called congeners. Migraine and cluster headaches are different from alcohol hangovers but may occur with a hangover because they can both result from drinking alcohol. Cluster headaches may start shortly after a drink is taken.

Caffeine. Too much caffeine can cause a headache. For people who habitually drink caffeine drinks or take caffeine pills, caffeine withdrawal can bring on a headache. Some coffee drinkers find that they will have a headache until their morning coffee, making it difficult to cut back or quit drinking coffee. Although some coffee and soda drinkers feel that caffeine stops the pain, it is a result of a withdrawal and rebound cycle. It is not a healthful habit to start. If you drink coffee, maintain moderate to low use and avoid dependency.

Sleep. A trigger for migraine is altered sleep schedules, such as sleeping later than usual. Napping with your head propped on the arm of the couch can trigger posterior (back-of-the head) headaches.

Sleep apnea, a sleep disorder where the sleeper stops breathing, sometimes hundreds of times per night, drops oxygen levels. Many physical problems result. People suffering sleep apnea have daytime sleepiness, and often wake up headachy from the many periods of oxygen starvation. Loud snoring and gasping are clues to sleep apnea, which occurs most often among very overweight people. (Refer to Chapter 27 for more on sleep apnea.)

Eyestrain. Close work, an eyeglass or contact-lens prescription that is not just right, and glare are some factors in starting a headache from eyestrain. Vision-correction surgery gives variable results. In the wrong hands, eye damage or faulty correction may result in ongoing strain.

To reduce chance of eyestrain, remember to regularly look up and at a distance away from your work. Let your eyes focus on different distances. If you wear glasses, have your glasses prescription checked. Make sure it is the right strength, and that all the other considerations of grinding the glass for your prescription have been met. Make sure that the distance between the pupils of your eyes was measured correctly, then ground correctly into your lenses. Ask your optometrist or optician to check the base curve and axis of your lenses. Make sure your glasses are the right distance from your eyes, and the earpieces do not squeeze your head. If you don't wear glasses, have a good eye exam to check the health of your visual system.

Tight Headwear. Wearing a tight hat, headband, earphones, swim goggles, earpieces of eyeglasses, headlamps, and other constricting objects on the head can produce a type of tension headache.

Carbon-Monoxide Poisoning. Headache is a common flag of an uncommon problem—carbon-monoxide poisoning. This poisoning can come from a faulty heating system at home, exhaust system in your car, blocked chimneys, or using kerosene lanterns, heaters, or stoves indoors, in tents, and in campers. People have been poisoned as a result of riding in trailered boats or in the back of recreational vehicles when exhausts are drawn inside. You can't smell, taste, or see carbon monoxide. Carbon-monoxide poisoning can be serious, even fatal. Small, inexpensive home carbon-monoxide detectors are available in stores, usually next to the smoke detectors. Make sure your home has good ventilation.

Drugs. Several prescription drugs cause headache, including blood pressure medicine, antidepressants, antibiotics, allergy medicines, antacids, sleep medicines, cholesterol-lowering medicines, and others. Regular use of pain-suppressing drugs, both prescription and nonprescription, lowers your own body's natural pain-suppressing ability. Withdrawal from these drugs can rebound you into a headache. Don't start unhealthful cycles of causing more pain with medicines. Get out of negative cycles you are in.

Breathing patterns. Sometimes, people breathe too quickly for any number of reasons, including fear and excitement, or from medicines or drugs. Overly quick, shallow breathing lowers blood carbon dioxide levels, sometimes enough to cause limb tingling, dizziness, light-headedness, headache, or other odd sensations. Other people may breathe too slowly, from reasons ranging from drug use to breath-control exercises for meditation or yoga, or during scuba diving, through trying to conserve air. Carbon dioxide can rise to levels causing headache.

Teeth and Jaw. Toothaches start some headaches. Biting, grinding, and clenching teeth at night during sleep can cause jaw fatigue and sometimes head and neck pain. Poorly fitting dentures can cause jaw misalignment and pain. Someone with a dysfunction of the jaw joint, called the temporomandibular joint (TMJ), may become headachy from chronic clenching at night, or even chewing food day after day.

Sinusitis. Sinusitis occurs when one or more of your sinus cavities fills with bacterial or viral fluid and becomes inflamed. Sinusitis may involve allergies to irritants, such as cigarette smoke, dust, ragweed, or animal hair, or may spread from an upper respiratory infection. According to the NIH, "Research scientists disagree about whether chronic sinusitis triggers headache." However, the pressure of swollen, inflamed sinuses is uncomfortable, and sinus pain occurring behind the eyes and nose is often thought of as a headache.

Nitroglycerin. People who get angina pectoris (meaning "chest pain" in Latin) are often prescribed nitroglycerin pills or patches to wear. Nitroglycerin dilates blood vessels, which improves blood flow and oxygenation, relieving chest pain. The nitroglycerin is important to relieving chest pain, but users often get headaches because brain blood vessels dilate, too.

Other Contributors. Headaches can come from high blood pressure, allergies, air pollution, sun glare, hunger, thirst, cigarette smoke, dust, and fumes from chemicals and paint. "Benign exertional headaches" can occur when starting physical activity, such as running, lifting, and even coughing, sneezing, or bending. These headaches are more common in men and rarely last more than a few minutes. Fatigue, glaring or flickering lights, even changes in the weather, can set off headaches.

Combinations of Things. Determining what triggers your headaches can take some thinking. Factors that singly would not be enough to start pain may combine. For example, you may hunch your shoulders and neck all day in an office chair or car seat, on a day with a high smog count, while listening to loud music, regularly drink coffee, eat junk food and unfermented soy protein snacks, drink soda or energy drinks with stimulants and artificial colorings, breathe shallowly because you mistakenly think you need to keep your abdomen tight (refer to Chapter 7 for healthier abdominal practices), and use chemical cleaners in the home, then have a meal with red wine, processed meat, and a chocolate dessert.

Treating Headaches

During the Stone Age, medical shamans treated headaches by cutting holes in the patient's skull with flints to let the demons out. The term for this practice is trephination. Not only did patients survive trephination, it seemed to be popular. Some skulls recovered from that period show more than one healed trephine hole. Trephining was

A Dynamite Headache Story

Nitroglycerin is an explosive used to make dynamite and blasting gelatin. It is also used in medicine to reduce chest pain. Who made such a connection, and what does that have to do with headaches?

The story goes that World War II dynamite-factory workers endured throbbing headaches as an occupational hazard. When they left their positions after the war, their headaches stopped, but some of them began dying of heart attacks. Why?

People whose blood vessels are narrowed by fatty deposits can't get enough blood to their heart, reducing their oxygen supply. Their heart must pump harder against narrowed areas, increasing oxygen demand. When oxygen supply doesn't meet oxygen demand, their heart cries out in pain, called angina pectoris. A physician may prescribe nitroglycerin, which dilates the blood vessels of the heart, restoring blood flow and relieving pain. It also dilates the blood vessels of the head. Headaches are a characteristic symptom of too much nitroglycerin.

Nitrates are the active ingredient in nitroglycerin. Munitions workers had been inhaling airborne nitrates on the job, sometimes causing headaches, but also dilating their coronary blood vessels. After discontinuing exposure, the vasodilatory effect was rapidly lost. Their blood vessels constricted to their previous size. Headaches vanished, but those workers with coronary vessels already diseased from the usual causes—high-fat diet and lack of exercise—fell victim to blocked blood flow to their hearts. By leaving the ordnance plants, they lost the protective vasodilatory effect of their workplace air.

Nitroglycerin is very explosive. Dynamite is close to 75 percent nitroglycerin. Because it is mixed with inert materials like sawdust, wood pulp, or diatomaceous earth, it will detonate only with a fuse or the kick of a blasting cap. But medicinal nitroglycerin will not blow up because it is only about 1 percent nitroglycerin and is packed in an absorbent, inert material that reduces its volatility. Just watch out for headaches.

practiced until the Middle Ages. By the ninth century, a headache remedy from the British Isles was to drink "the juice of elderseed, cow's brain, and goat's dung dissolved in vinegar." Understandably, headache sufferers often will do almost anything to relieve the terrible pain. Fortunately, better remedies are available today.

Tension-Type Headaches. Ordinary muscle-triggered headaches go away when you stop tensing your face, head, and neck. Acute muscle-contraction headaches can be relieved with a hot shower and moist heat packs, and getting outside in the sunshine and fresh air. Make sure you are breathing easily, rather than tensing. Training for better head and neck posture can reduce much of the pain that is common along the tops of the shoulders, the back of the neck, and around the shoulder blades. Some people have fierce tensing habits, triggering chronic headaches. They need to retrain their postural habits and learn not to tense their muscles. (Refer to Chapters 20 and 21 on back and neck pain.)

Migraines. According to neurologist and headache specialist Dr. William Young, the most commonly prescribed drugs used to relieve migraines are ergotamine tartrate, DHE, and sumatriptan. Various medicines for nerve pain are also used. Dr. Young stresses the importance of not overusing pain medications (more than two to three days a week), or a daily rebound headache may result.

During a migraine, it helps to seek a dark, quiet room, and use cold packs. Sometimes, it helps to press on the bulging artery in front of the ear on the painful side. Check the food you are eating in the interim to make sure you are not continuing to eat trigger foods.

Cluster Headaches. Medications commonly prescribed for cluster headaches include drugs like Cafergot®, DHE, and sumatriptan. Since one of the mechanisms proposed for at least one stage of cluster headache is enlarged and inflamed brain blood vessels, various treatments aim to reduce the size of the enlarged blood vessels using ice hats or oxygen. When you breathe pure oxygen, your body constricts brain blood vessels to protect your brain against too high levels of oxygen. Breathing 100 percent oxygen has been known to help relieve some cases of headache, but little data is available to back this assertion. Breathing oxygen at higher-than-usual pressures in a hyperbaric chamber is also under study. Most people with cluster headaches are put on medication. Pain medications rarely work, but more specific treatments are successful in many cases.

Trigeminal Neuralgia. Also called Tic douloureux (painful tic), this condition can cause brief "lightning bolts" of facial pain, set off by the smallest touch or movement of the face or mouth. It comes from a problem of a facial nerve called the trigeminal nerve. This nerve supplies your face, teeth, mouth, and nose with sensation, and also lets you chew. People with trigeminal neuralgia may fear chewing or brushing their teeth because those actions can set off the pain. Treatment for trigeminal neuralgia involves various medications, taken regularly for prevention. In other cases, procedures to quiet the trigeminal nerve can stop the episodes.

Acute and Chronic Sinusitis. Most people get rapid results in decongesting the areas by taking steamy showers and baths, using hot facial compresses, and eating spicy foods and chili peppers. Drinking hot peppermint tea or other warm, aromatic teas with lemon can be soothing. Reduce home allergens (rugs, cats, junk piles, cigarettes, or whatever concentrates trigger irritants). Medical treatment may involve allergy shots if the causes are allergic. A walk outdoors in fresh air and sunshine can help clear breathing and pain.

Avoid treatments that add to the original problem. Sniffing camphor inhalants can irritate the area. Sniffing salt-water mixtures can set up a cycle of irritation and rebound congestion. Pain relievers, and decongestants contribute to cycles of rebound as well. Antibiotics, formerly commonly prescribed, have been found not to help and can cause other problems. Avoid chronic use of inhaled steroids, which can cause bone loss and other problems.

When to See a Physician

Many headaches don't require medical care. Headaches from the occasional missed meal, muscle tension, or poor posture are easily remedied. But some headaches signal serious problems, such as head injury, stroke, or disease. According to the National Institutes of Health, you need prompt medical care for the following:

- Sudden, severe headache (reaching a maximum in less than one minute)
- Headache associated with convulsions
- Headache accompanied by confusion or loss of consciousness
- Headache following a blow to the head
- Headache associated with pain in the eye or ear
- Persistent headache in a person who was previously headache-free
- Recurring headache in children
- Headache associated with fever
- Headache that interferes with normal life

Preventing Headaches

To avoid tension-type headaches, good head and neck positioning is important. Check to see if you hold your head in a forward posture (refer to Chapters 20 and 21 on back and neck pain). Don't jut your chin forward when drinking, eating, looking upward, sitting driving, or any time. It is a bad forward-head posture. Avoid teeth clenching and grinding. Look in the mirror to see if you habitually purse your lips, furrow your brow, squint, or look surprised. Relax and enjoy your day. Some people keep a mirror at their desk to catch candid reflections when they are not "posing" for a mirror.

Common methods to prevent migraine headaches include medications, training to tell when you are approaching triggering circumstances, stress reduction, regular exercise, and eliminating trigger foods and activities. To find food triggers, stop eating the usual trigger foods. Keep a food diary. For one week, write down every food you eat, and the time of day. In the same space, note how you feel. Log the weather, what work and exercise you did that day, and anything else you think may relate. Review your food/headache list after one week (or longer if you did not have a headache during that time). Look for what happened in the 24 to 48 hours before your headache. Don't become a "migraine hermit," avoiding all activity.

Finding the cause is important to ending headaches. For example, for headaches from regular use of prescription medicine, consider stopping the need for the medicine, for example, changing to healthier movement habits to stop joint pain, and changing to healthier meals to stop the need for blood pressure and cholesterol medicines. For headaches from TMJ, problems may be corrected by retraining chewing habits. Chew on both sides, not one, which can load the temporomandibular joints unevenly.

Vitamin B2 (riboflavin) and other B vitamins have been shown to be effective for some migraine sufferers, with few reported side effects. Poor nutrition from regularly consuming fast food, soda, and junk food can create nutritional deficiencies. Do you use herbs, drinks, and supplements with stimulants or estrogen-promoting compounds? Better nutrition can solve headaches from these causes without supplements.

Take a look at your body positioning during sitting and movement, what junk food you eat, or if you eat foods with chemicals or dyes. Do you get enough healthy physical activity and daily fresh air and sunlight? Do you sit indoors in a stuffy environment with the windows closed? Do you use many chemical cleaning products in the home? Have your teeth and eyes checked. Have your furnace and chimneys checked. Find out if you tense your face and neck. Find out if you have allergies. Keep a list of what you eat to see if you have trigger foods. Then, as obvious as it sounds, avoid things that give you headaches, and seek healthful food and movement habits that prevent them.

Resources for More Information

National Headache Foundation
www.headaches.org
1-888-NHF-5552
info@headaches.org

American Council for Headache Education (ACHE)
www.achenet.org
19 Mantua Road
Mt. Royal, NJ 08061
1-856-423-0258

30

Leg Cramps, and What to Do About Them

For this, be sure, to-night thou shalt have cramps,
Side-stitches that shall pen thy breath up; urchins
Shall, for that vast of night that they may work,
All exercise on thee; thou shalt be pinch'd
As thick as honeycomb, each pinch more stinging
Than bees that made 'em.

—Prospero, in *The Tempest*, Act I, Scene II

What Are Leg Cramps?

Muscles contract to move your bones. It is their job. The muscles that move your bones around are voluntary muscles. You tell them when to contract. After you stop telling them, they relax. When a muscle contracts too much, too suddenly, and does not relax again, you get a cramp. It is a spasm. It hurts. Leg cramps usually occur in your calf, foot, or hamstring muscles, and occasionally affect the quadriceps muscles in the front of your thigh, or other muscles.

Calf Cramps. Your gastrocnemius, or calf muscle, is the prominent, fleshy muscle at the back of your lower leg, below your knee. It attaches from your knee to your heel. Its main job is to pull on your heel to point your foot down, an action called plantarflexion. Plantarflexion flexes your ankle toward the sole, or plantar surface, of your foot. You can (usually) easily see the "string" that your calf muscle attaches to your heel to pull with. The string is a tendon called the Achilles tendon. When your calf muscle cramps, it pulls your Achilles tendon more strongly than usual and won't let go, which pulls your foot downward into a pointed (plantar-flexed) position, and holds it there painfully.

Foot Cramps. Your foot muscles that curl your toes down extend along the bottom of your foot from your heel to your toes. When these muscles cramp, they pull your toes, usually your two middle ones, downward toward the sole of your foot—painfully—and hold them there in spasm.

Hamstring and Quadriceps Cramps. A hamstring cramp will hurt in the back of your upper leg, and contract your hamstring muscles enough to make your knee bend. A quadriceps cramp will tighten the front of your thigh, causing your leg to painfully straighten or partially straighten.

Why Do You Get Leg Cramps?

People get cramps in their calves and feet for one very common reason, which will be discussed in the next section. This section addresses several less common reasons for cramps in general.

People like to say that not eating enough salt, or bananas, or any particular food causes leg cramps, but that reason is unlikely. In Western societies, a deficiency of salt or potassium is hard to get. The average Westerner eats many times the amount needed. The body helpfully "pees" it all out until levels are normalized again. Biochemical reasons why an overstressed muscle may cramp are not pinned down. Scientists would love to know the chemistry, too. Some people may get cramps from too much salt or potassium loss because of disease, diuretics, or large fluid losses from prolonged vomiting and diarrhea. But it seems that in the general population, muscle cramps during exercise are not from large electrolyte disturbances.

An uncommon cause of constant, severe calf cramps is cirrhosis of the liver. A rare possibility is certain inherited disorders that specifically cause leg cramps. Sometimes, the pain is not muscle cramps at all, but from other conditions confused for cramps. Arteries of the leg can plug up for the same reasons blood vessels anywhere in the body plug up—vascular disease is not just of the heart. When a person with narrowed leg arteries starts activity, the legs need more blood than can fit through those vessels, and the leg cries in pain for oxygen. That process is called claudication, from a Latin word meaning "lameness." People at the highest risk include sedentary people, smokers, or people fond of high-fat diets. Pregnancy presses on vessels exiting to the legs, often causing leg pain and cramping. Certain prescription medicines have cramps as side effects.

The Most Common Reason for Leg Cramps

Foot and leg cramps are most often caused by holding your leg, ankle, and foot muscles tightly, rather than letting them swing fluidly when you walk around all day. Tight shoes that restrict your toes or the natural range of motion of your foot when walking change the way your legs need to move, and can shorten the muscles into being more cramp-ready. The extra work of tensing the muscle makes it overexert, another factor in cramping.

> You can get leg cramps from holding your leg, ankle, and foot muscles tightly, rather than letting them swing fluidly during walking.

Calf cramps during swimming are most usually caused by kicking with tight ankles, and holding the foot at a rigid angle. The muscle has to contract with too much force and gets "stuck" in a contraction cycle. Cramps at the bottom of the foot are usually from kicking with toes curled or hooked. Tightly hooked toes may be a habit, or a result of wearing fins that are too large or too small. Sometimes, a swimmer will bend the knees too much, too hard while finning, overstressing the hamstrings (the muscles at the back of the thigh), causing them to cramp as well. In a pool, pushing too hard off the wall to do a start or turn can contract the calf muscle too tightly, making it cramp.

> The most common reason swimmers get leg and foot cramps is kicking with tight ankles and hooked toes.

How to Release a Cramp

Relieving a cramp can be easy and quick. A cramp is a contraction of a muscle. To release it, pull the muscle to lengthen it. You pull in the opposite direction that the cramp is pulling. The following cramp releases work whether you are running, swimming, or lying in bed.

Calf Cramps. Calf cramps pull your foot downward. To release a cramp, pull your toes up toward the front of your leg and hold. Don't point your foot or start activity again too soon, or the muscle is likely to cramp again.

For calf cramps while swimming in shallow water, stop and stand on the non-cramping leg and stretch the cramping leg. In deep water, take a breath and float facedown. Grasp the cramping foot, and release the cramp while floating. This position is sometimes called a jellyfish cramp release because it makes you resemble a jellyfish with a body floating at the surface, and arms and legs trailing underwater like tentacles. Remember not to point your foot or to resume the bad kicking that caused the cramp. The muscle needs a short time to relax.

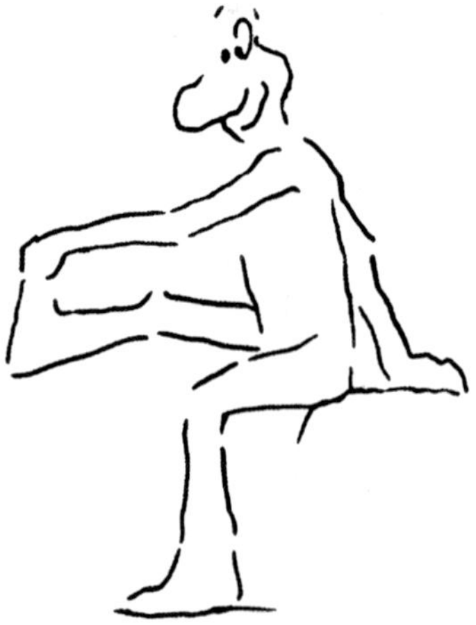

Figure 30-1. To stop a cramp, stretch the muscle in the opposite direction. To stretch out a calf cramp, pull your foot back and straighten your leg.

Foot Cramps. A cramp of the bottom of your foot pulls your toes downward. Grasp your toes, pull them back, and hold. While wearing fins, grab the fin tip and pull up and back just as you would for a calf cramp, as described previously, paying attention to pulling your toes back.

Hamstring Cramps. Hamstrings are the triple set of muscles in back of your upper leg. When they contract, they bend your knee. To uncramp the hamstrings, straighten your knee and hold.

Quadriceps Cramps. Your quadriceps are a set of four muscles (hence, the name "quad") in front of your upper leg. When they contract, they straighten your knee. To uncramp a cramping quadriceps muscle, bend your knee and hold. For more stretch on the thigh, you may need to pull the knee behind you.

Other Cramps. The principles are the same for any spasm your muscles may experience. A "stitch" in your side is a cramp of the diaphragm, your breathing muscle. A "stitch" may occur during a run or other active sport. One way to stretch out a "stitch" is to take a big breath and hold it while attempting to breathe out against the held breath. The pressure stretches things a bit and often releases the cramp. Other people find relief by raising their arms and straightening up, changing from the bent-over position, which contracts the muscles.

Back spasms can be painful and frightening. However, they are just cramps like all the others, and can often be quickly stretched out and relaxed with the proper stretch. They should not be left in spasm for any period of time. Like any other cramp, it makes the muscle more ready to continue the cramp cycle. (Refer to Chapters 20 and 21 on back and neck pain.)

What About Walking and Pounding?

Pounding the muscle is not effective to stop a leg cramp, but it can work coincidentally. Sometimes, pounding can push a muscle enough to lengthen it, but pounding is likely to make it contract more in defense. Standing up can functionally stretch and hold a cramp release for a foot or calf cramp. Walking can bend back the foot, lengthening the muscle enough to stretch out the spasm. The idea is to directly lengthen the muscle, rather than trying random actions without knowing why. Stretch a cramp.

Should You "Work Through" Extremity Cramps?

Do not ignore a cramp and allow it to continue cramping during whatever you are doing. Allowing a muscle to remain in spasm perpetuates a negative cycle. Spasm itself makes the muscle more electrically "irritable" and prepared to remain in spasm. You don't need to stay in pain when cramps are so easily reversed. Directly stretch the cramp out.

For a short time after releasing a cramp, it usually feels like it wants to cramp again. If you point your foot just after relieving after a calf cramp, for example, it will contract the calf muscle again, and the calf is likely to cramp again. Don't keep contracting the muscle. Let it release by holding the cramp release stretch.

How to Prevent Leg Cramps

Daily Habits. Don't walk around holding your leg, ankle, and foot muscles tightly. Don't wear tight, uncomfortable shoes, or shoes that you may think are comfortable but that restrict your toes or the natural range of motion of your foot when walking. Take time to exercise, relax, and regularly stretch your legs and feet.

Leg and Foot Stretches. Stretch your feet and the back of your legs. It has been noted by some muscle-dynamics scientists that in societies without sit-down toilets, the habitual squatting stretches the appropriate muscles, making calf and foot cramps rare. For functional stretching, every time you bend for things around the house using the half-squat with feet side by side, keep both heels down (Figure 8-1, right). Doing so will stretch the back of both legs at once every time you bend. When walking, face your feet and knees straight ahead. Turning your feet outward loses the natural stretch on the bottom of the foot with each step. When going up stairs, keep the heel down on the upper step, for better muscle use and a built-in Achilles stretch. Built-in functional stretches are important to normal leg- and foot-muscle function. Don't wear tight shoes that push the toes together, gradually tightening them. Pull your toes apart with your hands every day.

Proper Kick When Swimming. The most effective prevention for leg cramps from kicking while swimming is not to kick with rigid ankles or curled toes. Kicking this way is a bad habit. Many people who kick this way do not know how to kick with loose ankles and floppy feet. The hallmark of people who hold their ankles tightly while kicking in a pool is that they make little forward progress when using a kickboard without fins, no matter how hard they kick. Their legs often sink, and kicking is tiring. Don't hold your foot in any one position, and don't deliberately bend it up and down with your kick. Allow it to flop loosely, independent of your leg. Loose kicking is one of the most important aspects to kicking properly.

Exercise to Retrain Muscle Use. The most effective exercise if you get leg cramps is a drill to retrain your foot to relax (be separate from muscular control) while using the rest of your leg.

- Sit with your lower legs dangling. At a pool, sit at the rim of the pool, with your lower legs dangling free underwater.
- Grasp your lower leg near your ankle with both hands. Shake your leg up and down, paying attention to how your foot moves. It should flop freely as you shake it. Don't hold it rigidly angled at the ankle. Don't hook or curl your toes. To do so may take some work and practice. Let it be as loose and floppy as a rag doll.
- Carefully observe that as you shake your leg downward, your foot should flop upward, and as you quickly pull your leg up again, your foot flops downward loosely. It should not yank upward as a unit. If you shake side to side, your foot should also swing freely.

Doing this exercise until you are successful is crucial for anyone who gets leg cramps while swimming. You can practice this exercise anytime you are sitting comfortably. Someone else can shake your leg, too. Do this exercise until you have retrained your legs' neuro-muscular patterns so well that you can flop your feet by quick, small knee movements without using your hands.

The test of a good, loose kick is when you can go into a pool without fins, take a kickboard, and kick with easy forward progress. Most people who have tight ankles make little (or sometimes no) headway. People with tight, hooked ankles, who also use a large deep swinging kick, can find themselves traveling backward. Think of tight ankles, held rigidly at an angle from your leg, as airplane flaps. Trying to move forward with tight ankles is like trying to accelerate with your flaps down. With practice, you can loosen your ankles, develop an easy, powerful kick, and eliminate the majority of your leg and foot cramps while swimming.

No More Leg Cramps

Get regular, built-in leg and foot stretches by bending properly with both heels down (Figure 8-1, right) in your daily activities. Strengthen and regularly use the muscles of your feet and legs so they can handle exertion better. Leg cramps are not something you have to put up with.

31

Funny Physical Facts

Laughter is a form of internal jogging. It moves your internal organs around. It enhances respiration. It is an igniter of great expectations.

—Norman Cousins

Why Does It Hurt and Tingle When You Hit Your Funny Bone?

Why do they call it the funny bone? It is called the funny bone because it's the humerus. Why isn't it funny at all when you hit it?

The humerus is the long bone in your upper arm, extending from shoulder to elbow. A nerve called the ulnar nerve runs from your spine through your shoulder and elbow to your hand. Your ulnar nerve passes closest to your skin's surface just under the knob of bone at the elbow end of your humerus. When you ding your elbow there, you abruptly compress your ulnar nerve against the bone, causing acute, temporary pain and numbness.

Your ulnar nerve runs through your elbow in a passageway called the cubital tunnel. In medicine, the word cubital refers to the elbow. A person taking your blood pressure will position their stethoscope in the "antecubital space," in front of your elbow. Cubital comes from an ancient word that you've probably heard before. If you know the story of Noah's Ark, you remember "cubits," a unit of measure that Noah used to build the Ark. A cubit is the distance from fingertips to elbow. A dinged funny bone is called transient cubital tunnel syndrome.

How Much Blood Do You Have to Cut Off Before Your Foot Falls Asleep?

None. The phenomenon of "falling asleep" is not related to blood, but to nerve. When you compress a nerve for long enough, you can temporarily cause the numbing and pins-and-needles tingling that is popularly called "falling asleep" and medically called neuropraxia (nur-uh-PRAKS'-ee-ya). One common, short-duration example is banging your funny bone. Sudden compression of the ulnar nerve in your elbow is responsible for the tingling funny bone, explained previously.

Another well-known, longer-duration example is the phenomenon occurring in one or both legs after sitting too long at the edge of a bench, particularly in the bathroom. This phenomenon is called "toilet-seat neuropathy" in medical jargon. In this occasion, after sitting too long, you try to stand up but fall over or hop around on tingling feet. It usually reverses quickly.

Where Did the Expression "Knee-Jerk Reaction" Come From, and What Does It Really Mean?

You've probably had a physician or someone else tap you just below your kneecap. Your lower leg jumped without you thinking about it. A knee-jerk reaction is one you don't think about. In other words, it doesn't use your brain.

Just below your kneecap is the tendon connecting your four thigh muscles (quadriceps) to your lower leg. When the tendon is hit, it stretches slightly, but suddenly. The stretched tendon sends a sensory signal, which is a signal about what you felt, up your leg to the part of your spinal cord just above your behind. The signal says, "We're being stretched too fast, and it may mean trouble. Send help to contract us." The signal is reflected (which is why it's called a reflex) to a motor nerve.

Motor nerves control movement. The motor nerve in your spinal cord sends a signal to your thigh muscles, the quadriceps. The signal says, "Contract." Your quads contract to counter the stretch. Your leg jumps without any input at all from your brain. By the time a separate sensory signal gets all the way up to your brain to tell you that your tendon was stretched, your quads already contracted quickly, making your leg jump. The simple sensory-to-motor loop that needs no more than your spinal cord to function is called a stretch reflex. You can elicit other stretch reflexes by tapping behind your ankle on your Achilles tendon, or near the crease of your elbow on your biceps tendon.

You have other kinds of reflexes. They vary in complexity, but none needs your brain to operate. Sneezing is a reflex reaction to upper-respiratory irritation. Coughing is a reflex reaction to lower-respiratory irritation. The "wink" reflex closes your eye when something tries to fly in. The "hot-stove" reflex yanks your hand away from high heat in the same "sensory-in, motor-out" reaction that, like other reflexes, does not involve conscious thought to initiate action. The simplest reaction in your body is the reflex, and the "knee jerk" is the simplest of reflexes—only two nerves and no brain.

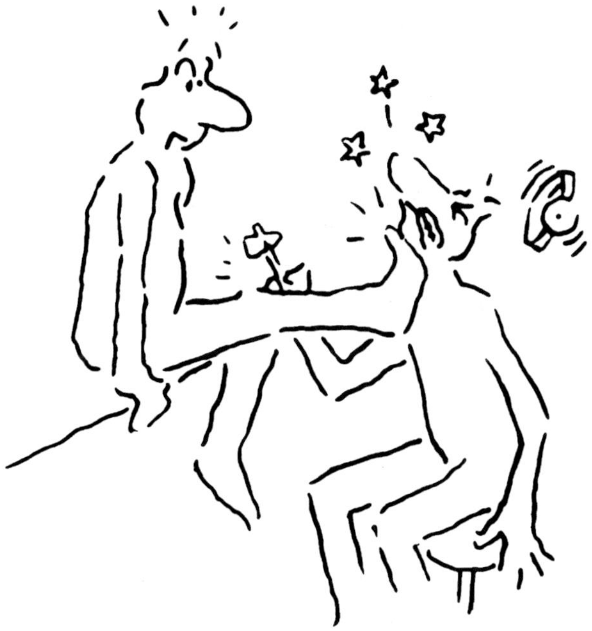

Figure 31-1. A knee jerk is a reflex that doesn't use your brain.

What Makes You Feel "Pumped Up" After Lifting Weights? How Does the Muscle Grow That Fast?

Your muscles don't immediately grow in the sense of adding lean weight or splitting muscle fibers. The size increase that occurs right after lifting and inflates muscles (and egos) is only fluid, and temporary fluid at that. When you lift heavy weights, your working muscles contract, compressing the blood vessels in them. Circulation is temporarily reduced, or even stopped, with extreme muscular contraction.

After you lift weights, a larger-than-normal volume of blood and fluid rushes back into your muscle, in reaction to the previous deficit. The extra blood puffs up the muscle. A fancy technical term is dedicated to this phenomenon of extra blood puffing up muscles when they react to being contracted. The prefix for an amount greater than normal is "hyper-". The suffix "-emia," for blood, comes from the Greek haima (from which we get the words hemorrhage, hemophilia, hemoglobin, and even hemorrhoid). Speaking technically, pumping up is called reactive hyperemia.

Is It True That if You Put Sleeping People's Hands in a Glass of Water, They Will Wet Themselves?

No. It is not true, but it is always worth a try for the sake of science. Merely dipping the hand or fingers is ineffective. When you fully immerse your body in water, a real physiologic need to "go" occurs. However, even then, if you are potty-trained, the signals will not override your training. If you were immersed fully during sleep, this result would still be so, as long-duration immersion experiments show.

Due to the effects of making you want to go, the increased output occurring with immersion may be called the "P phenomenon," or PP for short. The P phenomenon happens because immersing your body in water shifts blood away from your arms and legs to the area of your chest called the thorax. Because of buoyancy, fluids just float into the thorax. Being in a cold environment also shifts blood volumes to the thorax, which is why you often notice the P phenomenon when stepping into a cold shower. Volume detectors in the heart notice the increase in fluid and, to normalize thoracic volume, helpfully signal your body to voluntarily show some fluid the way out.

In warm or hot water, however, the phenomenon is reduced. Blood vessels expand in your arms and legs in response to the heat. This peripheral vasodilation shifts blood to your limbs and reduces thoracic blood volume, reducing the physiologic cascade responsible for the P phenomenon. The fact that warm water reduces the response offers even more evidence against the glass-of-water story, when the claim is that the water has to be warm.

The P phenomenon occurs in the microgravity environment of space travel. Fluids float away from the legs and into the upper body, just as during immersion in water. Astronauts have a technical term for this condition. They call it the "Fat-Face, Chicken-Legs Effect."

What Does Your Stomach Say When You Lie?

Preliminary research from the University of Texas shows that people who lie could be caught by the reaction of their stomachs. Researchers developed a new test that uses a device called an electrogastrogram (EGG). The EGG determines the speed of a person's stomach contractures, or "beats," which are normally at three per minute. Preliminary findings show that the stomach's rate does not increase if the person is telling the truth, no matter how nervous he may be. In contrast, a person's heartbeat can increase whether the person is telling a lie or the truth. Researchers hope the new technique could improve accuracy of polygraphy, which relies on heart-rate response. Research team leader Pankaj Pasricha stated: "The heart is unreliable because it's affected by not only by your brain, but by many other factors, such as hormones. The gut has a mind of its own—literally. It has its own well-developed nervous system that acts independently of almost everything except your unconscious brain."

Kevin Murphy, a psychologist at Penn State University, recently headed a panel for the U.S. National Academy of Sciences to analyze the science behind polygraph devices. He stated, "Polygraph detectors, whatever their ilk, measure stress and not lying. No accepted scientific model links the body's stress reactions to lying. So, while there may be experimental data for a correlation between the two, the lack of a known causal link leaves room for uncertainty in polygraph tests. This new test might give more, potentially very useful, data."

Why Do You Sometimes Get Dizzy When You Stand Suddenly?

When you stand and sit, some of your blood volume pools in the veins of your legs because of the pull of gravity. Sometimes when you stand suddenly, the rush of pooling blood in your legs from gravity briefly lowers the blood supply and blood pressure to your head. You may feel light-headed. When this sensation occurs, you just need to bend over safely to lower your head. Lowering your head allows gravity to restore blood, relieving dizziness. Extreme pooling has caused occasional cases of fainting when standing suddenly, when standing long periods at attention, and when climbing out of the water, especially hot water in spas and hot tubs. Pooling has been fatal to beached whales.

After sitting for long periods at work and on a plane, your feet may swell with pooling fluids. Contracting your leg muscles while sitting, and by getting up and moving around pumps blood upward, reducing pooling and your risk of clots. Before standing, lightly contract leg and arm muscles to reduce chance of dizziness upon rising.

What Can Your Fingerprints Reveal About You?

Fingerprints contain a mixture of skin cells, lipids, sweat, and substances acquired on the person's hands. People leave traces of proteins, salts and fatty acids on everything they touch. People differ in the amount of their different kinds of secretions. Forensic techniques may determine if the person leaving a particular fingerprint is a smoker, what cosmetics they wear, and possibly, if they handled substances like drugs or explosives. Although individuals can't be specifically identified, suspects can be ruled out. Sue Jickells, an analytical chemist at Kings College in London, stated: "We have found you can detect cotinine, made when someone metabolises nicotine, in fingerprints. This tells you if that person is a smoker, and this kind of additional information could be useful if you don't have a suspect." She has also shown that traces of cosmetics and aftershave can be found in prints. Remaining questions are whether each person's prints are truly different, how much prints are changed by what was last touched, and whether sweat profiles could tell when the print was made, on the premise that characteristic chemicals evaporate or break down at different rates when exposed to air.

Can You Tell Human DNA by Looking?

In the movie *Mission to Mars*, actor Gary Sinise's character is sitting at a computer monitor observing a short section of DNA (about two full twists). He exclaims, "This DNA looks human." However, all DNA, regardless of the organism, has the same characteristic double-helix and is made up of the same bases. All mammals have at least 90 percent of their DNA in common. Unless Sinise's character sequenced the entire fragment and compared it to a DNA sequence known to be human, he couldn't conclude that it was human.

What Is the Popping Noise When Your Joints Crack?

Joints pop in several ways. The interesting story starts with bubbles. A certain amount of nitrogen from the air around you dissolves in your body fluids, including joint fluids called synovial fluids. When pressure is decreased, the gas can come out of its dissolved form. If that happens quickly, bubbles form. This process can happen in easy ways (for example, popping your knuckles or squatting down and cracking your knees.) Even scuba divers can do so by coming up from a dive too fast. It does not make noise, but can cause decompression sickness, where bubbles come out of solution in their bodies, get stuck, and cause pain and other problems in all the various places that they get stuck. The diver may then make a lot of noise. Cracking your knuckles doesn't cause or relate to decompression sickness, although the bubble formation can be similar. Exactly how and why is complex. A summary of a few of the basics follows.

Gases like carbon dioxide and nitrogen are present in dissolved form in your bodily fluids. They are held in solution by the pressure of air around us and by gas pressures in your body. If you pull your finger joint so that it enlarges briefly, the slight vacuum formed creates a temporary low-pressure cavity. The low pressure pulls gas molecules out of solution, forming bubbles in a process called vacuum cavitation. The bubbles quickly collapse. Pop. It takes time for the gas to redissolve before the joint can crack again. Another way bubbles can form besides enlarging the joint space is crushing the muscle against bone, as during some kinds of knuckle and knee cracking. Pop.

Studies have also looked at body tissues (in a laboratory) that are full of dissolved gas (the tissues, not the laboratory). These tissues had no bubbles, even after experimentally subjecting them to large pressure reductions. However, when energy was added by moving the tissue (as happens with muscle contraction), bubbles readily formed. *Pop. Pop.*

Not all joint cracking is due to bubbles. Often, it involves tendons moving quickly over adjacent bony knobs, making a distinctive noise. *Pop*. Tendons are tough, inelastic fibers that connect a muscle to a bone. Snapping tendons occurs routinely in many people's shoulder, elbow, hip, back, and ankle joints. Occasionally, tendon snapping occurs in the knee. This kind of snapping, unlike knuckle popping, can be repeated within short intervals, sometimes during every step when walking. *Pop. Pop. Pop*. Tight muscles can cause it, and specific stretching exercises can relieve it. Sometimes popping is so painful, constant, and detrimental to sports activity that people are told they need surgery to move the tendon to a slightly different position to avoid the snapping. Such surgeries can usually be skipped with muscle-retraining techniques.

Another reason for joint popping can come from using bad sitting, standing, and lifting postures all day. As muscles tighten and contract unevenly, tendons or ligaments can get pulled slightly away from their accustomed track. People often learn that they can "crack" their back to restore a more comfortable position. *Pop*. Although it often feels good, it is not a miracle cure. It is better to learn to identify and minimize the muscle stress that caused the need in the first place.

How detrimental knuckle and other joint cracking may be to your joints depends on degree. It's probably safest to avoid any vigorous trauma to your joints. Joints are important parts of your body. Joint deterioration is related to the extent of abuse, genetics, and other not-well-identified factors. Although not a certainty, chronic, traumatic joint stress may be a contributor to early wear and tear that may lead to arthritic degeneration.

Not All "Knuckle" Popping Is in Your Body

Marine propellers cavitate bubbles by similar mechanical forces as knuckle popping. The rotating propeller blade rapidly forms low-pressure areas. Dissolved gas cavitates out of the water near the blades. When these many tiny bubbles suddenly form and then collapse with great vigor against the blade, they make noise and eventually pit the blade. *Pop. Pop. Pop.* Anticavitation devices are important tools to extend the life of propellers and minimize submarine noise.

How Much Does a Human Head Weigh?

The average adult human head weighs around 4.5 kilograms (10 pounds), varying with body size. Another question is how do you weigh it? You can cut off someone's head and weigh it, but how can you weigh someone's head without cutting it off? One way to weigh body parts is to measure the volume of the part by immersing it in water to see the volume of water it displaces. To measure the displacement of someone's head, they must lower their head into a tub of water vertically and crown downwards until the water reaches the base of the chin. The water needs to be as near to 0 °C as the volunteer could bear (to know the water density). The water that spills over the sides of the experimental tub is collected and its volume measured. It is also good to repeat the immersion several times to make sure you have a repeatable result. You can then estimate the weight of the head from the volume of water displaced. This estimate is also based on charts and tables of average body weight compared to displaced water. Modern computer analysis can make estimates without putting someone's head in a bucket of water.

Is It True That Time of Death Is Predictable From Body Temperature or Cooling?

After death, the metabolic processes that make heat in the body stop, and the body cools. Algor mortis is an old term for cooling of the body after death. It comes from two Latin words meaning, "the chill of death." Algor mortis is one of the three changes observed soon after death: algor mortis, livor mortis, and rigor mortis.

Cooling does not follow predictable time intervals as once thought. Although forensic temperature measurement of the body is done, the phenomenon of algor mortis is often too imprecise to estimate time since death. In 1710, English physician John Davey first used the then-new invention of the thermometer in a human body at autopsy. Davey's experiments on the bodies of British soldiers were published based on his work that took place in the high heat of Malta. Later pathologists following Davey's published descriptions apparently did not place the thermometer inside the body, but in the armpit. Their publications of the inaccurate information of cooling became widely popularized and passed from school to school. It turns out that the widely held dogma that body temperature drops at a precise and steady rate of 1.6 degrees an hour (later rounded to 1.5 for ease of calculation) was never the case. The old term algor mortis is becoming uncommon, and usually replaced by "body cooling."

Is It True That Time of Death Is Predictable from Skin Discoloration—Livor Mortis?

A dark purplish discoloration of the skin after death, livor mortis occurs from blood pooling in body parts lower than others. It comes from two Latin words: *livor* meaning "darkening," and *mortis* meaning "death." Common synonyms are hypostasis (stuff stagnating below), postmortem hypostasis, postmortem livedo, and postmortem lividity (black-blue-gray discoloration). Livor mortis usually develops within a few hours of death and reaches a maximum after about twelve hours. Postmortem lividity is eventually hidden by even more intense discoloration that happens as the body putrefies.

Development time for livor mortis is so variable that it is not useful to estimate time since death. Its use in forensics lies in color and distribution. Pink lividity (rather than purple) suggests poisoning by carbon monoxide or cyanide, or hypothermia as possible causes of death. Distribution of lividity that is different than that expected by blood pooling due to gravity may suggest that body has been turned after death.

Is It True That Time of Death Is Predictable from Body Stiffening—Rigor Mortis?

The term "rigor mortis" comes from two Latin words meaning "stiffening" and "death." The stiffening is caused when the usual chemicals that govern muscle contraction, primarily calcium ions, can no longer leave the muscle to relax it. After death, an initial period of loss of all muscle tone occurs, then rigor mortis develops over hours, gradually stiffening the body in whatever position resulted from the influence of gravity. Rigor mortis does not change the position of the body. It is not true that rigor can make a body sit up or clench its fists. As putrefaction occurs, rigor diminishes. When a body in rigor is found in a position not expected by gravity, it suggests the body had been moved after death. Onset, development, and loss of rigor are so variable that rigor mortis is not useful to determine time since death.

Can Bugs Tell Exactly When Someone Died?

As a body decomposes, many species of flies and beetles colonize it in an ordered progression. Insect analysis is frequently used for estimating time of death. Accuracy is claimed within months or weeks, even days if the body has been dead less than a month.

However, in multi-year experiments by Melanie Archer of the Victorian Institute of Forensic Medicine in Melbourne, Australia, variations occurred from one year to the next, varying with weather, how temperatures in the environment surrounding the corpse were estimated, and changes in insect numbers. No previously published studies on reference corpses had been repeated over successive years.

Archer concluded: "The estimates are not as tight as some forensic scientists imply in court. We need to introduce some rigour." Forensic entomologist Lee Goff at Chaminade University of Honolulu, Hawaii, agrees that many lawyers and forensic scientists are unaware of the limitations. "The legal community want things to be precise, but they have to remember that we are dealing with estimates." Insect corpse analysis is often flawed.

Can You Really Turn Into Soap?

A brown, fatty, waxy, soap-like substance can form on dead humans and animals that are buried in moist places with favorable temperature. This substance is called adipocere. *"Adipo-"* comes from the word meaning soft animal fat. The word root *"cere"* comes from the Latin word for wax. Adipocere is mostly insoluble salts of fatty acids, such as oleic, palmitic, and stearic acids. It is also called "grave wax." The Philadelphia Mutter Museum has a specimen of an adipocere body that is popularly called "The Soap Lady."

Do Hair and Nails Grow After Death?

When you are alive, fingernails grow an average of about a tenth of a millimeter per day. Toenails grow about a half to a third more slowly. Head hair grows about half an inch each month. In his novel, *All Quiet on the Western Front*, Erich Remarque imagines a dead friend's nails growing in corkscrews after his burial. In the 1959 movie *The Tingler*, Vincent Price's character states that hair and nails grow after death. However, hair and nails no longer grow after death. It is a myth. A body dehydrates after dying. The flesh dries and retracts away from nails and hair. Also, the tiny muscles surrounding each hair follicle stiffen. Although hair and nails remain the same length as before death, they protrude more prominently. These changes can appear as an increase in length. To combat skin shrinkage, funeral homes put moisturizing cream on bodies, particularly on the faces of men with heavy beards.

Does Hair Grow Back Thicker and/or Darker When You Shave It?

It doesn't. Hair seems to change when it really doesn't. All body hair is thicker, and usually darker, at the base than the tip. When you shave, you cut off the thinner, lighter tips. When the rest of the hair shaft starts growing past the skin line again, you see only the thicker, darker part of the hair you cut. When that decapitated hair finally reaches the end of its cycle and falls out, the hair growing to replace it is not altered from its original shape or genetically determined color. If you shave again before this happens, you will feel the stubby growth again soon enough. As far as boys shaving for the first time, the beard typically becomes coarser with the passing years of manhood–shaved or not. Hair change with maturation should not be confused with effects of shaving.

Why Are the Areas on the Side of the Head Called Temples?

The word "temple" comes from the Greek word for "time." The sides of the face near the ears are usually the first to go gray, evidencing the inevitable passage of time.

Is Oxygen a Feel-Good Drug?

Breathing oxygen is popularly thought to help football players, make you feel good, cure headaches, and work as an aphrodisiac. All of these claims have been disproven—except one.

It used to be a practice by American football players to breathe oxygen, believing it would help performance and recovery. Breathing oxygen will not help. The sprints and tackles in football are so short that the body fuel that is used is quick and ready-stored fuel, not oxygen. Football may be a hard sport, but it is not an aerobic one. Football moves do not use oxygen to make energy. Players use anaerobic fuel stored in their muscles. Oxygen supplementation increases blood levels only minimally since blood already carries almost all the oxygen it can hold. To put it technically, your oxygen saturation is usually around 97 to 98 percent. Any small increase in blood oxygen saturation with bottled oxygen will be gone by the time players get back to the field and aligned in formation.

Studies by the Department of Internal Medicine at Baylor University, reported in the *Journal of the American Medical Association*, found no advantage to breathing 100 percent oxygen on recovery from exhaustive bouts of exercise, no difference in performance during a second bout after breathing 100 percent oxygen, and that the professional athletes who served as subjects could not identify whether they were breathing 100 percent oxygen or room air. In other studies, a percentage of subjects who were told they were breathing oxygen but received room air reported elevated mood.

Breathing supplemental oxygen benefits exercise if breathed during long duration, heavy exercise. Heart rate and blood levels of lactic acid decrease, and time to exhaustion increases. Still, carrying oxygen tanks while jogging or biking presents interesting practical problems. If you want to get more oxygen to your cells for greater long-distance ability, you can do it yourself in another way. Regular aerobic training enhances your body's entire oxygen-carrying and -using system.

For effect on libido, no evidence suggests any physical aphrodisiac capability of oxygen. The placebo effect is potent in this area.

Where oxygen seems to work is in relieving some kinds of vascular headache. Breathing 100 percent oxygen constricts blood vessels in the brain. One of the mechanisms proposed for at least one stage of cluster and migraine headache is enlarged brain blood vessels that inflame and hurt. Oxygen is under study as a treatment for cluster headache (refer to Chapter 29).

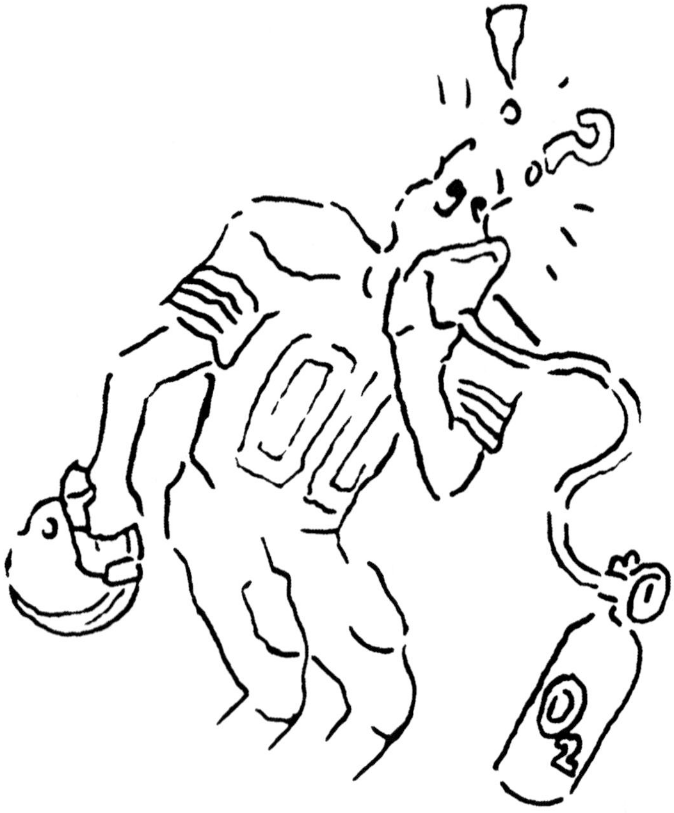

Figure 31-2. American football players do not play better by breathing supplemental oxygen.

Glossary

A

Acetabulum [From Latin *acetum*, "vinegar," the origin of the term acetic acid. Acetabulum is a shallow vinegar vessel or cup.] Cup-shaped hollow in your hipbones, where the head of your upper leg bone (femur) fits. The socket of the ball and socket joint. Your acetabulum is located at the junction of the three hipbones, the ilium, ischium, and pubis bone. See Femur, Ilium, Ischium, and Pubis.

Acromion [From Greek *akros*, "extreme," or "tip" + *omion*, diminutive of *omos*, "shoulder."] The bone of the outer end of your shoulder, formed by your shoulder blade (scapula) winging around to the front of your shoulder. Your collarbone attaches in front.

Adenosine Triphosphate (ATP) (uh-DEN'-oh-sin try-FOS'-fate) [Named for its adenosine base plus three phosphates.] The molecule made in your body that supplies energy to your cells for all your biochemical processes. It has two phosphates held on by low-energy bonds, and a third with a high-energy bond. ATP releases energy by breaking off the phosphate with the high-energy bond, becoming adenosine diphosphate (ADP). In extreme situations, ADP loses another phosphate to become adenosine monophosphate (AMP), but little more energy is gained, as it is a low-energy bond. You have three systems that make ATP—one is aerobic, and two are anaerobic. See Aerobic Metabolism, Anaerobic Metabolism, and Creatine Phosphate (CP).

ADH See Antidiuretic Hormone.

Aerobic Capacity See Endurance, Cardiovascular.

Aerobic Exercise Activities that are long and intense enough to benefit your cardiovascular system. Sitting in a chair uses aerobic metabolism for about 100 percent of your energy needs, but it is not an aerobic exercise.

Aerobic Metabolism System of making ATP (an energy molecule) using oxygen with stored carbohydrate, fat, and protein. Aerobic metabolism goes on all day and night, even when you're sitting around or sleeping, making a distinction between aerobic metabolism and aerobic exercise. In animals, it takes place in the cells' organelles, called mitochondria. Your aerobic system has two pathways: the Krebs cycle and the electron transport chain. You make most of your ATP in the electron transport chain. When you exercise aerobically, oxygen carries off hydrogen ions, transforming lactic acid back to pyruvate, which can be used to make ATP. It also means that lactic acid does not get a chance to build up as it does when you are anaerobic. Your aerobic system allows you to generate energy for long, low- to moderate-intensity activities. Your aerobic metabolism can supply much energy, but can't do it very fast. Your anaerobic systems allow you to do quick, high-intensity activities. The combination of systems makes your exercise capacity versatile. See Adenosine Triphosphate (ATP), Anaerobic Metabolism, Electron Transport Chain, and Krebs Cycle.

Aldosterone (al-DOHS'-tur-own) [Named for its chemical structure containing an aldehyde and a sterol.] Steroid hormone secreted by your adrenal gland and regulated by your kidney. Helps you retain salt and water, and excrete potassium, to maintain their healthy balance in your body.

Allergy [From Greek *allos*, "other" + *ergon*, "action."] Condition where a person may react with sneezing, itching, and skin rashes to things like pollen, foods, or microorganisms, which cause no reaction in other people. Term coined by Austrian physician Pirquet, around the early 1900s.

Amenorrhea (ay-men-or-REE'-ah) [*a*-, "without" + Greek *men*, "month."] Long-term cessation of menstruation due to various causes. A risk factor for osteoporosis.

Amphetamines [Composite word from A(lpha) + M(ethyl) + PH(enyl) + ET(hyl) + amine.] A group of stimulant drugs, sometimes used to increase athletic performance, to reduce fatigue, or to reduce hunger as an ingredient in diet pills. They are sympathomimetic, as they mimic the activation of your sympathetic nervous system, primarily by releasing nerve transmission chemicals called catecholamines, especially epinephrine (adrenaline) and norepinephrine (noradrenaline) from nerve endings. See Catecholamine, Ergogenic Aid, Sympathetic Nervous System, and Sympathomimetic.

Anabolic Steroids Drugs capable of increasing muscle growth. Not all steroids are anabolic (for example, the anti-inflammatories prednisone and cortisone, and Vitamin D). Anabolic steroids have several damaging effects along with their muscle-building properties. Harmful effects are sometimes permanent. Bodybuilders sometimes try to find unregulated sources from veterinary and overseas suppliers. Products may sometimes be counterfeit or of varying quality. Certain health food store products that are regular food have labels suggesting that they have anabolic effects. This practice is not illegal. Become educated to watch out for misleading claims. See Ergogenic Aid.

Anaerobic Capacity Ability of your body to use special stored fuel, not oxygen, for rapid-onset, short-duration, intense activity. Because it is not an oxygen-using (aerobic) system, it is called anaerobic. You use your anaerobic system for sprinting, swimming against hard currents, lifting heavy weights, and any short, intense activity. You can improve your anaerobic capacity by exercising anaerobically, by practicing short, intense exercises. See Anaerobic Metabolism, and compare to Aerobic Exercise and Aerobic Metabolism.

Anaerobic Metabolism Two systems of making ATP, a special energy molecule, without using any oxygen. The first system is your ATP-CP system of stored ATP. Your second anaerobic system is glycolysis. It is important for you to have systems of making energy without using oxygen for the many activities that begin so quickly—and are so high intensity—that your oxygen system is not able to supply needs. Your anaerobic systems allow you to do quick, high-intensity activities. Anaerobic metabolism can't make much ATP, but can make it very quickly. Your aerobic system allows you to generate energy for long, low- to moderate-intensity activities. The combination of systems makes your exercise capacity very versatile. See Adenosine Triphosphate (ATP), Aerobic Metabolism, and Glycolysis.

Anorexia Nervosa [From Greek *an*, "without" + *orexis*, "appetite," from *oregein*, to reach out for.] An abnormal loss of appetite and refusal to eat, resulting in emaciation and malnutrition. A risk factor for osteoporosis.

Anthropometrics (an-throw-poh-MET'-tricks) [From Greek *anthrapos*, "human being" + *metrikos*, from *metron*, "measure."] Science of identifying and comparing human body measurements, such as lengths and widths of segments, to measurements of other segments, and to measurements of other people. One use of anthropometrics is to measure bone lengths and widths at specific joints to tell the size of your body's frame—small, medium, or large—which helps determine optimum weight. Another use of anthropometrics is to predict the sport you might excel in, based on your specific body size and other anthropometric measurements.

Antidiuretic Hormone [From Greek *anti*, "opposite or against" + *diourein* "to pass urine" (*ourein*, to urinate).] Abbreviated ADH. A hormone made in the back (posterior lobe) of your pituitary gland that makes smooth muscle contract, particularly in all your blood vessels. ADH raises blood pressure and reduces excretion of urine. Also called vasopressin (from Latin words meaning an agent that presses down blood vessels).

Antihistamine [From Greek *anti*, "opposite" + *histamine*.] An agent that reduces effects of an inflammatory chemical called histamine. Both histamines and antihistamines are naturally produced in your body, but you occasionally need a "boost" of an oral or injectable antihistamine. Antihistamines work by blocking or displacing histamine at its sites of action. See Histamine.

Apnea (AP'-nee-uh) [From Greek *a-*, "without" + *pnoia*, "breathing."] Temporary halt to breathing. Examples are voluntary breath holding while swimming underwater, controlling amount of breathing while singing or blowing up balloons, and involuntary lapses from sleep disorders involving snoring. See Sleep Apnea.

Apples and Pears Body-classification system to predict, in a very general way, a tendency toward cardiovascular risk and obesity-linked disease. People who store fat primarily in their upper body and abdomen have bodies that resemble an apple shape, while pear-shaped people store fat mostly around the hips and thighs. Apple shape is associated with higher disease risk than pear shape.

Arrhythmia [From Greek *a-*, "without" + *ruthmia*, "rhythm."] Irregular heartbeat. Arrhythmias occur normally now and then among normal heartbeats, without ill effect or you being aware of them. Too many arrhythmias, occurring too often, can be harmful.

Arteries Muscular, elastic, branching system of thick-walled tubes carrying blood away from your heart to your body. See Veins.

Arthritis [From Greek arthron, "joint," + itis, "inflammation."] Inflammation of a joint, or joints, with pain, swelling, loss of function, and sometimes deformity of the joint. Arthritis manifests in various forms. Degenerative, or osteoarthritis, involves wearing away the smooth cartilage on bone ends (articular cartilage). Osteoarthritis can be because of, or along with, trauma to the joint or habitual wear and tear from poor positioning habits. Other kinds of arthritis, like rheumatoid arthritis, are thought to be an autoimmune attack by the body against itself. Arthritis pain can be reduced with good exercise, sunlight, and changing body-movement habits to healthful positioning.

Atherosclerotic Plaques [From Greek *athero*, "gruel-like," + *sclerosis*, "hardening."] Irregular deposits of lipid in the lining of medium and large arteries. Associated with cardiovascular disease.

B

Ball-and-Socket Joint Type of joint, found in your shoulder and hip, allowing rotary motion in every direction. The ball is a rounded knob of one bone that fits into a cavity or socket of the other. Also called enarthrosis. See Acetabulum and Femoral Neck.

Body-Mass Index (BMI) Pen-and-paper test for obesity, obtained by taking your weight in kilograms divided by height in meters squared. If BMI is above 25, you are considered by this test to be fat. If over 30, you are considered obese.

Bone Semi-stiff connective tissue that holds up and gives form to soft, tissue. Bones in different parts of your body have varying amounts of a dense, compact, outer layer, called cortical bone, and an inner, loose, spongy trabecular bone. The central part of your long bones is filled with marrow. Bones are covered by the periosteum.

Your bones are not all hard, inorganic mineral. Bone is about 75 percent inorganic material and 25 percent organic material. The protein, or collagen, portion of bones gives them flexibility and resiliency. If you remove the calcium from a bone by soaking it in vinegar, the bone would become as flexible as a dog's rubber plaything. See Cortical Bone, Periosteum, and Trabecular Bone.

Bradycardia [From Greek *brady*, "slow" + *kardia*, "heart."] Slow heart rate in an adult human, usually fewer than 60 beats per minute.

Bronchi (BRON'-kai) [From Greek *bronkhos*, "windpipe."] Plural of bronchus. The two branches of your windpipe leading to your lungs.

Bursa [From Greek, "wineskin," "purse."] A little sac containing viscous lubricating fluid, located where a tendon passes over a bone, or at points of friction between moving body structures. You have over 70 bursas in various places in your body. Chronically irritating a bursa can result in inflammation, called bursitis. Shoulder bursitis can result from bad shoulder exercises. Knee bursitis can result from too much kneeling, what used to be called "housemaid's knee" Bursitis is becoming more common from exercises done kneeling instead of using stronger positions off the knees.

C

Cadaver Fat Analysis Body-fat-determination technique of cutting a body open to directly measure fat stores.

Calcium Balance Amount of body calcium gain versus loss. Positive calcium balance occurs when more calcium is absorbed from your diet than excreted. Excess calcium deposits in your skeleton. When loss exceeds absorption, calcium will mobilize (be taken) from your bone, a process called negative calcium balance.

Calipers [Alteration of caliber.] Small instrument used for measuring diameters. Calipers used for body-composition analysis measure the thickness of your folds of fat. Caliper measurement is painless, except by overenthusiastic testers. The error of measurement can often be large, varying greatly with tester experience. Calipers are often misused in health clubs. If, for example, you are measured at 25 percent the first time, and 22 percent the second time, it is incorrect to state that you lost 3 percent fat. Because of error of measurement, it is impossible to tell.

Carbohydrate [From Latin *carbon* + Greek *hudro*, "water," because they are made of carbon, hydrogen, and oxygen.] Organic compounds including sugar, starch, and cellulose. Found in nutritional quantities only in plants, they are a major energy source. Animals (including humans) store a carbohydrate called glycogen in their muscles and liver. See Glycogen.

Carbohydrate-Loader Drink Beverage containing carbohydrate, used to replace fluids and delay fatigue in long-endurance events. Commercial products containing refined sugar sources can be considered junk food, not health food. See Carbohydrate, Carbohydrate-Replacer Drink, and Electrolyte.

Carbohydrate-Replacer Drink High-carbohydrate drink, used both to replace fluids and restock your body's carbohydrate supply after long-endurance events. Commercial products containing refined sugar sources can be considered junk food, not health food. See Carbohydrate, Carbohydrate-Loader Drink, and Electrolyte.

Catecholamine (cat-eh-COAL'-uh-meen) [Named for its chemical structure derived from a catechol and an amine.] Important family of nervous-system chemicals that work as both neurotransmitters and hormones to transmit signals in your body. Some of your important catecholamines are dopamine, norepinephrine, and epinephrine. Your body makes them in sequential steps, starting with the amino acid tyrosine. Each step turns each catecholamine into the next. First, you make tyrosine into dopa. From dopa, you make dopamine. From dopamine, you make norepinephrine. From norepinephrine, you make epinephrine (same as adrenaline).

Cervical Vertebrae [From Latin *cervic*, "neck."] The seven bones of your neck. They are named sequentially down from your head as C1 through C7. If you feel the back of your neck, your most prominent bump is your C7 vertebra. Your other six cervical vertebrae are above it. Below C7 begin your 12 thoracic vertebrae, which are the bones of your upper back. See Lumbar Vertebrae, Thoracic Vertebrae, and Vertebra.

Cholesterol [From Greek *khole*, "bile" (because it was first found in gallstones) and the origin of words like gall and gold, + Greek *stereos*, "solid."] Made in your liver, cholesterol is an important constituent of all your cell membranes, and a precursor to steroid hormones. Cholesterol circulates in your blood plasma, carried around by proteins of various densities (lipoproteins). Cholesterol is the most abundant steroid in animal tissues, but not found at all in plants. See High-Density Lipoprotein Cholesterol and Low-Density Lipoprotein Cholesterol.

Claudication [From Latin *claudico*, "to limp."] Leg pain from clogged blood vessels in your legs.

Coca Leaves [Coca is Spanish, from the *Quechua kúka*.] Dried leaves of certain small shrubs or trees, genus *Erythroxylum*, especially E. coca. The leaves contain alkaloids and the raw materials that can be processed into cocaine, and are chewed for a stimulating effect by people of the Andes to help tolerate hunger, fatigue, and altitude, or harvested and purified for making cocaine. See Ergogenic Aid.

Coccyx (KOKS'-icks) [From Greek *kokkyx*, "cuckoo," from its resemblance to a cuckoo's beak.] Tail bone. Small, triangular bone at the end of the spine in human beings and tailless apes. Made of four fused rudimentary vertebrae. See Cervical Vertebrae, Lumbar Vertebrae, Thoracic Vertebrae, and Vertebra.

Coenzyme A body chemical that you need to enhance or promote action of an enzyme. Coenzymes are smaller than the enzymes they work with. Usually contains a vitamin or mineral combined with a specific protein. Sometimes, coenzymes are misrepresented as able to improve physical ability if taken orally, which is not the case. Like all proteins, they are broken down into component parts to digest and pass through your intestinal wall. They will not automatically reassemble into the original coenzyme on the other side. See Enzyme and Ergogenic Aid.

Cortical Bone [From Latin *cortex*, "bark."] Also called compact bone. Dense, strong bone forming the outside shell or wall of your long bones. When bone loss occurs with normal (and accelerated) aging processes, cortical bone loss occurs later than trabecular bone loss. See Bone, Periosteum, and Trabecular Bone.

Cramp [Possibly from Middle Dutch *crampe*, "hook," to restrict or prevent from free action or expression.] Sudden, involuntary, painful muscle spasm, or shortening. Stretching your muscle to lengthen it releases the cramp. Cramp releases on leg, foot, back, and side cramps can be easily done yourself, or by orthopedists, osteopaths, and trained massage therapists and physical therapists.

Creatine Phosphate (CP) [Named for its composition of creatine with phosphoric acid.] Organic compound in your muscles that stores and provides energy for muscular contraction. Breaking down creatine phosphate provides the phosphate you need to make ATP, the bottom-line energy molecule for all your body processes. Also called phosphocreatine. See Adenosine Triphosphate (ATP).

D

Disc [From Greek *diskos,* "to throw."] Round, flat, fibrocartilage cushion between certain bones. You have small discs between your jawbone (mandible) and your head bone (temporal bone). Sometimes, these discs wear out, causing pain at the joint between those two bones called the temporomandibular joint (TMJ), causing TMJ pain. Your vertebral discs lie between the bones of your spine (vertebrae). Vertebral discs are commonly injured over time by bad sitting, standing, and lifting postures, particularly discs of your lower back (lumbar vertebrae). You usually impose the greatest stresses on the lumbar vertebrae when lifting, sitting, and standing improperly. See Disc Herniation and Lumbar Vertebrae.

Disc Herniation Also referred to as slipped discs. Protrusion of a vertebral disc beyond its normal place. Can cause pain by itself, and also by pressing on nerves and other structures, which causes pain away from the site of herniation. Discs are pushed out of place over time by bad sitting, standing, and lifting habits, usually involving bad forward bending. Pain from slippage and herniation can usually be quickly stopped without surgery, by stopping bad forward bending, and instead using good bending, sitting, and exercise habits. Simply doing back exercises or taking pills or having surgery does not stop the source of the pain, and damage can continue.

Dorsiflex [From Latin *dorsum*, "back" + *flex*, "to bend."] Turning your hand or foot toward the upper side. To bend the ankle so your toes point backward toward the top of your foot. See Plantarflex.

Dowager's Hump Curved, hunched appearance of the upper back in both men and women, caused by osteoporotic crush fractures of the thoracic vertebrae (bones of the upper back). See Osteoporosis.

E

Electrolyte [From Greek *electro* + *lytos* and *lysis*, "soluble" or "loosening," the origin of such words as dialysis, electrolysis, and analysis.] Any substance that, when dissolved in a liquid, becomes electrically conductive because it breaks up into ions. Ions are atoms or molecules with at least one electron more or less than normal for it, giving it a negative or positive charge. For example, table salt (sodium chloride) breaks down in water into the positive sodium ion and the negative chloride ion. In physiology, the term electrolyte usually refers to the ions, rather than the original substance. Your cells use electrolytes to regulate processes, such as flow of water across your cell membranes. Ions propagate signals along nerves for all the thousands of functions that nerves control to keep you alive, moving, and thinking. Two of your principal positively charged ions (electrolytes) are sodium and potassium. Magnesium and calcium are also positive ions. Two important negatively charged ions are chloride and bicarbonate.

Electrolyte Drink Beverage containing electrolytes and, usually, carbohydrates to supply water, electrolytes, and carbohydrate before, during, or after exercise. Commercial products containing refined sugar sources can be considered junk food, not health food. Drinking sugar water is not a healthy habit in the long run.

Electron Transport Chain A sequence of reactions that are part of how you make ATP energy aerobically. Electrons from the Krebs cycle get transported to oxygen by small electron carriers. The electrons pass through a series of iron-containing proteins called cytochromes (close relatives of hemoglobin). Each player in the series is increasingly fond of electrons, so that the entire series runs "downhill," and energy is produced. Energy not used for chemical work dissipates as heat. The electron transport chain is also called the respiratory chain and the cytochrome system. See Adenosine Triphosphate (ATP) and Krebs Cycle.

Endorphin [Composite word from endogenous ("made from within") + "morphine-like substance."] A class of hormones produced by a number of processes, including extended, hard exercise. Not confirmed, but, along with other opioid chemicals produced in your body, associated with positive mood after good workouts.

Endurance, Cardiovascular [From Latin *indurare*, "to harden."] Ability of your heart and lungs to get oxygen and nutrients to your body for fuel during exercise. Determines how long you can go at a given pace. Needed for continuous, mid- and low-intensity walking, running, skiing, swimming, cycling, and so forth. Also called cardiorespiratory endurance, aerobic capacity, or functional capacity. See Aerobic Metabolism, Anaerobic Capacity, and Anaerobic Metabolism.

Endurance, Muscular [From Latin *indurare*, "to harden."] Ability of muscles to move a relatively light weight repeatedly. Walking, swimming, finning, cycling, running, and even sitting and standing up straight all day require muscular endurance.

Enzyme [From Greek *en-*, "in" + *zume*, "yeast," the origin of the word zymurgy, the branch of chemistry dealing with fermenting and brewing alcohol. From Greek zein, "to boil."] A protein that speeds up chemical reactions. Enzymes function by holding other molecules in just the right way so that they can put the molecules together or break them apart. Examples of enzymes that help break apart other molecules include lactase, which breaks down lactose in milk; amylase in your saliva, which starts breaking down carbohydrates you eat; papain, a plant enzyme used in meat tenderizer that breaks down meat protein; and zymase, the enzyme in yeast that breaks down sugar into alcohol and carbon dioxide. The various synthetase enzymes help put molecules together. With notable exceptions, names of most enzymes end in the suffix "-ase." All enzymes are proteins. Enzymes that you eat are destroyed by digestion before they can pass into your bloodstream and reach your body tissues. Digesting means breaking down to components small enough to pass through your intestinal wall. It will not automatically reassemble into the original enzyme on the other side of your intestinal wall. Eating enzymes, promoted as health foods (except digestive aids), will not raise your body's enzyme levels. See Coenzyme.

Ergogenic Aid [From Greek *ergon*, "work" + *gen*, "producing" or "generating"]. Products that enhance physical ability. Ergogenic aids may be nutritional, psychological, or physical. Not everything claimed to be ergogenic is ergogenic. Many sham products can be found on the market. Not all products sold as dietary and ergogenic aids are completely healthful or non-habit-forming, such as the several stimulant herbs on the market, or products containing caffeine. See Amphetamines, Anabolic Steroids, Coenzyme, Ginseng, Ma Huang, Minerals, and Vitamins.

Extension Increasing the angle of a joint. Elbow extension is when you straighten a bent arm. Knee extension is straightening your knee. Neck and back extension involve moving your head or torso, respectively, away from a bent-forward position. Hyperextension is extending your joint past a straight line, or 180 degrees. See Flexion.

F

Facets, Vertebral [From Old French *facette*, "little face."] Small, smooth areas on your spine bones (vertebrae), where one vertebra fits together with the next. If injured over time with bad back posture, can be a cause of back pain. Usually associated with chronic, excessive, arching postures.

Fat A greasy substance found in adipose tissue of animals, and in seeds and nuts. In animals, fat is the principle storage form for energy. As a food, fat gives you 9 calories per gram. Carbohydrate and protein, by comparison, give you 4 calories per gram. See Carbohydrate and Protein.

Femoral Neck Slender part of your upper thigh bone (femur) near your hip between the long bone of your femur with the "ball" part of your femur (the femoral head). Your femoral head fits into the "socket" of your hip, called the acetabulum. The femoral neck is a common site of osteoporotic fracture. See Acetabulum, Ball and Socket Joint, Femur.

Femur [From Latin for "thigh."] Thigh bone (upper leg bone) between your hip and knee. It is the largest and strongest bone in your body.

Flexibility [From Latin *flexibilis*, "to bend."] Ability to move safely and comfortably through a range of motion to do the things you want to do.

Flexion [From Latin *flectere*, "to bend."] Decreasing the angle of a joint. Elbow flexion, for example, is bending your elbow. Knee flexion is bending your knee. (Genu is the Latin word for "knee," as in the word genuflection, also meaning, "knee bending.") Neck and back flexion involve curling your head or torso, respectively, toward a bent-forward position. Too much flexion in your lower back, usually from poor posture when sitting and bad bending habits, contributes to disc degeneration and herniation, and back pain. See Extension.

Folic Acid [From Latin *folium*, "leaf," for its common occurrence in leafy vegetables.] Substance from the Vitamin B complex group, occurring in green plants, fresh fruit, and yeast. Also called folacin, folate, and Vitamin Bc. Deficiency of folic acid is known to be associated with birth defects, and more recently with heart disease and stroke. Eating more green, leafy vegetables adds folic acid to your diet.

Food Pyramid Any of the several schematics of various food groups and relative amounts considered right or adequate for nutritional health. The various food pyramids replace the previous "four food groups." Fruit and vegetables form the large, solid base of the newer pyramids. Middle groups of protein include beans, grain, and nuts. Small sugar and fat group at the top point, indicates to eat only a small amount of them. Food pyramid recommendations stress vegetables as main dishes, with meat as side dishes if you eat meat—not the other way around.

Four Food Groups An obsolete system of grouping foods into four categories to be eaten at every meal. It was found that diets based on the four categories were high fat, stressed too much meat and dairy, and had only about half of the minimum daily-required amounts of needed nutrients.

Free Radical An atom, molecule, or macromolecule existing temporarily with at least one unpaired electron. Electrons usually prefer to be paired. Being unpaired makes them reactive and eager either to acquire another electron or to lose the unpaired one. Some free radicals are beneficial, such as those involved in muscle contraction and in your immune response, while others are involved in disease processes. Free radicals occur normally as a by-product of breathing, and in increased numbers during exercise, in smog, from cigarette smoke, and in high-pressure oxygen environments. In 1954, Rebecca Gershman and her colleagues, in a theory now widely accepted, proposed that the damaging effects of oxygen toxicity are caused by oxygen free radicals. Because it has one unpaired electron, oxygen free radicals strongly want to take an electron from other molecules, particularly from your fatty acids and proteins. When oxygen free radicals grab electrons from your hemoglobin, cell membranes, or protein enzymes, they can't do their jobs, and become free radicals themselves, going on to grab electrons from others, in a destructive game of tag. Your body produces various antioxidant substances to neutralize many free radicals.

G

Gastrocnemius [From Greek *gastro*, "belly," referring to the largest part of a muscle + *kneme*, "leg."] Large, prominent muscle of the calf of your leg. Attaches to your Achilles tendon and pulls on the tendon to pull your foot downward (plantarflex).

Ginseng [From Mandarin Chinese *ren*, "person" + *shen*, collective name of a variety of herbs with fat, fleshy roots sometimes resembling the form or outline of the human body.] Any of several plants, or roots of plants, of genus *Panax*, particularly *P. pseudoginseng*, of eastern Asia, or *P. quinquefolius* of North America. Stimulates your nervous system, raising your heart rate and blood pressure. See Ergogenic Aid.

Glycogen [From Greek glukos, "sweet" + gen, "making" or "producing."] The form in which glucose (sugar) is stored in your body, mostly in your liver and muscles. Glycogen is converted to glucose through a series of enzymatic steps to meet your body's rapid energy needs. See Glycolysis.

Glycogen Loading An exercise and diet procedure to increase the amount of glycogen you can store. Greater stores of glycogen extend your exercise capacity.

Glycogen Sparing Body process of using more fat as an exercise fuel, and less glycogen, and so "sparing" your glycogen. Glycogen sparing allows more time until your glycogen stores are exhausted, allowing you to exercise longer. Being in better shape "teaches" your body better glycogen sparing.

Glycolysis [From Greek *glukos*, "sweet" + *lysis*, "breaking down" or "loosening," seen in such words as dialysis, electrolysis, and analysis.] Metabolic process of breaking down carbohydrates and sugars, typically glucose, to generate ATP, your "bottom-line" energy molecule. Occurs in almost all living cells. In humans, the last product generated by glycolysis while making ATP aerobically is pyruvic acid (aerobic glycolysis). When you are anaerobic, the process goes one more step to lactic acid (anaerobic glycolysis). When you have enough oxygen, lactic acid can be changed back to pyruvic acid. This series of reactions was described by Gustav Embden and Otto Meyerhof in the 1930s, and so it is sometimes called the Embden-Meyerhof cycle. Glycolysis can make only two molecules of ATP from a molecule of glucose, while your aerobic metabolism can make 36. Being aerobic makes more energy, which is why your aerobic system lets you exercise longer than your anaerobic system. See Adenosine Triphosphate (ATP), Glycogen, Lactic Acid, and Pyruvic Acid.

H

Hamstring Muscles Triple set of muscles on the back of your upper leg. Your hamstring muscles work to bend your knee and straighten your hip. Your two innermost hamstrings, or medial hamstrings, are the semimembranosus and semitendinosus muscles. Your outside, or lateral, hamstring is the biceps femoris muscle. The term hamstrings is also used to refer to the tendons of the three muscles, readily felt as stringy cords on either side of the hollow of the back of your knee.

Hemochromatosis [Greek *haima*, "blood" + *khroma*, "color" + *osis*, "condition."] A hereditary disorder of iron metabolism, where you absorb and keep too much of the iron you eat. Iron deposits in the tissues, particularly the liver, pancreas, and skin, where it causes a bronze coloration and constant fatigue. Eventually, heart and liver failure may occur.

High-Density Lipoprotein Cholesterol Popularly called "good cholesterol." Compound containing lipid (fat) and protein. HDL removes cholesterol from your bloodstream, and does not collect on or stick to the inner linings of your arteries. You can increase your levels of HDL with exercise and healthy meals. See Cholesterol and Low-Density Lipoprotein Cholesterol.

Hip Flexors Muscles that bend (flex) your hip into a sitting position. Many people confuse hip-flexor exercises that bend the hip, like sit-ups and leg lifts, for abdominal exercises that, when functionally done, would involve holding your spine in neutral position. Three major hip flexors are the iliacus, psoas (SEW'-as), and rectus femoris. The iliacus and psoas, often lumped together as the iliopsoas, are your "filet mignon" muscles. Cattle raised for the mass production of beef are prevented from exercising so that their hip flexor muscles become soft and fatty for humans to eat. Tight hip-flexor muscles in humans contribute to poor bent-forward posture, lower-back pain from the resulting overarch when the hip is tilted forward by tightness, and (surprisingly) shoulder injuries when your shoulder has to overrotate to reach overhead because tight hip flexors do not allow your torso to straighten fully. Standing with your body bent forward at the crease where the leg meets the body is often from tight hip flexors. Being unable to lie flat face up or down without lower-back pain is often from the tight flexors that do not allow fully straightening at the hip and instead overarch the lower back.

Histamine [Named because it is an amine derived from histidine, and so hist (idine) + amine.] An amine released from cells of your immune system as part of an allergic reaction. Histamine powerfully stimulates gastric secretions, constricts bronchial smooth muscle that restricts breathing, and dilates small blood vessels. Sometimes, this dilation is extensive enough to cause a drop in blood pressure. See Antihistamine.

Homeostasis [From Greek *homos*, "same" + *stasis*, "standstill."] Continuous regulation of all your body's goings-on, using physiologic checks and balances to maintain your system at its set equilibrium. Body temperature, oxygen levels, pH, water balance, plasma ion regulation, calorie utilization, and many other processes are all tightly regulated. The principle was first described by French physiologist Claude Bernard, and later given its name by Walter Cannon, a Harvard physiologist.

Homeotherm (HOME'-ee-oh-thurm) [From Greek *homos*, "same" + *therme*, "heat."] Animals who generate and regulate heat internally to maintain a largely constant body temperature that is independent of, and typically above, surrounding temperature. Birds and mammals are homeotherms. Sometimes called endotherms. See Poikilotherm.

Hormone [From Greek *horman*, "to urge on."] Chemical messengers, usually peptides or steroids, produced in one body tissue and traveling through your blood to stimulate or suppress activity in another tissue. Examples, among many, are insulin, adrenaline (epinephrine), and antidiuretic hormone (ADH). Hormones regulate body processes as diverse as growth, metabolism, and reproduction, and they can modify behavior.

Hydrostatic Weighing Also called underwater weighing. Body composition analysis technique to determine body fat, called the "gold standard" because it has a low error of measurement, and other tests of body composition are often compared in percentage error to hydrostatic weighing. To be weighed hydrostatically, you sit on a scale in a vat of water, and then exhale all you can while keeping your entire body underwater.

Hypertonic [Prefix *hyper-*, "more" or "above" + Greek *tonos*, "tension."] In chemistry, a solution containing a higher concentration of dissolved particles compared to a reference solution, usually blood or body tissues. For example, seawater is hypertonic to your blood (about three times more concentrated, contrary to popular belief that they are similar). See Hypotonic and Isotonic.

Hypotonic [Prefix *hypo-*, "less," or "under" + Greek *tonos*, "tension."] In chemistry, a solution containing a smaller concentration of dissolved particles compared to a reference solution, usually blood or body tissues. For example, fresh water is hypotonic to your blood. See Hypertonic and Isotonic.

Hypovolemic Thirst. One of your two thirst mechanisms. Stimulated by low body-water stores. See Osmotic Thirst.

Hypoxia [Prefix *hypo-* + *oxa*, "oxygen."] Condition in which insufficient oxygen reaches body tissues. Distinct from (but usually related to) hypoxemia, which is insufficient oxygenation of blood.

I

Ilium [From Latin *ilium*, "groin" or "flank."] Widest and uppermost of three bones that make up each side of your pelvis. The ilium on each side of your hips can be felt as the "shelf" that you can rest a bundle on. See Ischium and Pubis (your other two pelvic bones).

Inflammation [From Latin, *in* + *flammare*, "to set on fire."] Response of body tissues to an injury, bite, sting, or infection. Characterized by warmth (calor), redness (rubor), swelling (tumor), and pain (dolor). Inflammation attracts immune cells, which secrete free radicals to kill bacteria and other invaders. Most back and neck pain is not inflammatory in nature, which is why taking anti-inflammatory medicines is not a helpful or healthful course of treatment. See Free Radical.

Insensible Perspiration Sweat that evaporates before you are aware of it. The term sometimes includes evaporation from your respiratory tract.

Insulinogenic [Insulin + Greek *gen*, "producing."] Substance that encourages insulin production. Sometimes, carbohydrate products are misrepresented in health-food stores as special foods that stimulate insulin. Because one function of insulin is to encourage protein storage, advertisers lead people to believe that eating such food will build muscle. But just about any food is insulinogenic, and another function of insulin is to aid fat storage. Conversely, a popular high-protein diet promotes the idea that you must avoid non-protein foods because they stimulate insulin, leading to more fat storage, and eat only high-protein foods. It also seems to be misleading (and potentially unhealthy). High-protein diets "work" because they are low-calorie, not for any insulin-stimulating or suppressing quality.

Insurance Tables Predetermined values in insurance-company tables of ranges of "acceptable" weights for various heights and frame sizes. Usually, if you are more than 20 percent over this weight range, you are considered by the particular tables to be obese. Sometimes used to determine approximate risk of some cardiovascular diseases, and thus eligibility for certain kinds of insurance.

Ischemia (is-KEE'-me-uh) [From Greek *iskhein*, "to hold back" + *haima*, "blood." Haima is the origin of words like hemoglobin, hemorrhage, and hemorrhoid.] Decrease in blood supply to your cells due to constriction or obstruction of your blood vessels, for example, during heart attack or muscle spasm. Pain and loss of function follows ischemia.

Ischial Tuberosity [From Greek *iskhion*, "hip."] "Sit bones." Protuberance at the base of your lower-hip (ischial) bones, where muscles—notably your hamstrings—attach. You can feel your ischial tuberosities as the bumps of bone that you sit on. The ischium is the lowest of the three bones that, together, make up each half of your pelvis. The other bones are the pubic bones, which fuse in front to become your anterior hip bone, and the ilium, whose crests on either side of your hip you can feel as the two "shelves" that you can rest a package upon.

Ischium [From Greek *iskhion*, "hip joint."] The lowest of the three bones that make up each half of your pelvis. At the bottom of each ischium is a bump, called the ischial tuberosity. These bones are the bony bumps you sit on. See Hamstring Muscles, Ilium, Ischial Tuberosity, and Pubis.

Isotonic [From Greek *isos*, "equal" + *tonos*, "tension."] In chemistry, a solution containing the same total concentration of dissolved particles as a reference solution, usually your blood or body tissues. For example, many commercial electrolyte sports drinks are isotonic to your blood. A popular myth is that your blood is isotonic to seawater. However, it is much less concentrated, or hypotonic.

Even many sea creatures have different tonicities than the sea—some higher and some lower.

J

Jiggle Test An informal test of body composition to see general lack of tone from insufficient muscle and excess fat. See Apples and Pears, Body-Mass Index, Calipers, and Hydrostatic Weighing.

K

Krebs Cycle [Named for Sir Hans Adolf Krebs, who won the Nobel Prize in 1953 for this important discovery.] A cyclic series of reactions that are part of how you use oxygen to make the energy-yielding molecule ATP. It is a cycle, as the last step in the chain of reactions is making the chemical you started with (citric acid). Each of the steps in the cycle needs a specific enzyme. Electrons removed during the Krebs cycle enter your second major aerobic pathway to make ATP energy, called the electron-transport chain. The Krebs cycle is also called the citric-acid cycle or tricarboxylic-acid cycle (TCA). See Adenosine Triphosphate (ATP), Aerobic Metabolism, and Electron Transport Chain.

L

Lactic Acid or Lactate [From Latin *lact,* "milk," named because bacteria in milk produce it from the milk sugar lactose in the process of making their energy. They excrete the lactic acid into the milk, which sours it.] Molecule formed by metabolizing glucose for energy, when not enough oxygen is present (anaerobic metabolism). Lactic acid is associated with the burning feeling of muscles that occurs during anaerobic metabolism. Lactic acid has good functions, such as serving as a fuel for the heart. When enough oxygen is present, lactic acid changes back to pyruvic acid, which can be used in aerobic metabolism. See Adenosine Triphosphate (ATP), Anaerobic Capacity, Anaerobic Metabolism, Glycolysis, and Pyruvic Acid.

Ligament [From Latin *ligare,* "to bind."] Tough, fibrous bands connecting bones to each other, connecting cartilage at a joint, or supporting an organ.

Low-Density Lipoprotein Cholesterol Popularly called "bad cholesterol." Compound containing lipid (fat) and protein. Dietary cholesterol and cholesterol made in your liver are transported to your blood vessels and muscles by LDL. Too much LDL can be a risk factor for cardiovascular disease. See Cholesterol and High-Density Lipoprotein Cholesterol.

Lumbar Vertebrae or Lumbar Spine [From Latin *lumbus*, "loin."] Five spinal bones of your lower back. They are named, from top to bottom, L1 through L5. The intervertebral discs most often involved in lower-back pain are between L4 and L5 and particularly between L5 and S1. S1 is your first sacral vertebra. Degeneration and herniation is most common from bad sitting and bending habits, not aging or disease. See Cervical Vertebrae, Disc, Sacrum, and Thoracic Vertebrae.

M

Ma Huang [From Mandarin Chinese *ma*, "hemp" + *huang*, "yellow."] Asian plants of the genus Ephedra, particularly E. sinica, which contains the stimulant ephedrine. Ma huang is often sold in health-food and Eastern-medicine stores in various drinks and pills for its stimulant effects on your nervous system, heart, and blood vessels. It can be dangerous in high amounts and when mixed with various common drugs and medicines, other stimulant drinks, and alcohol. See Ergogenic Aid and Sympathomimetic.

Meniscus [From Greek *meniskos*, diminutive of *mene*, "moon," for its shape.] In anatomy, menisci are flat cartilaginous discs that act as cushions between the ends of your knee bones. In each knee, you have two menisci, side-by-side between your upper leg bone (femur) and lower leg bone (tibia). The meniscus on the inner side of each knee is your medial meniscus. The one on the outer side is your lateral meniscus. Menisci can be torn by twisting your knee, and worn out by poor leg postures when walking. See Disc.

Menopause [From Greek *meno*, "month" + Greek *pausis*, "cessation."] Phase of life after menstrual and reproductive functions. Twenty-five percent of American women reach menopause by age 47, half by 50, three quarters by 52, and 95 percent by age 55. Menopause, particularly surgically caused, is a risk factor for osteoporosis. A physical corollary occurs in men, where hormonal functions taper and bone loss accelerates, among other effects.

Metabolism [From Greek *metaballein*, "to change."] The total of all physical and chemical processes in cells and living systems as a whole, necessary for energy synthesis to maintain life.

Minerals [From Latin *mineralis*, pertaining to mines and mining.] Dietary minerals are inorganic elements essential to the health of humans, animals, and plants. Examples include iron, calcium, potassium, sodium, and zinc.

Mole [From German *mol*, short for *Molekulargewicht*, "molecular weight."] A unit of measure to manage large numbers of atoms, molecules, ions, and so forth. One mole is 6.0225×10^{23}, or Avogadro's number. Also called gram molecule.

Muscle Spindles [Named for their thin, spindle-like shape.] Small, thin, sensory organs in your muscles (and the muscles of all vertebrates). Muscle spindles are sensitive to the stretch of the muscle they are in. Also called neuromuscular spindle, stretch receptor, and Kühne's spindle. Named for Wilhelm (Willy) F. Kühne, German physiologist and histologist (1837–1900) who first identified them. See Myotatic Reflex and Proprioceptors.

Myotatic Reflex [From Greek *myo*, "muscle" + *tasis*, "a stretching."] Quick muscle contraction in response to a sudden stretching force on your muscle. Initiated by stimulation of muscle proprioceptors called spindles—stretch receptors in your muscles. Also called the Liddell-Sherrington reflex, the muscular reflex, and the stretch reflex. See Muscle Spindles and Proprioceptors.

N

Neurotransmitter [Neuro is from the Greek *sinew*, meaning "string" or "nerve" + "transmitter."] Group of chemicals your body produces to send nerve impulses from one nerve ending to the next, across a tiny space called a synapse. Examples of neurotransmitters, among many, are acetylcholine, serotonin, and catecholamines, such as dopamine, norepinephrine, and epinephrine.

O

Ondine's Curse (or Undine's Curse) Literary term from Greek mythology for sleep apnea. Ondine (or Undine) was a water spirit who cursed a deserving villain with being able to breathe only voluntarily. When he fell asleep, he stopped breathing, and suffocated. See Sleep Apnea.

Oophorectomy (oo-for-EK'-tuh-mee) [From Greek *oon*, "egg," + *phoros*, "bearing," + *ectom*, "excising" or "removing."] Surgical removal of the female gonads, the ovaries. Sometimes done in conjunction with hysterectomy—removal of the uterus. Equivalent in hormonal effect to male castration. A risk factor for osteoporosis and various serious health problems.

Osmotic Thirst One of your two thirst mechanisms. Stimulated by high blood-electrolyte content, regardless of your body's total water volume. It is why salty things make you thirsty, even when you are drinking (and why bars serve salty food). Drinking ethanol-containing fluids also makes you thirsty because ethanol increases urination and water loss by suppressing the hormone ADH. See Antidiuretic Hormone and Hypovolemic Thirst.

Osteomalacia [From Greek *osteon*, "bone" + *malakia*, "softness."] Gradual softening and bending of bone, usually from Vitamin-D deficiency. Associated with varying amounts of pain.

Osteopenia [From Greek, *osteon*, "bone" + *penia*, "poverty."] Any decrease in bone mass below normal. Among the causes are osteomalacia and osteoporosis.

Osteoporosis (ah-stee-oh-pore-OH'-sis) [From Greek *osteon*, "bone" + *poros*, "passage," *"pore"* + *osis*, "a condition," from the Greek word for "suffering."] Decreased bone mass leading to porous and fragile bones that fracture easily. High-risk sites are your upper back, hip, and wrist. Healing is difficult and slow. Occurs mainly in postmenopausal women and elderly men, and from certain medicines. Prevention includes getting adequate sunlight, avoiding unnecessary medicines, weight lifting, and resisting your own body weight during walking, dancing, tumbling, running, skating, and skiing.

Overload Principle Term to describe the need for higher-than-accustomed loads to improve exercise capacity. The type of overload required is specific to the system; for example, to increase strength, you need to lift heavier weights (your muscles must contract at tensions close to their maximum). To increase endurance, you need to cover longer distances. To increase your flexibility, you need to regularly take your joints through greater ranges of motion.

Oxygen Debt A term used as if synonymous with oxygen deficit. Refers to the extra oxygen you use during recovery from exercise to "repay" the oxygen needed but not available at the time of high intensity exercise (breathing hard). When energy stores decrease and lactic acid builds during your "debt" phase, you have to slow or stop exercise, and gasp for more oxygen while your limbs burn with lactic acid. The oxygen you take in during your "debt-paying" phase is used to make energy and remove lactic acid. See Anaerobic Capacity and Lactic Acid.

P

Parasympathetic Nervous System Part of your autonomic nervous system. Works to decrease heart rate, decrease blood pressure, dilate blood vessels, and stimulate digestive secretions. Inhibits or opposes your sympathetic nervous system. Your parasympathetic nervous system nerves originate in your brain stem and the lower part of your spinal cord. See Sympathetic Nervous System.

Perfusion [From Latin *perfundere*, "to pour."] Blood flow.

Periosteum (per-ee-OSS'-tee-um) [From Greek *peri*, "around" + *osteon*, "bone."] Membrane that covers your bones except at your bone ends. At bone ends, you have cartilage called articular cartilage. The periosteum is an attachment for your muscles and tendons. In young bones, the periosteum has two layers—the inner layer makes new bone tissue, and the outer layer is the tough, fibrous connective-tissue layer that conveys blood vessels and nerves supplying your bones. As you get older, your inner, bone-producing (osteogenic) layer gets thinner. See Bone, Cortical Bone, and Trabecular Bone.

Physiology [From Greek *phusis*, "nature" + *ology*, "study."] Study of the functions of living beings and their parts.

Pickwickian Syndrome Informal, literary name for sleep apnea in obese people, named after the "fat boy" in Dickens' The Pickwick Papers, who was obese with daytime sluggishness. See Sleep Apnea.

Plantarflex [From Latin *plantaris*, from *planta*, "sole of your foot."] To bend your ankle so that your foot points toward your sole, or bottom. See Dorsiflex.

Plasma [From Greek *plassein*, "to mold."] Clear, yellowish, non-cellular, fluid part of blood. Makes up about 55 percent of blood volume. Plasma without the clotting protein fibrinogen is called serum.

Poikilotherm (POY'-kill-oh-thurm) [From Greek poikilos, "various" + therme, "heat."] Animals, such as fish and reptiles, whose body temperature varies depending on surrounding temperature. Sometimes called ectotherms. See Homeotherm.

Postmenopausal After menopause. A woman is considered postmenopausal when she has had no menses for one year. See Menopause.

Power [From Latin *potere*, "to be able."] In exercise physiology, power is a measure of how fast you can be strong. Exercise power is the combination of speed and strength. Someone who can lift a weight in two seconds has twice the power of someone who needs four seconds to move that same weight.

Premenopausal Before menopause. See Menopause.

Prime Mover Muscle or muscles mainly responsible for a particular movement.

Proprioceptors [From Latin *proprius*, "one's own" or "self," + *ceptors*, "receiving information."] Sensory receptors in muscles, tendons, joints, and your inner ear. Proprioceptors detect changes in your position or movement. Your most abundant proprioceptors are your muscle spindles, which notice stretch in your muscles. When suddenly stretched, or stretched too far, your spindles send a signal that stimulates another signal that comes back to tell your muscle to contract. Proprioceptors help you keep your balance, and prevent muscle tears from too much stretch. Also called mechanoreceptors. See Myotatic Reflex.

Protein [From Greek *pratos*, "first."] Large, complex, organic molecules of one or more chains of amino acids. Proteins are fundamental components of all living cells, and necessary for proper functioning. Proteins contain carbon, hydrogen, oxygen, nitrogen, and usually sulfur. Many important body components are proteins, such as enzymes, hormones, and antibodies.

Pubis or Pubic Bone [From Latin *pubes*, "groin."] The front, lower part of your hipbones that form the front arch of your pelvis. Your left and right pubic bones come together in front at your pubic symphysis. The pubic bone is distinct at birth and later fuses together with your other two hipbones, the ilium and ischium. See Ilium and Ischium.

Pyruvic Acid or Pyruvate [From Greek *pyr(o)*, for "fire," "heat," or "derived from acid" + Latin *uva*, "grape" (from being produced by the dry distillation of racemic acid, originally derived from grapes).] Molecule produced from breaking down glucose to make energy (glycolysis). When enough oxygen is present for the intensity of exercise (aerobic glycolysis), pyruvate can change into another substance called acetyl CoA, which feeds into your aerobic metabolism where you can make much more energy. When enough oxygen is not present (during anaerobic glycolysis), pyruvate turns to lactate (or lactic acid). In this case, energy is limited, and the lactate building in your working muscles causes a burning feeling. See Aerobic Metabolism, Glycolysis, and Lactic Acid.

Q

Q_{10} Effect The enzyme reactions in your cells that produce energy and control body functions speed up as your body temperature rises. A 10-degree C rise would double the rate of enzyme reactions. This is called the Q_{10} Effect. Your internal temperature could never change 10 degrees without severe health consequences, but the two to four degrees that a warm-up raises your temperature uses the Q_{10} Effect to boost athletic performance, make stretching safer, and soothe arthritic joints.

S

Sacrum [From Latin *sacrum*, "sacred" (bone).] Broad, slightly curved, triangular bone forming the back wall of your pelvis. Made of five fused vertebrae. The sacrum joins your lowest lumbar vertebra from above, your coccyx below, and your hip bones on either side.

Scoliosis [Greek *skolios*, "crooked" + the suffix *-osis*, "a condition."] Sideways curving or twisting of the spine. Scoliosis may involve one or more curves, and may be due to muscle and/or bone deformity, or chronic unequal muscle contractions. Associated pain can often be reduced with good back exercises.

Sleep Apnea Sleep disorder involving snoring, where the snorer stops breathing during sleep because of upper airway obstruction, causing repeated shortages of oxygen to the brain. Sleep apnea sufferers are often overweight, heavy-necked males, but heavy females are also affected. Sleep apnea raises the incidence of stroke and cardiac irregularities. The repeated awakenings from the apnea, sometimes hundreds per night, result in chronic daytime sleepiness. This sleepiness is documented to greatly raise the risk of serious automobile accidents. Sleep apnea can be stopped, but not cured, using high-pressure air that opens airways, delivered by a facemask worn during sleep. The machine is called a Continuous Positive Air Pressure (CPAP) machine. For long-term treatment, losing weight is often effective.

Somatotyping Body classification system according to three characteristics—thinness (ectomorphy), fatness (endomorphy), and muscularity (mesomorphy). Nobody is only one type, but a combination of them, usually with one or two predominating.

Spondylolisthesis (spon-di-lo-lis-THEE'-sis) [From Greek *spondylo* + *olisthsis*, "slipping and falling."] Slipping, resulting in abnormal forward movement, of one of the vertebrae on the vertebra below it from overarching the lower spine. Sometimes associated with lower-back pain. Holding neutral spine relieves symptoms in many cases.

Spot Reducing Any method thought to remove fat only from specific body areas. Although many products and potions on the market promise spot reduction of body fat, only liposuction or other medical procedures removes deposits at specific locations.

Sprain Partial or complete tear of a ligament, from stretching past its limit of range. Usually painful.

Strain [From Latin *stringere*, "to extend" (and possibly the origin of the word perestroika.] To injure a muscle, sometimes from overuse, sometimes from stretching past its limits, or for long periods in bad posture.

Strength [From Old English *strang*, "strong."] Ability to move a heavy weight one or few times.

Stroke Volume Amount of blood ejected from your heart with each beat. Stroke volume (SV) times heart rate is cardiac output, or SV x HR = Q. If stroke volume increases with increased venous return, as with immersion or lying down, heart rate decreases to keep cardiac output constant.

Swimmer's Ear Painful infection or inflammation of your outer ear, which is the part you can see (the auricle) and stick your finger into (the canal). Cotton swabs and scratching your canal contribute to swimmer's ear by removing protective cerumen (ear wax). Earplugs rarely keep water out, and often create conditions good for swimmer's ear by rubbing away wax and holding water in your canal. Swimmer's ear usually is easily prevented and treated with white vinegar or Otic Domeboro drops. Swimmer's ear is not related to middle-ear or inner-ear injuries caused by pressure, or to congestion of your middle ear, so decongestants do not help. Swimmer's ear does not automatically require stopping swimming or diving, just drying your ears afterward. Serious and recurring cases need medical intervention.

Sympathetic Nervous System [From Greek *sympatheo*, "to feel with."] Part of your autonomic nervous system. Works to increase heart rate and blood vessel constriction, and reduce digestive secretions. Opposes and balances your parasympathetic nervous system. Your sympathetic nervous system nerves originate in the thoracic and lumbar regions of your spinal cord. See Parasympathetic Nervous System and Sympathomimetic.

Sympathomimetic (sim-path-oh-my-MET'-ik) [From *sympatho*, for the sympathetic nervous system + *mimikos*, "imitating."] A substance that mimics the action of your sympathetic nervous system by releasing nerve transmitter chemicals called catecholamines (especially epinephrine and norepinephrine) from nerve endings. Commonly known sympathomimetic substances are amphetamines, ephedrine (found in "health-food" stimulants and certain allergy medicines), phenylephrine (powerful vasoconstrictor used in preparations to relieve nasal congestion and maintain blood pressure during anesthesia), and phenylpropanolamine (used as a nasal decongestant, a bronchodilator, and appetite suppressant). The term adrenomimetic has been proposed to replace the term sympathomimetic, which some feel to be less accurate. Adrenomimetic (add-REE'-no-my-MET'-ik) means having an action similar to that of your body chemicals epinephrine and norepinephrine. In general, the term sympathomimetic is used rather loosely, but should be used only when discussing drugs that actually produce effects that mimic activation of your entire sympathetic system, not just central nervous system stimulation. Not everything that is a central-nervous-system stimulant is sympathomimetic (for example, caffeine, nicotine, strychnine, and picrotoxin). Strychnine and picrotoxin are such strong central nervous system stimulants that they are considered convulsants. See Amphetamines, Ergogenic Aid, Ma Huang, and Sympathetic Nervous System.

T

Tendon [From Latin *tendere*, "to stretch." This derivation is interesting, as tendons don't stretch greatly except with injury.] Tough, fibrous, inelastic modification of the ends of muscle, which connect your muscles to your bones.

Thoracic Vertebrae [From Latin *thorax*, "breastplate" or "chest."] Twelve upper-back bones, named T1 through T12, from upper to lower. A pair of ribs attaches to each thoracic vertebra, 12 pairs of ribs in all. Both men and women have 12 paired ribs, 24 total. Men do not have one less rib.

Trabecular Bone (tra-BECK'-you-lar) [From Latin, diminutive of *trabs*, "beam."] Spongy, branching, supporting meshwork of bone found mostly in your vertebrae and the ends of long bones. Decreased density first occurs in trabecular bone.

U

Undine's Curse Alternate spelling for Ondine's Curse. See Ondine's Curse and Sleep Apnea.

V

Vasoconstriction [From Latin *vas*, "vessel" + Latin *constrict*, "to compress."] Decrease in diameter of blood vessels, usually arterioles.

Vasodilation [From Latin *vas*, "vessel" + Latin *dilatare*, "to enlarge."] Increase in diameter of blood vessels, usually arterioles.

Veins Membranous Branching system of thin-walled tubes that carry blood from all areas of your body back to your heart for transport to your lungs. See Arteries.

Vertebra (plural: vertebrae) [From Latin *verto*, "to turn."] Spine bone. Humans usually have 33 vertebrae—seven cervical (C1 to C7), 12 thoracic (T1 to T12), five lumbar (L1 to L5), five sacral (fused into one bone, your sacrum), and four coccygeal (fused into one bone, your coccyx). Each vertebra bears the weight of all your body above it.

Vitamins [From Latin *vita*, "life" + *amine*, so called because they were originally thought to be amines.] Any of various organic substances essential for normal growth and activity. Deficiencies may cause various diseases and problems, but taking more than a needed amount has not been shown to have beneficial effects. It is often difficult to determine a "needed amount," making the topic difficult to study.

VO_{2max} (pronounced vee-oh-tu-max) VO_2 is how much oxygen you consume. Max VO_2 is the maximum amount of oxygen your system can extract and use to do exercise.

W

Waist-to-Hip Ratio A simple, general test of physical status. Take your waist and hip measurements. Divide your waist by your hip measurement. For health, stay below 0.8 for women and 1.0 for men.

Warm-Up Raising body temperature until it is more energy efficient, and safer for your joints and cardiovascular health to exercise. Although often thought to be only accomplished with slow, gradual increase in physical activity of your large limbs, as with walking, cycling, and slow jogging, warming can quickly be achieved with a dozen or so push-ups and lunges. Can also be assisted by passive heating with hot baths and local heat packs.

Weight-Bearing Activity Exercise where body weight provides the resistance, as in walking, running, dancing, skiing, skating, and hiking. Regular weight-bearing exercise is known to increase bone density and reduce risk of osteoporosis in your hip and back. You need to add weight lifting (or push-ups) to increase bone density at the third site that is also at risk for osteoporosis, your wrist.

Weight-Loading Activity Exercise where external weight provides the resistance, as in weight lifting and carrying packages. Regular weight loading is known to increase bone density and reduce risk of osteoporosis.

About the Author

Dr. Jolie Bookspan is a sports medicine specialist and physiologist known around the world for innovative research to make medicine, fitness, and injury rehabilitation healthier. As a researcher for university and military aerospace, warfare, and medicine divisions, she studied human performance and survival in extremes of exercise, heat, cold, altitude, immersion, hyperbarics, high G-forces, weightlessness, nutrition, forensics, and injury.

Far from the ivory tower, she has carried gear up and down the mountains and deserts of India, Nepal, Asia, and Northern Africa, swam to work in an underwater laboratory, breath-hold dived with the Ama diving women of Japan, and was professor of anatomy at a college in the mountains of Mexico.

She has written 13 medical textbook chapters and nine books on healthier exercise, hyperbarics, and diving medicine. She writes the health column Fitness Fixer for Healthline.com, and is the science officer for The Vidocq Society, a forensic organization allowing only 82 members worldwide. Harvard clinicians have called her "The St. Jude of the Joints" in her private practice in sports medicine.

Bookspan is a fourth-degree black belt, and was an undefeated full-contact ring boxer and Muay Thai fighter, competing in the Netherlands and Thailand, and studying with the monks of Japan, Nepal, and Thailand. She is happily married to Paul, also a ranking black belt. They were inducted into the Eastern USA International Black Belt Hall of Fame with several awards–including 2004 Martial Arts Man and Woman of the Year.

Left paralyzed in an accident, she rehabbed with her own methods while doctors insisted that she accept she would never walk again. Two months after recovering, a second accident left her paralyzed, even more seriously than before. She walked again, against all expectations.

Bookspan says her most important awards and achievements are the notes she gets from patients and readers who use her methods to stop years of pain that they were told they "just had to live with." Bookspan invites you to use all she has worked for to make your health and life better than you ever thought possible.